MEDICINAL HERBS OF CANADA

Text and art by
BRENDA JONES

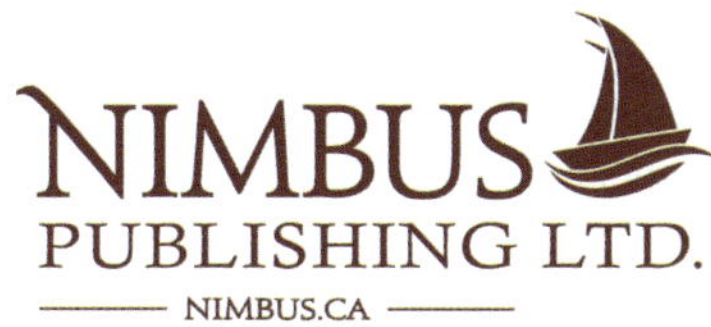

Nimbus Publishing Limited
3660 Strawberry Hill Street, Halifax, NS, B3K 5A9
(902) 455-4286 nimbus.ca

Nimbus Publishing is based in Kjipuktuk, Mi'kma'ki, the traditional territory of the Mi'kmaq People.

Printed and bound in Canada
NB1828

Editor: Penelope Jackson
Editor for the press: Claire Bennet
Cover Design: Heather Bryan
Interior Design: Brenda Jones & Heather Bryan

Library and Archives Canada Cataloguing in Publication

Title: Medicinal herbs of Canada : a pictorial manual / Brenda Jones.
Names: Jones, Brenda, 1953- author, illustrator
Description: Includes index.
Identifiers: Canadiana (print) 20250333198 | Canadiana (ebook) 20250335379 | ISBN 9781774715277 (softcover) | ISBN 9781774715284 (EPUB)
Subjects: LCSH: Medicinal plants—Canada—Identification. | LCSH: Medicinal plants—Canada—
Identification—Handbooks, manuals, etc. | LCSH: Herbs—Therapeutic use—Canada. | LCSH: Herbs—
Therapeutic use—Canada—Handbooks, manuals, etc. | LCSH: Herbals—Canada. | LCSH: Naturopathy. | LCGFT: Field guides.
Classification: LCC QK99.C3 J65 2026 | DDC 581.6/340971—dc23

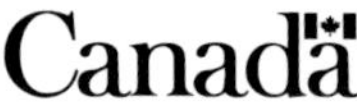

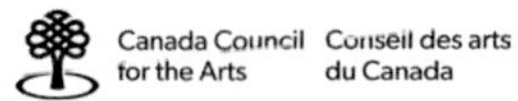

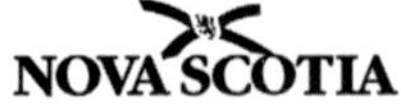

Nimbus Publishing acknowledges the financial support for its publishing activities from the Government of Canada, the Canada Council for the Arts, and from the Province of Nova Scotia. We are pleased to work in partnership with the Province of Nova Scotia to develop and promote our creative industries for the benefit of all Nova Scotians.

TABLE OF CONTENTS

Disclaimer

The information provided in this book is intended for educational purposes only. Every effort has been made to ensure the accuracy of this information through extensive research; however, I make no guarantees regarding errors or omissions and assume no legal responsibility for injuries resulting from the use of remedies in this book. The suggestions included are not intended as a substitute for professional medical care.

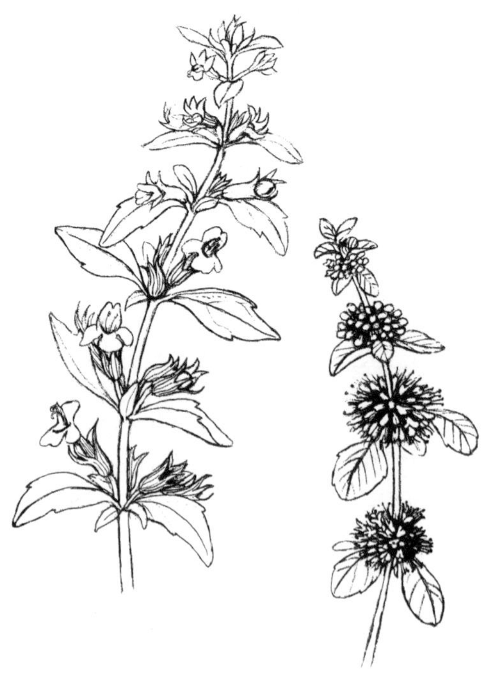

INTRODUCTION

Since ancient times, herbs have played a major role in healing in every culture around the world. Traditional remedies were passed down from one generation to another, using local plants and trees to cure disease, heal wounds, or ease pain. Particularly in Indigenous cultures, shamans, healers, and midwives played an important role in society, and their knowledge was gifted to future generations through word of mouth.

Unfortunately, over the last hundred years much of this knowledge has been lost due to the takeover of modern science and the pharmaceutical industry, attempted genocide of many Indigenous cultures, and the destruction of rare species and their habitats. However, with the increase in chronic diseases and superbugs and the difficulties accessing healthcare in recent years, there has been a resurgence of interest in medicinal herbs as people attempt to find relief for themselves. Although drugs will always play a major role in the healthcare industry, they are not the only answer. There is room for a more gentle, holistic approach to healing and for working with nature and all the gifts the earth has given us.

Having grown up in Prince Edward Island, I learned how important it is to spend time in wild places. Nature has been a source of grounding for me ever since I was a child, whether through planting my own garden and digging my fingers into the sweet-smelling soil, or just roaming the forests and countrysides. There is a quiet, healing energy in the earth, and the further we are away from it, the more disconnected we are from our own spirit. I learned to appreciate this connection after spending thirty years in a big city. Every cell in my body was trying to tell me to return to my roots. I had a good job, friends, and family in the city, but my soul craved the water and the open fields and cool forests, where I could see the horizon and the stars, watch the sun rise

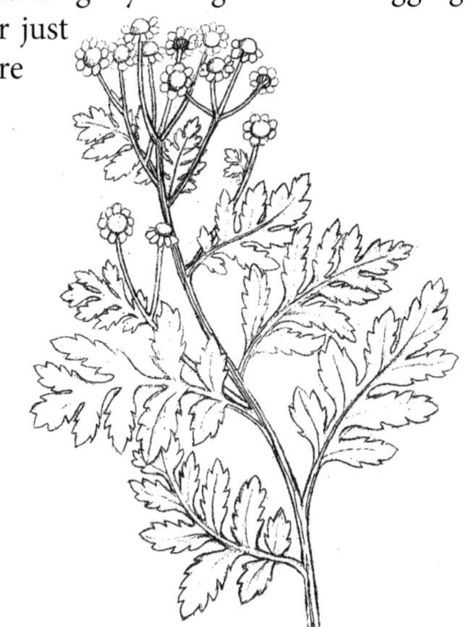

and set, and observe storms rolling in. By the time I reached my mid-fifties, I had chronic insomnia and digestive problems, and I was burnt out. I had to make a change. So, without any real plan, I moved back to the Island.

My interest in plants grew when I began searching for solutions to my own health problems, and I soon developed a fascination for the traditional herbal remedies that had been used across this country for centuries. But I was frustrated trying to accurately identify the herbs growing in my area. There was very little information available at the time, and none of the books I found had detailed photos or drawings, so I began doing my own research. I took workshops and online courses, consulted online databases, and bought every book I could find on the subject. My career in illustration was put to use; I drew and painted each plant as accurately as I could, and after a number of years I had compiled a collection of illustrations and remedies that eventually turned into *Medicinal Herbs of Eastern Canada* and, several years later, *Medicinal Herbs of Western Canada.*

This new cross-Canada edition has ultimately brought the two books together, with updated scientific research and 25 new additions to create a complete guide for foragers and amateur herbalists across the country, making it easy to identify, gather, and use over 130 herbs safely.

It is important to note that if you are wildcrafting your herbs, you should be conscious of where you pick them and how abundant they are. Never use plants that grow along a busy highway or next to farmers' fields that are sprayed with pesticides or anywhere that might be contaminated. Always use plants that are healthy and strong, not eaten by insects or diseased, and make sure there are enough plants left behind that you won't be depleting the local population. Only take what you need, and if using the top of the plant, leave the roots intact so it can grow back. If there are only a few, or the species is endangered, leave them alone; you can probably order them online and grown sustainably. I have gotten into the habit of leaving a pinch of tobacco when I take something from the environment; it reminds me that the plants are a gift and we should leave something in return. Indigenous Peoples have always been conscious of this, giving thanks for everything that is taken from the land; it is never taken for granted or wasted. We would all be better off learning from these teachings.

I have included a section at the end of the book to help identify the most common poisonous plants, particularly the ones you should not touch. I urge you to consult it when gathering herbs or foraging in the wild, and to teach your children which ones to avoid. I can't stress enough that if you're not sure, do not eat it! There are many berries, not all included here, that might look tasty to a small child but may result in a nasty bellyache or are even deadly when consumed. Also, be aware that a plant may be medicinal in small doses but could become toxic if not used properly, so please heed the warnings provided.

Research has shown that immersion in nature is both pleasurable and highly beneficial to our health and well-being. It can lower blood pressure, reduce anxiety and stress, and even improve immunity to disease. I can only hope this book will encourage people to do more "forest bathing" and learn more about all these amazing plants on their journeys, what they can use to improve their health, and what they should avoid. When approached with care and respect these plants can teach us a great deal about ourselves and the world around us.

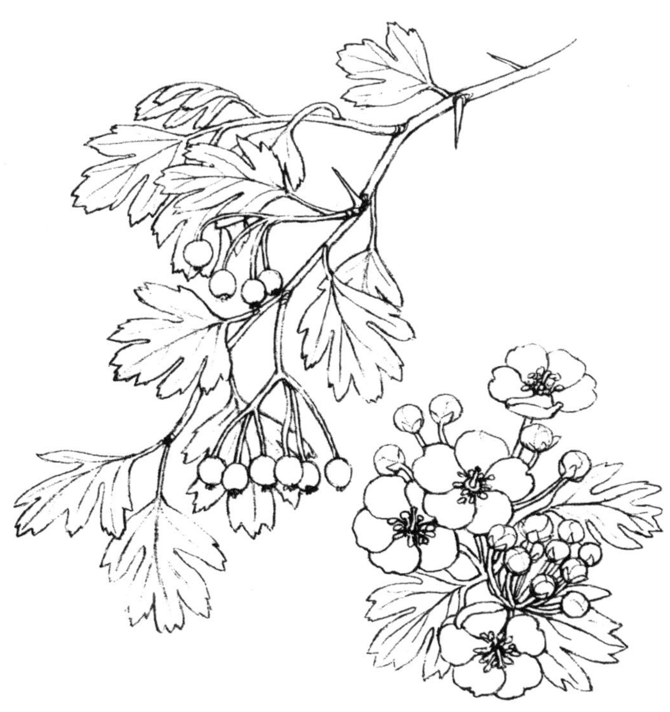

HERBAL PREPARATIONS

These are some of the most common methods for preparing herbs.

INTERNAL REMEDIES

Infusions

Probably the simplest way of using herbs, infusions are simply teas made from a herb or mixture of herbs in order to extract the healing properties. This method is best for the leafy parts and flowers of the plant, and they should be chopped fine to expose as much surface as possible. Since fresh herbs contain more water, we usually double the amount. A standard infusion consists of:

- 1 tsp. dried herbs or 2 tsp. fresh
- 1 cup boiling water
- Let infuse for 10–15 minutes, preferably in a covered teapot, particularly if the herb is fragrant, to retain the volatile oils. Strain into a cup and drink hot or cool.

Decoctions

This method is used for more woody parts of the herb, like stems, bark, roots or rhizomes, and sometimes berries. They require a bit more steeping to extract the medicines and should be chopped as finely as possible before decocting. A standard decoction consists of:

- 1 tsp. to 1 tbsp. fresh or dried herbs, chopped or finely ground
- 1 cup cold water
- Place in a pot, cover, and heat on the stove until it comes to a boil. Reduce heat and simmer 20–40 minutes. Cool slightly and strain. You may make a larger batch, but leftovers should be refrigerated and used within 48 hours.

Tinctures

Standard tinctures are made by macerating fresh or dried herbs in 40% alcohol, preferably vodka or brandy. (Other solvents like apple cider vinegar or glycerine may be used, but these are technically not tinctures). This method extracts more of the medicinal qualities and preserves them longer than if they were simply dried. The standard folk method for making alcohol tinctures is:

- For fresh herbs, fill a mason jar about ⅔ full.
- For dried herbs, fill jar about ½ full.
- For roots, bark or berries, fill jar about ⅓ full.
- Make sure they are clean and dry, and chop or grind to increase surface exposure. Fill up the jar with alcohol. For a more precise measure, weigh the plant material so that there is a ratio of 1 part (in grams) to 2 parts alcohol (in millilitres) for fresh plants, and 1 part to 5 parts alcohol for dried plants.
- Cover and seal the jar. Check after a while to make sure the herbs are still covered, as some will expand and may spoil. Add more alcohol if necessary. Store in a cool, dry place for about 6 weeks, shaking the bottle periodically.
- After 6 weeks, strain the mixture into a measuring cup covered with several layers of cheesecloth. Gather up the cheesecloth with the plant material in it and squeeze out as much liquid as possible to get the maximum amount, as this is where it is more concentrated. Let settle and strain again if necessary. Pour through a funnel into an amber tincture bottle, label and date, and store in a dark cupboard.

NOTE: Some plants require a stronger alcohol in order to extract their medicines, particularly herbs containing resins, like cannabis or balsam. For these it's best to use pure, organic grain alcohol at 85–95%. Deviations from the standard tincture instructions are explained in the individual profiles.

Syrups

Syrups are a good way to make herbal concoctions more palatable, particularly if they happen to be strong and/or quite bitter. The sweetener, usually sugar or honey, also helps preserve the medicine for a longer period of time. Here is a basic recipe for cough syrup:

- ⅓ cup dry herbs
- 2 cups cold water
- ½ cup honey or sugar
- Place woody herbs or roots and water in a saucepan and bring to a boil (if you have leaves or flowers, add them at the end of simmering time). Allow to simmer until liquid has reduced by about half. Cover the pan and let sit for an hour or so. Strain out plant matter and return the liquid to the pot. If adding honey, heat very gently, just enough to soften the honey, and remove from heat. If sugar is added, heat just long enough to dissolve the sugar. If you wish, you can add up to 3 tbsp. of brandy or other alcohol.

EXTERNAL REMEDIES

Infused oils

Herbs can easily be infused into oils for use as massage oil, to relieve itchiness, soreness or inflammation, as a bath oil, or for culinary use. We typically use organic cold-pressed virgin olive oil, but sweet almond, grapeseed, jojoba, or coconut oils can also be used. They will last up to a year if kept in a cool, dark place.

Make sure herbs are clean and dry. If using fresh herbs, do not wash them, as you want the least amount of moisture possible in the jar. Leave on the counter for a couple of days to let bugs escape and any moisture to evaporate, then chop and pack into a sterilized mason jar, up to ¾ full. I prefer to use dried herbs as they are less likely to spoil.

Cover with oil, leaving ½ inch of space at the top and making sure that plant material is completely submerged. Use a knife to release any air bubbles in the liquid. Cover with wax paper and screw on lid. Leave in a dark place for 4–6 weeks, shaking occasionally.

Strain into a bowl covered with cheesecloth and squeeze out as much liquid as possible. If you used fresh herbs, check after a few hours to see if any water has settled to the bottom before pouring into the bottle as you'll want to leave it behind. Using a funnel, pour oil into a clean, dry, sterilized bottle and label.

Ointments and salves

These are a great way to protect and soothe inflamed skin and to heal sores and wounds. They contain oils or fats but no water, so they form a layer on top of the skin rather than sinking into it like a cream. Any kind of infused oil may be used in this basic recipe.

- 20 grams beeswax
- 100 ml. herb-infused oil
- 1 small (120 ml.) mason jar, sterilized
- Gently warm the beeswax and oil together in a double boiler or Pyrex bowl set into a pan of water. When wax has melted, place a drop on a saucer and place in the freezer for a minute to test the consistency. If it's too hard, add a little more oil; if too soft, add more beeswax. Remove from heat, cool slightly, and add a few drops of essential oil if desired.

Liniments

A liniment is basically a mixture of a strong herbal decoction and alcohol, which is readily absorbed into the skin to relieve the pain of sprains, sore muscles, or broken bones. The addition of alcohol adds to the shelf life of the decoction and aids absorption of the herbs. Here is a basic recipe:

- 1 part vodka or rubbing alcohol
- 2 parts decoction (should be well strained before adding alcohol)
- You can also make a good liniment by placing a mixture of herbs in a sterilized jar and adding enough Witch Hazel or rubbing alcohol to cover. Screw on lid and let the mixture sit for 4–8 weeks. Strain and pour into a sterilized bottle or spray bottle and label to remind you that it is NOT to be taken internally. It will keep for about a year.

Poultices

A poultice consists of solid fresh plant material that has been mashed or bruised to release the medicines, or dried herbs that have been ground and made into a paste by adding warm water. This paste is placed directly on to the skin and can be covered with a hot water bottle if desired. They are usually made from warming and stimulating herbs, vulneraries, astringents, or emollients.

Compresses

Compresses or fomentations are clean cloths like gauze or cotton that have been soaked in a hot infusion or decoction. They are placed on the affected area and kept as hot as possible to enhance the action of the herbs. A hot water bottle can be placed on top of the compress to keep it warm for a longer period of time. Vulnerary herbs, stimulants, and diaphoretics make good compresses.

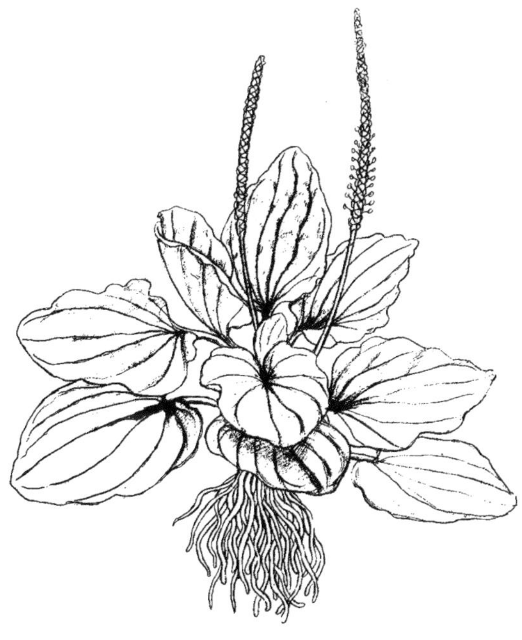

AGRIMONY

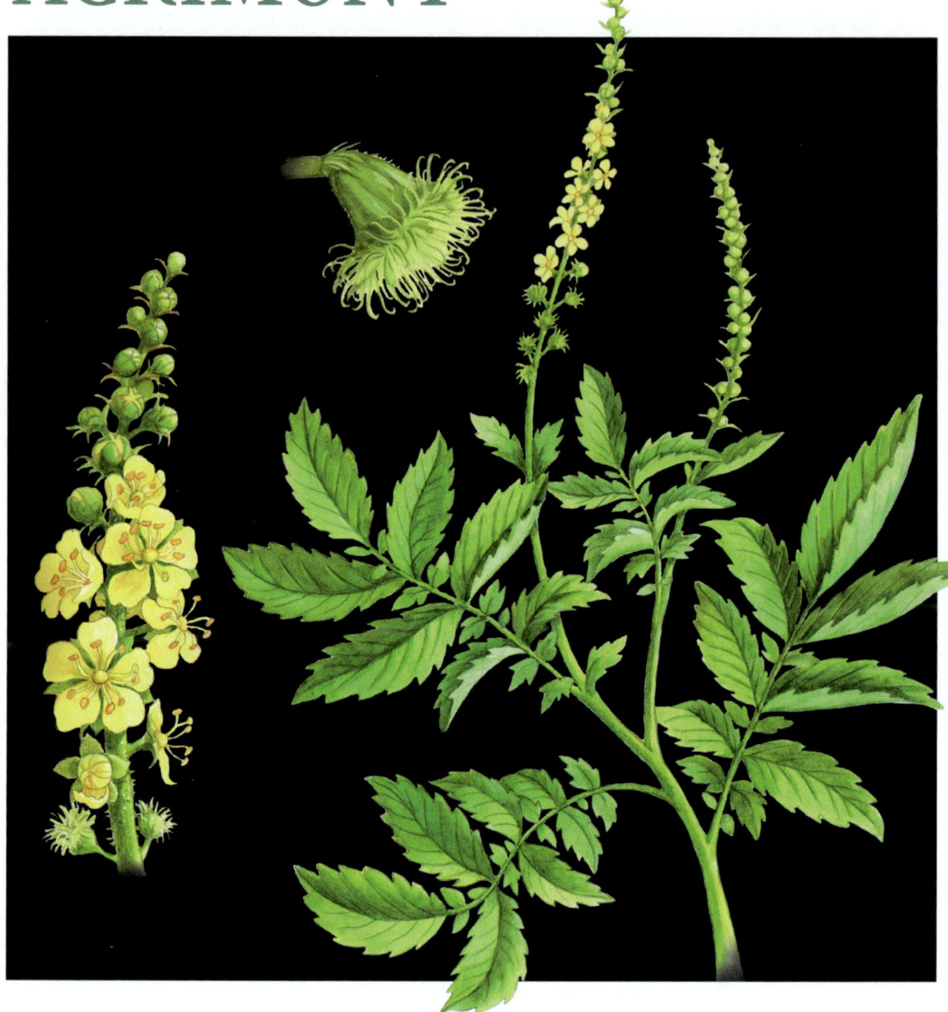

Agrimonia eupatoria; Agrimonia gryposepala; Agrimonia striata

FAMILY: Rosaceae (Rose)

OTHER NAMES: Tall Hairy Groovebur, Woodland Agrimony, Grooved Agrimony, Cocklebur, *Fr.* Aigremoine

PARTS USED: Aerial in bloom, roots

CHARACTERISTICS: Neutral, drying, bitter, slightly sweet, and sour

ACTIONS: Anti-inflammatory, antispasmodic, antiviral, antidiabetic, anticancer, astringent, alterative, antibacterial, tonic, diuretic, vulnerary, cholagogue, hepatic, relaxant

RANGE: *A. eupatoria* introduced in Ontario; *A. gryposepala* native to British Columbia, Manitoba to the Maritimes; *A. striata* native from British Columbia to Newfoundland and Labrador

Agrimony actually consists of several different species that grow in Canada, typically in woodlands, around the edges of fields, and along roadsides. Once called "Fairy's Wand," the European variety (*A. eupatoria*) is the one usually used in medicine, although our native varieties have similar properties. It grows to a height of 1.2–1.8 m., has an erect, hairy stem with alternate compound leaves composed of many unequal leaflets, smooth above, hairy underneath, and strongly serrated. The tiny yellow 5-petalled flowers are slightly aromatic and grow on slender branched erect spikes, which bloom between July and September. The fruit are seeds with little hooks that attach themselves to anything that passes by—usually animal fur. The upper stems of the plant should be gathered early in the summer and dried in the shade, not above 40°C.

MEDICINAL USES:

Liver problems, indigestion, diarrhea, wounds, urinary infections, kidney pain, kidney stones, incontinence, bedwetting

- Contains tannin, so its bitter, astringent properties stimulate the liver and increase digestive secretions, flushing out toxins. It relieves symptoms of diarrhea and mucous colitis, indigestion, gallbladder inflammation, jaundice, and gout. Its action on the liver may relieve other symptoms of liver congestion such as dry, brittle hair, dysmenorrhea, or (in Traditional Chinese Medicine) inner anger or frustration.
- Infusion makes a good spring tonic.
- Eases urinary inflammation and cystitis, bedwetting, incontinence, kidney pain and stones.
- Antibacterial, infusion used as a gargle soothes mucous membranes, eases sore throats, laryngitis, and mouth ulcers, and taken internally helps lung inflammation.
- Ointment or infusion from seeds and leaves used topically can help heal burns, slow-healing wounds, inflammation, varicose veins, bruises, eczema, and psoriasis. Stems external bleeding.
- On an energetic level, it helps relieve emotional tension and frustration.
- May be effective in lowering blood-sugar levels, but more study is needed.

FOLKLORE: When placed under a person's head at night, Agrimony was said to induce a deep dreamless sleep.

INFUSION: Add 1 cup boiling water to 1 tsp. dried herb, infuse 10 minutes, drink 3 times a day until symptoms dissipate.

TINCTURE: Dried herb, 1:5, 40% alcohol, 1–3 ml., 3 times a day.

CAUTION: Do not exceed recommended dosage. Do not use if pregnant or breastfeeding. Patients with excessive bleeding should use with caution. May cause photodermatitis. May cause nausea or mild digestive upset if taken in large quantities or over a long period of time. Use with caution if you have liver or kidney disease.

ALFALFA

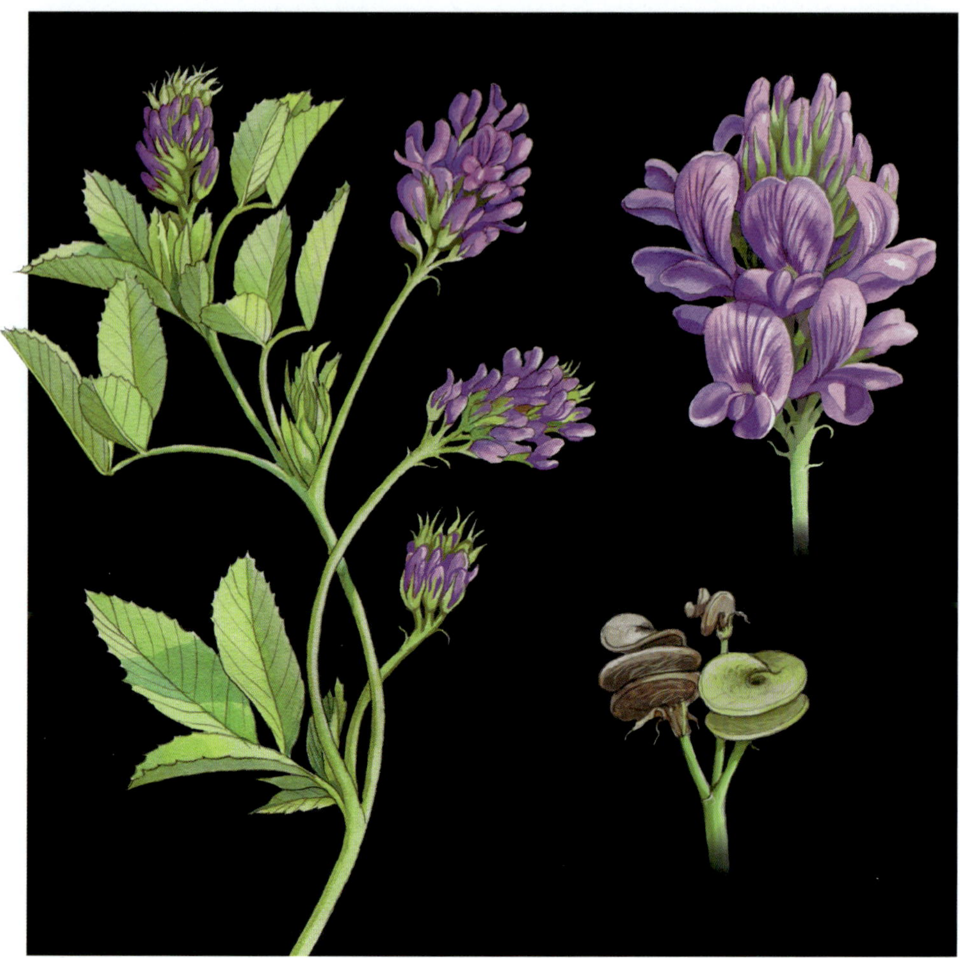

Medicago sativa

FAMILY: Leguminosae or Fabaceae

OTHER NAMES: Lucerne, *Fr.* Luzerne

PARTS USED: Aerial

CHARACTERISTICS: Sweet, salty, bitter

ACTIONS: Alterative, antioxidant, anti-inflammatory, aperient, restorative, cooling, diuretic, antihemorrhagic, galactagogue

RANGE: Introduced across Canada

This colourful perennial has been cultivated as a forage crop for hundreds of years. At full size it may reach a height of up to 1 m. It somewhat resembles Clover, but its leaves grow more elongated as it matures and are notched at the tips. The flowers that appear in June or July range from pink to mauve or purple and are pollinated by bees or butterflies. Grown for fodder, it also increases milk production in livestock and fertilizes the fields, its long roots fixing nitrogen in the soil after a couple of years of growth, making it one of nature's best green manures. It grows in sunny locations and well-drained soil and can be picked during the summer and dried for later use.

MEDICINAL USES:

Wasting diseases, lack of appetite, anemia, hemorrhage, cystitis

- Leaves and young shoots are edible, raw or cooked. Very nutritious, rich in chlorophyll, vitamins A, B, C, K, protein, and minerals.
- Restorative tonic, helps build weight and improve digestion during convalescence, warms the stomach, increases appetite, restores strength and vitality. Tonic for the weak and emaciated, where there is poor assimilation of nutrients, despondency, and chronic indigestion. Good for peptic ulcers and slow peristalsis.
- Relieves chronic and acute urinary tract infections, with backache and sparse urination. Diuretic, it helps with prostate irritations.
- Nourishes the blood, helps anemia, slows hemorrhaging. Estrogenic properties may help ease menopausal symptoms and PMS. Increases milk production in lactating women. May help lower cholesterol.
- Works slowly and penetrates deep into the body where chronic problems originate. Should be taken regularly over long periods to correct chronic problems.

OTHER USES:
- Young shoots, flowers, and sprouts are good in salads.
- A yellow dye can be made from the seeds.
- Fibre from the plant has been used to make paper.

INFUSION: 1–2 tsp. dried herb in 1 cup of boiling water. Infuse 5–10 minutes. Drink 3 times a day.

COMBINATIONS: May be combined with Stinging Nettle for use as a blood tonic, Red Clover as a nutritive tonic, or add Ginseng and Ashwagandha for anemia. When combined with Sage, may help in the treatment of hot flashes and night sweats during perimenopause and menopause.

RESEARCH: One study on rats that received varying doses of nicotine and Alfalfa showed it may reduce the risk of toxicity in the liver and heart, proving that it could have applications in the future to reduce damage on the body due to smoking.

CAUTION: Contains saponin-like substances. Do not eat in large quantities. Avoid during pregnancy, and with hormone-sensitive cancers. May trigger attacks in people with systemic lupus erythematosus; avoid in autoimmune diseases and gout. Seeds should not be eaten, as they contain canavanine, a toxic amino acid. Avoid use if taking Warfarin.

AMERICAN ASPEN

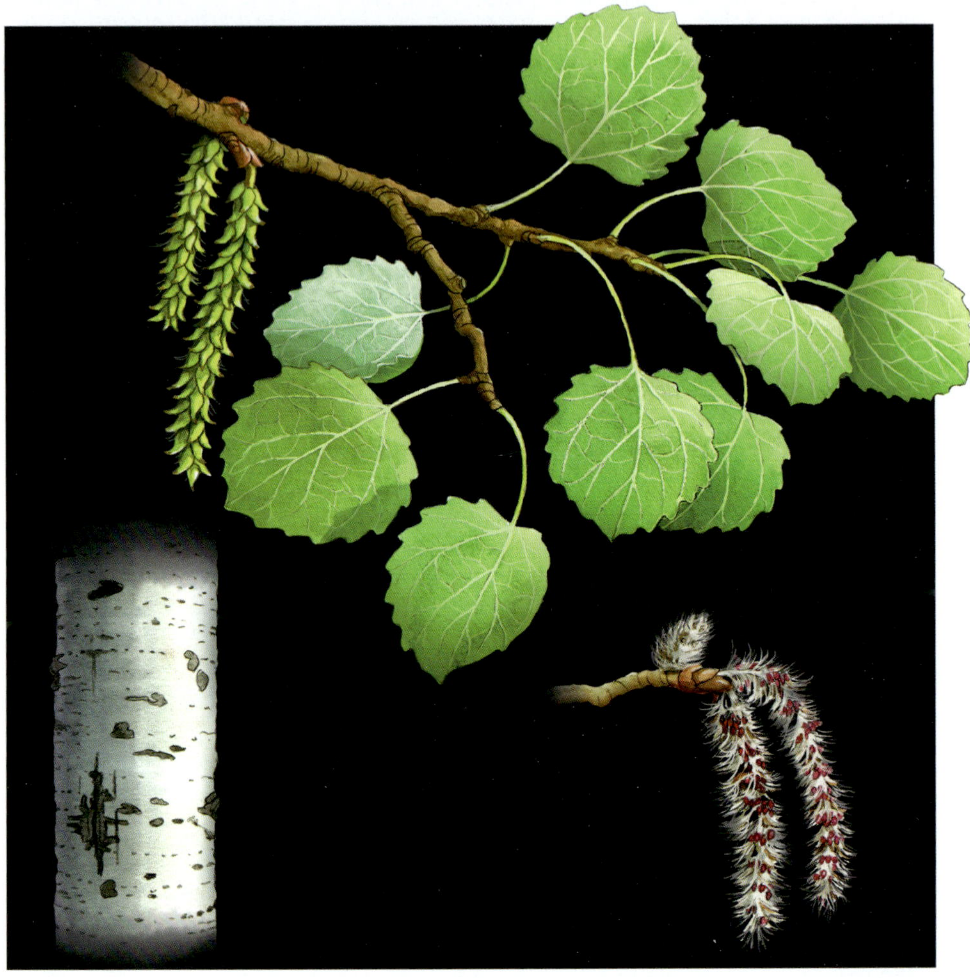

Populus tremuloides

FAMILY: Salicaceae

OTHER NAMES: Quaking Aspen, Trembling Aspen, Poplar, *Fr.* Peuplier faux-tremble

PARTS USED: Inner bark, root, leaf buds

CHARACTERISTICS: Bitter, astringent, dry

ACTIONS: Antimicrobial, analgesic, anti-inflammatory, astringent, diuretic, diaphoretic, febrifuge, nervine, vermifuge, antiscorbutic, expectorant, purgative

RANGE: Native across Canada

Quaking or American Aspen has been so-named because of the gentle rustling noise made by its leaves in even the slightest of breezes. It's a native deciduous tree from the Willow family found across Canada, usually under 15 m. tall, and, like the Willow, has been used for centuries for its pain-relieving properties. Short-lived and fast-growing, it is dioecious, meaning male catkins (grey and fuzzy) and female catkins (green and smooth) grow on separate trees. Leaves are alternate and oval or heart-shaped, shiny green on top and dull or silvery underneath, turning yellow-orange in the fall, with rounded teeth. The bark of younger trees is creamy white, grey, or greenish white with dark markings and covered in a powdery coating, where older bark is dark grey to greenish brown, rough, and furrowed. The trees multiply by sending out rhizomes, forming large groves. Bark should be taken from recently fallen trees or branches or lateral branches so as not to weaken the tree. Peel off the outer bark and dry for later use.

MEDICINAL USES:

Pain, digestive and liver disorders, menstrual cramps and excessive bleeding, urinary infection, anorexia, arthritis, wounds

- Dried inner bark contains salicin, from which aspirin is derived, and is analgesic, antiseptic, and antimicrobial. Buds can also be used, but are not very soluble in water so should be macerated in oil or alcohol. Makes a great salve or oil for arthritis or muscle pain, as well as for an irritated nose in colds. It reduces inflammation and encourages healing.
- Relieves digestive upsets due to sluggishness and liver disorders. Tonifies the digestive tract, relieves chronic diarrhea, and stimulates bile production. May stimulate appetite and help with anorexia, stomach pain, and worms.
- Warm tea is good for coughs, colds, and fever, and can be gargled for sore throat. Also useful for urinary tract infections that are chronic and slow to heal.
- Decoction taken to relieve cramps, excessive bleeding, and leukorrhea. Tones the uterus.
- Taken internally to help arthritic pain, rheumatism, fibromyalgia, gout, and lower back pain.
- Light powder on bark used to stop bleeding, prevent hair growth, and mixed with jojoba oil can be used as sunscreen.
- Bark or leaf may be chewed and packed around a tooth to relieve toothache.
- Poultice from mashed bark or root relieves hemorrhoids, skin inflammation, rashes, wounds, burns.

OTHER USES:
- Inner bark is sweet and edible raw, added to soups and flour for bread. Catkins also edible and high in vitamin C, but bitter.
- Sap may be tapped and drunk as a beverage.

DECOCTION: Simmer 1 tsp. dried bark in 1¼ cups water for 10–15 minutes. Let steep for 1 hour, take ¼–½ cup up to 4 times a day.

TINCTURE: 1 part dry bark to 2 parts vodka/distilled water mix (1:1). Take 15–20 drops before meals to aid digestion, 1–10 drops to relieve anxiety.

COMBINATIONS: Combine with *Uva-ursi* (Bearberry) to make an excellent tonic for bladder infections.

CAUTION: Avoid use internally if sensitive to aspirin.

AMERICAN GINSENG

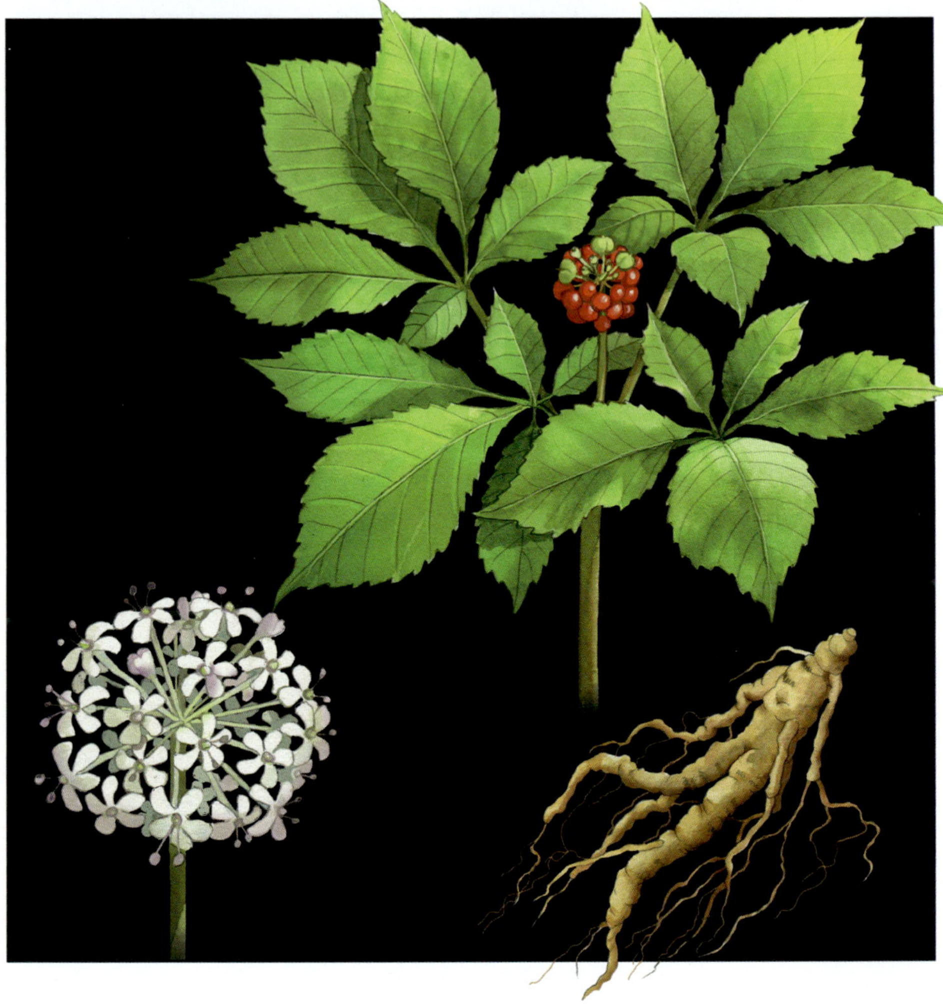

Panax quinquefolius

FAMILY: Araliaceae

OTHER NAMES: Five-leaved ginseng, Redberry, *Fr.* Ginseng à cinq folioles, Panace à cinq folioles

PARTS USED: Root, berry

CHARACTERISTICS: Sweet, cool, moist

ACTIONS: Adaptogen, adrenal tonic, alterative, antioxidant, anti-inflammatory, antimicrobial, anticancer, cardiotonic, demulcent, hypertensive, sedative, stimulant, stomachic

RANGE: Native to southwestern Quebec and southern Ontario

This slow-growing native plant is a close relative of Asian Ginseng (*Panax ginseng*), and has similar properties; however, American Ginseng has a stronger antioxidant activity, is cooling and a Yin tonic, and is less stimulating, whereas the Asian Ginseng is warming and nourishes Yang. Because it is highly valued in China, much of it has been exported there over the last hundred years, which has led to it being overharvested and endangered in this country. A mature plant grows up to 60 cm. in height with leaves composed of 5 leaflets radiating from a single stem. At the centre of this whorl of leaves is a cluster of tiny white flowers which turn into bright red berries. The root resembles a parsnip or a human being, however you want to look at it, with scars on the root neck that indicate its age. It takes 5 years for the root to mature, doubling in size and weight. Note that although it grows wild in southern Ontario and Quebec, it's considered an endangered species and is illegal to harvest from the wild. Most commercially available Ginseng is now cultivated.

MEDICINAL USES:

Stress, chronic coughs, debility and aging, memory problems, impotence, nervous stomach, high cholesterol, diabetes, cancer

- A favourite for problems related to aging, it enhances memory and clears brain fog when taken over a long period of time, regulates arterial tension and decreases cholesterol levels. Contains ginsenoside saponins, which are responsible for its anti-inflammatory, antioxidant, vasorelaxant, and anticancer properties.
- Alterative and adaptogenic, it helps the body adapt to stress, shock, and fatigue; calms nerves; relaxes a nervous stomach; and strengthens the adrenals to better deal with stress.
- For diabetics, it increases the effects of insulin and regulates glucose.
- Treats chronic coughs, increases stamina, enhances the immune system.
- It may work as an aphrodisiac and counteract male impotence. May have an effect on erectile dysfunction.
- Because of its cooling actions, should not be used in cases where there is coldness, such as colds, chills, or cold extremities.

DECOCTION: ½–2 tsp. in 1 cup of boiling water. Simmer 10–15 minutes. For debility or to recover from illness, take for 2 or 3 days.

TINCTURE: Dried root 1:5, 70% alcohol. For cultivated roots, take 20–40 drops, 1 to 3 times a day. Reduce dosage if insomnia or nervous overstimulation occurs.

RESEARCH:

- Effects such as cognitive enhancement are attributed to a group of saponins specific to Ginseng known as ginsenosides. It was found to improve cognitive performance and increase calmness in a group of healthy young adults. A study of older adults in 2018 showed that regular consumption for at least 5 years improved memory later in life. There is also potential in treatment of Alzheimer's disease and anxiety.
- Some studies have shown that American Ginseng lowered blood sugar levels in people with type 2 diabetes. Increases insulin sensitivity and inhibits formation of fatty tissue.
- It has an anticancer effect by inducing apoptosis (death of tumour cells) and reducing inflammation and has been shown to inhibit spreading of breast, liver, and prostate cancer cells. It also has an antimicrobial effect on several pathogenic strains of bacteria.
- Studies indicate its antioxidant properties reduce hypertension and lower heart rate, improving cardiovascular disease, and may have a preventative effect against nerve damage due to stroke.

CAUTION: Avoid if taking anticoagulants such as Warfarin, do not take for at least 7 days before surgery. Avoid if pregnant or nursing, or if there is impaired liver or kidney function. Large doses may cause headaches or raise blood pressure. Avoid taking with other stimulants like coffee or alcohol. Regular large doses may cause insomnia or overstimulation. Avoid if taking immunosuppressant medications, statins, antidepressants, or diabetes medications. Because of its cooling effect, it is advisable to take during the summer.

ANGELICA

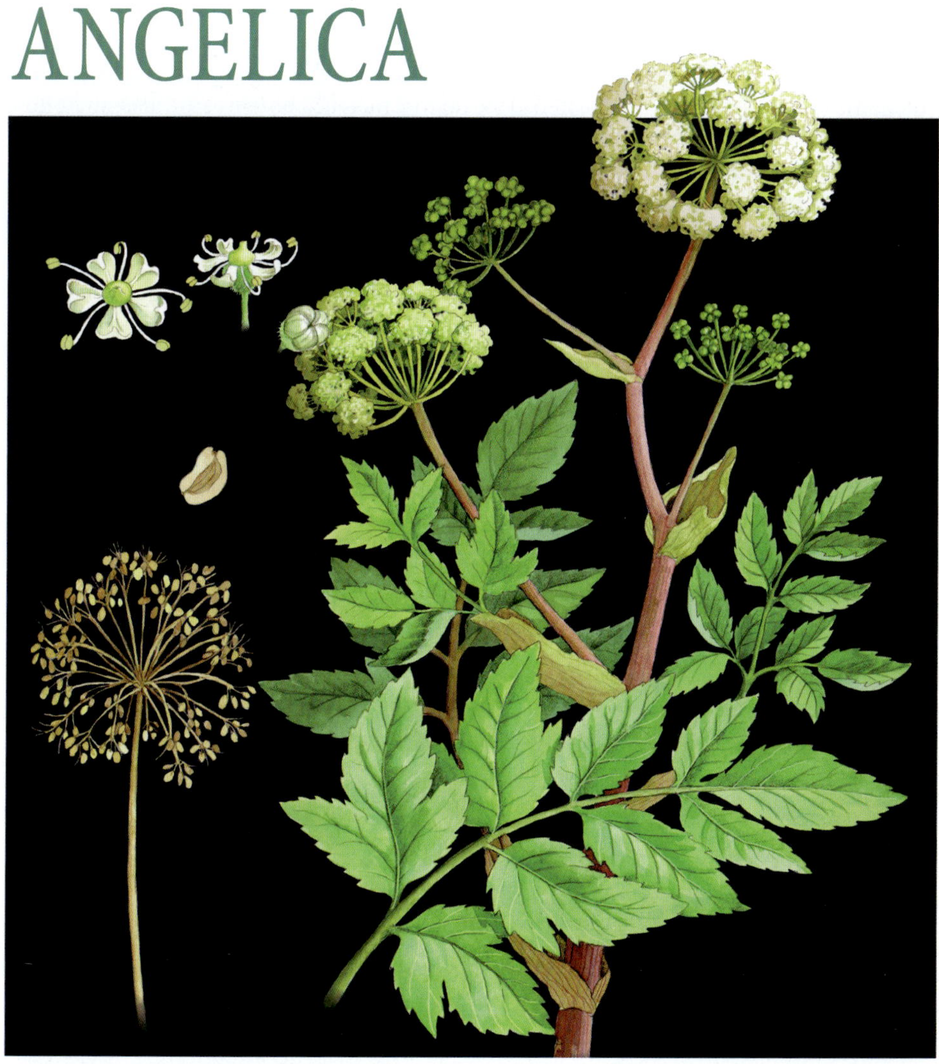

Angelica atropurpurea

FAMILY: Apiaceae

OTHER NAMES: Purplestem Angelica, Great Angelica, *Fr.* Angélique

PARTS USED: Root, leaves, seeds

CHARACTERISTICS: Spicy, bitter, warm, sweet, drying, stimulating

ACTIONS: (Mostly root) carminative, stimulant, emmenagogue, antibacterial, diaphoretic, expectorant, diuretic, tonic, antispasmodic

RANGE: Native from Ontario to Newfoundland and Labrador, Nunavut

Angelica, a large, robust perennial, resembles its European relative, *A. archangelica*, both physically and medicinally, although it's less aromatic and perhaps not quite as potent. Its hollow, purplish stems often grow up to 2 m. tall. The leaves are also on hollow footstalks, which are covered in a sheath at the base, and are composed of numerous bipinnate leaflets with finely toothed edges, the veins ending on the tips of the notches. The yellowish-green to white flowers are grouped into large round umbels and pleasantly aromatic. Dig roots up in the fall of the first year, slice longitudinally to speed drying, and store in an airtight container. Angelica is most potent when tinctured in alcohol. Collect leaves in early summer before flowering. This plant contains furocoumarins, which may increase photosensitivity or cause dermatitis; gloves are recommended.

Since this plant, along with others in the carrot family, closely resembles Woodland Angelica, Poison Hemlock, Water Hemlock, Cow Parsnip, and Giant Hogweed—all of which are highly toxic—it is imperative to correctly identify the plant before even touching it! The safest way to use this plant is to grow it in your garden from certified seeds, and do not harvest if any of the above are growing in the area.

MEDICINAL USES:

Rheumatic complaints, digestive weakness, gas, menstrual irregularities, coughs, and colds.

- A warming herb, Angelica acts as an expectorant, and helps relieve symptoms of colds, flu, bronchitis, and other upper-respiratory complaints where there is a thick, sticky mucus and unproductive cough that requires soothing. It relaxes the cough reflex and encourages the production of loose, thin mucus that is more easily coughed up. Promotes perspiration and movement of stagnant fluids including lymph and mucus, draining and drying dampness. Infusion can be used as a gargle to ease sore throat.
- Tea stimulates appetite and digestive process, as it encourages gastric and pancreatic secretions; helps with anorexia. Relieves gas, heartburn, flatulence, stomach upsets, and colic.
- Poultice of mashed roots warms and stimulates circulation, helps with gout, arthritis, and rheumatism, as well as swelling and pain from broken bones.
- Tea balances female hormones, relieves menstrual cramps, eases the symptoms of menopause, brings on menstruation (but not to be used when pregnant).

OTHER USES:
- Young shoots and stems are sweet and can be cooked or eaten raw.
- Essential oils from seeds and root are used in perfumes and as flavouring for gin, vermouth, and Chartreuse.

FOLKLORE: Angelica was given its name in 1665 by a monk who claimed he dreamt of an angel who told him the plant had the power to prevent and cure bubonic plague. It has always been purported to have special powers against poison, plague, and contagious diseases, as well as warding off evil spirits and spells and prolonging life. A decoction mixed with bathwater is said to remove negativity and hexes.

INFUSION: 1 tsp. powdered seeds, dried root, and/or leaves per 1 cup boiling water. Steep 10-15 min.

TINCTURE: Dried herb 1:5 in 50% alcohol. Take 1–3 ml. up to twice a day.

COUGH SYRUP: Boil 2 tbsp. root in 4 cups of water for 3 hours. Strain and add honey. Take 2 tbsp. as needed.

COMBINATIONS: Used with Bearberry or Gravel Root for stones or urinary problems.

CAUTION: Not for use during pregnancy—can cause miscarriage. Avoid getting juice of the plant into eyes. Use gloves to handle. Do not use fresh roots; they must be dried. Can increase photosensitivity. Avoid if you are diabetic, as it can increase blood sugar. May increase blood clotting, so avoid if you are at risk of stroke. Not recommended for women who have heavy periods or if you are trying to conceive. Avoid if you have chronic intestinal inflammation.

ARNICA

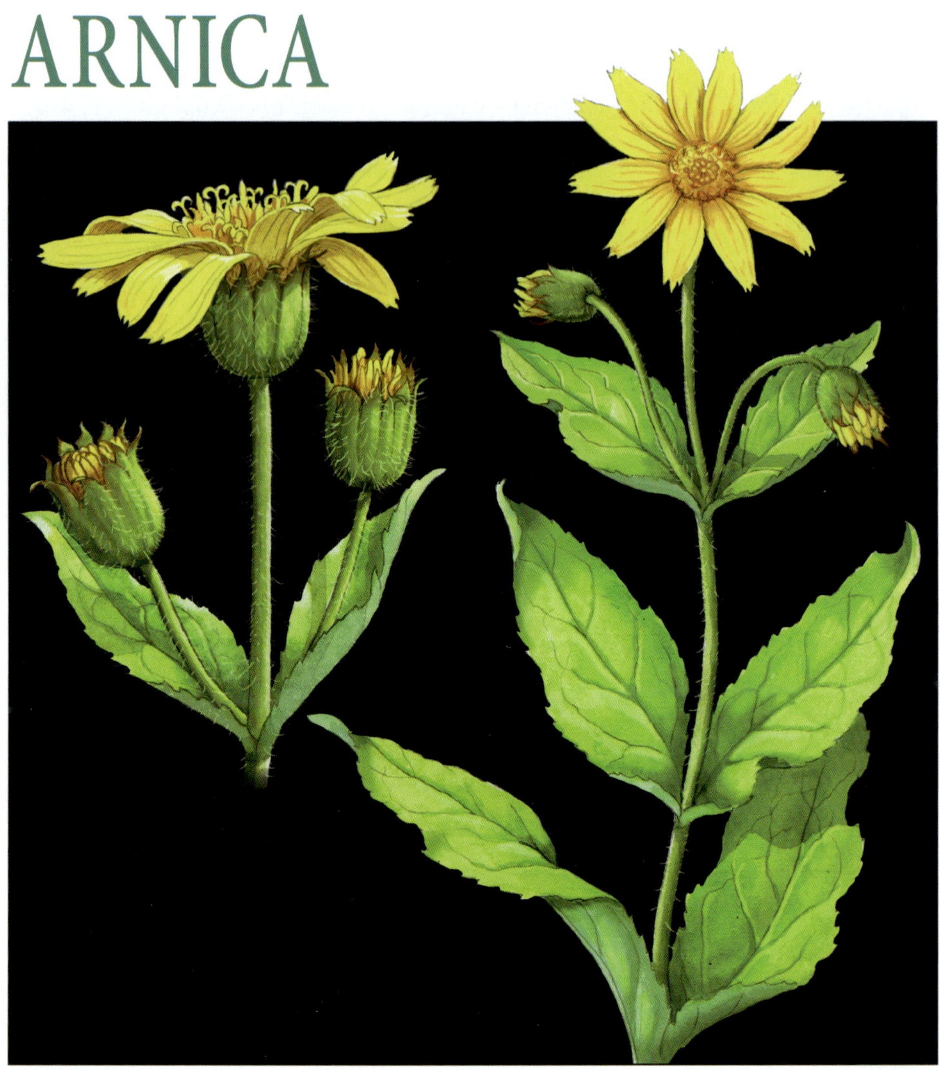

Arnica mollis

FAMILY: Asteraceae

OTHER NAMES: Hairy Arnica, *Fr.* Arnica douce, Arnica moelleux

PARTS USED: Flowerheads

CHARACTERISTICS: Warm, drying, bitter, acrid

ACTIONS: Stimulant, analgesic, anticoagulant, nervine, vasodilator, anti-inflammatory, vulnerary, antifungal, rubefacient, lymphatic, antimicrobial

RANGE: Native across Canada

Similar to the European variety *Arnica montana,* this species, among others, grow mostly across northwestern Canada. Arnica is mostly found in meadows, fields, and foothills, spreading in thick mats by underground rhizomes. Most of the plant is hairy, depending on the species. The erect stem grows from 15 to 61 cm. tall and has 2–4 pairs of opposite leaves, which can be up to 18 cm. long and are irregularly toothed and lance-shaped. Basal leaves are smaller and elliptical, and may be on separate shoots. The bright yellow composite flowers appear throughout the summer, with 10–20 petals that are grooved lengthwise and toothed at the tip. Typically one flower emerges at the top, followed by two others below on shorter stems. Gather only the flowerheads, preferably just after opening, and dry for later use.

MEDICINAL USES:

Sprains, swellings, bruises, sore muscles, soft tissue injuries, osteoarthritis, fractures, dental surgery pain

- Although once used internally for chest pain, acute cardiac debility, and angina, it is now strongly discouraged as an internal medicine due to its potentially lethal side effects. It is now only used topically in creams, liniments, and salves.
- Pain relief is due to its rubefacient action, which is caused by volatile oils creating a mild irritation on the skin. This causes dilation of the blood vessels and draws blood to the area, bringing warmth and increased circulation, reducing fluid stagnation and pain.
- Rubbed on to sore muscles, arthritic joints, sprains, myalgia, fractures, and swellings. If applied immediately after injury, a bruise might not even appear. Do not use if skin is broken.
- After dental surgery, when rubbed on the skin along the jawline, can decrease pain and stiffness.
- Eases symptoms of carpal tunnel syndrome.

INFUSED OIL: Fill a mason jar ⅔ full with dried flower petals. Cover with olive oil, seal, and place in a dark place and let macerate 4–6 weeks. Strain through several layers of cheesecloth, bottle, and label.

POULTICE: Place a handful of flowerheads into boiling water, cover, and let steep until room temperature. Wrap flowers in cheesecloth and apply to skin to relieve bruising, arthritis, or inflammation.

COMBINATIONS: Comfrey, St. John's Wort, or Cayenne may be added to oils or salves.

RESEARCH:

- *Arnica montana* was tested in comparison to ibuprofen on patients with osteoarthritis of the hands, and after 21 days there was no difference between the two groups. This confirms that Arnica relieves pain and improves function to the same degree as NSAIDs.
- Other studies were conducted to assess the effectiveness in bruising, ankle sprains, and muscle pain and Arnica was proven effective at reducing pain and speeding recovery.
- A clinical study was conducted on sixty patients who underwent surgery to remove impacted molars. Standard therapy of antibiotics and NSAIDs was used on all patients, however, one test group applied Arnica to the jawline for 10 days. It decreased pain and stiffness in the jaw to a greater degree than standard therapy alone.

CAUTION: Toxic if taken internally. Stomach irritation may occur if used internally. High doses may cause dizziness, tremors, tachycardia, arrhythmia, and collapse. May cause skin irritation; do not use on broken skin.

ARROWLEAF BALSAMROOT

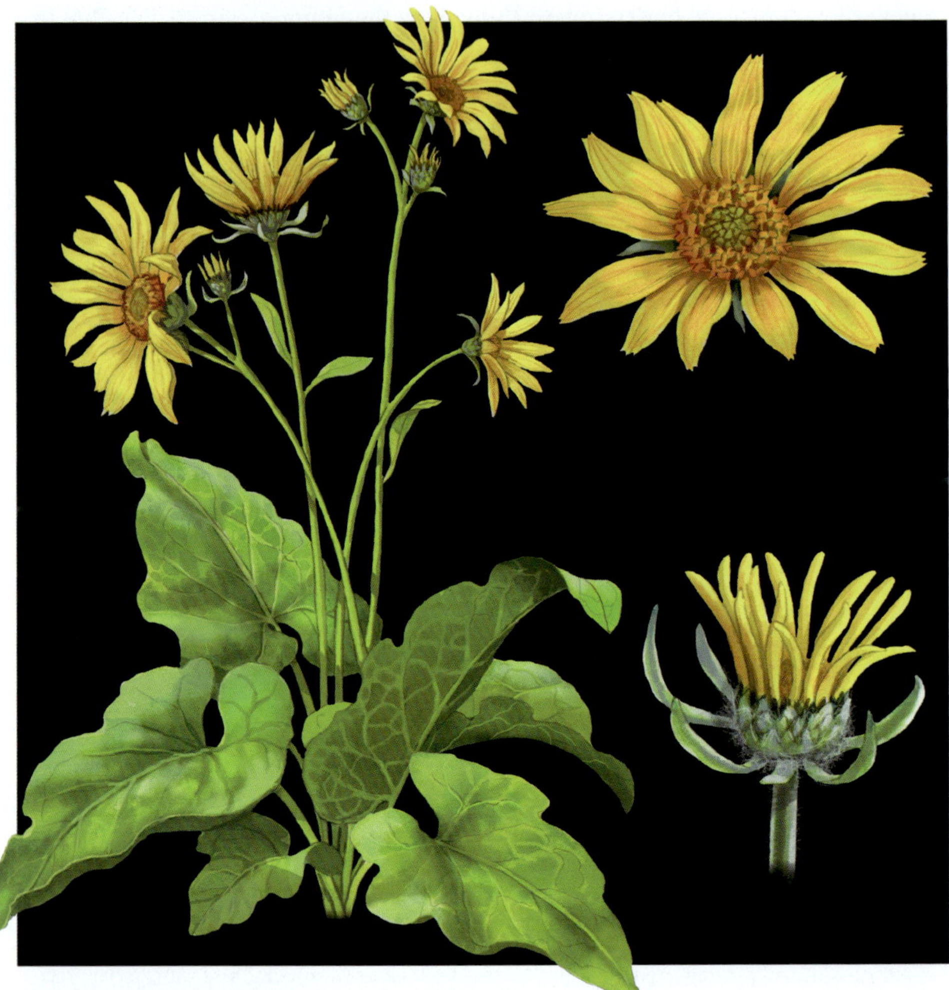

Balsamorhiza sagittata

FAMILY: Asteraceae

OTHER NAMES: Oregon Sunflower, Breadroot, *Fr.* Balsamorhize à feuilles sagittées

PARTS USED: Whole plant

CHARACTERISTICS: Pungent, warm, dry

ACTIONS: Antirheumatic, antimicrobial, diuretic, diaphoretic, febrifuge, vulnerary, expectorant, stomachic, antifungal, stimulant

RANGE: Native to British Columbia, Alberta, and Saskatchewan

One of the most important plants for Indigenous Peoples of British Columbia, this large perennial was once a major food source, its long taproot, young shoots, and seeds providing nourishment and medicine throughout the year. Growing on rocky hillsides and grasslands, the woody root of these plants may reach 1.5–2.4 m. deep as they get older, is pungent and resinous in taste, and is usually the part used in making medicines. Several leaf stems arise from the hairy crown; the soft basal leaves are heart-shaped, pointed at the tip, and often up to 60 cm. long. Other small lance-shaped leaves grow on the flower stems, which are 15–81 cm. and topped with one or several yellow sunflower-like blooms from April to June. The whole plant smells resinous when rubbed. It provides food and shelter to wildlife and is of great benefit to the environment, the long roots holding soil together and preventing erosion. Harvest roots in the fall when they're about the size of a large carrot, as they are easier to break apart. Use a hatchet or machete to chop it up into small pieces for tincturing.

MEDICINAL USES:

Stomach problems, colds, fevers, lung congestion, sore throat, skin irritations

- Used medicinally by the Indigenous Peoples of the Pacific Northwest for lung infections, stomach complaints, and toothaches, but the root was also an important food staple, providing nutrition throughout the year.
- Infusion or tincture of the whole plant is used for stomach pains, colds, coughs, fevers, and headaches. It promotes the flow of mucous in the respiratory tract, releases mucous in the sinuses, and soothes inflammation. Contains antibacterial compounds that stimulate white blood cells and aid the immune system to fight infection.
- Root may be chewed for sore throat, mouth sores, or toothaches. A syrup of the roots soothes coughs and sore throat.
- A decoction of the root is used at the onset of labour to ease pains and delivery.
- The root or leaves can be pounded to use as a poultice on wounds, burns, blisters, bites, swellings, poison ivy rash, or sores. Infused oil eases pain of rheumatism, sore muscles, and arthritis.
- A few drops of tincture may relieve Seasonal Affective Disorder (SAD) and lift the spirits.

OTHER USES:

- Young shoots can be eaten raw or steamed, flower stems and young leaf stalks eaten raw or cooked. Traditionally, the root was usually roasted for several days in fire pits to make it sweeter and more digestible.
- The seeds can be dried and roasted and pounded into a meal.
- An infusion of the root was sometimes used to promote hair growth.

TINCTURE: Dried root, 1:5 in 65% alcohol, 15–50 drops up to 4 times a day in hot water.

COMBINATIONS: Tincture may be combined with Cottonwood bud tincture and honey for sore throats.

CAUTION: May cause kidney irritation in large doses, but generally the whole plant is safe to use.

BALSAM POPLAR, BLACK COTTONWOOD

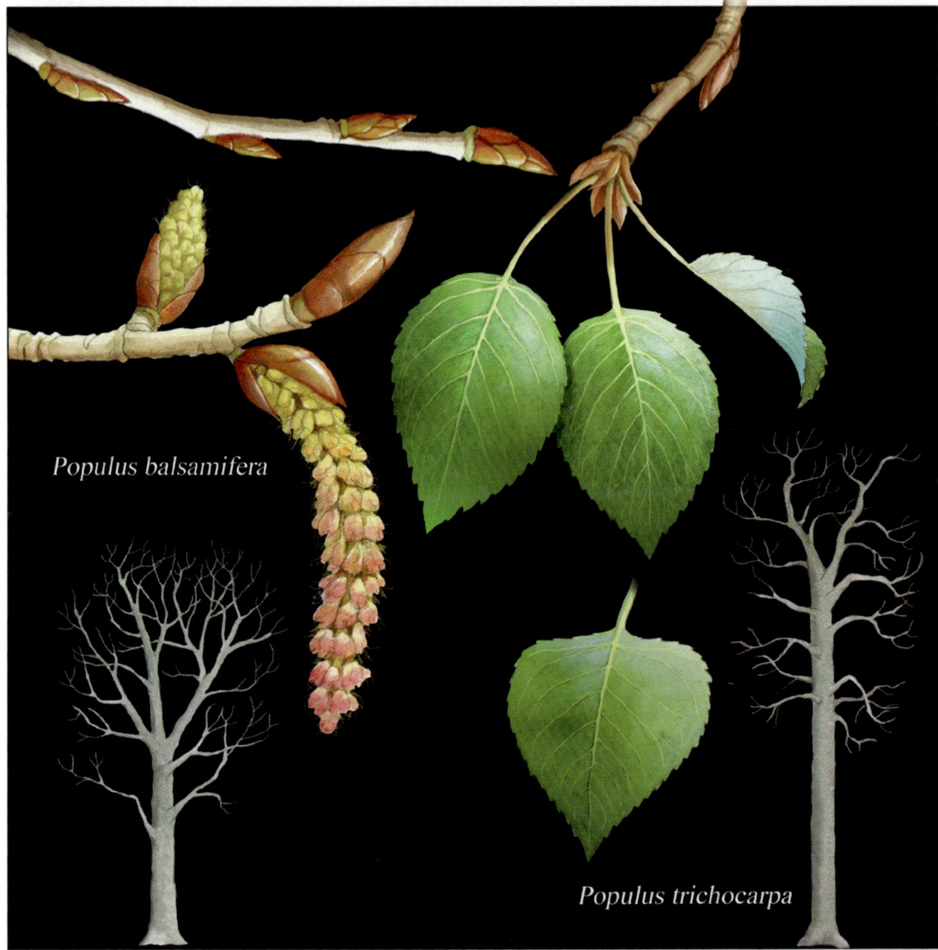

Populus balsamifera (Balsam Poplar)
ssp. Populus trichocarpa (Black Cottonwood)

FAMILY: Salicaceae

OTHER NAMES: *P. balsamifera*: Balm of Gilead, Hackmatack, Tacamahac, *Fr.* Peuplier baumier; *P. trichocarpa*: Western Balsam Poplar, *Fr.* Peuplier de l'Ouest

PARTS USED: Buds, twigs, inner bark

CHARACTERISTICS: Resinous, bitter, warming, astringent, drying

ACTIONS: Analgesic, anti-adipogenic, antimicrobial, antioxidant, antirheumatic, antiseptic, antifungal, anti-inflammatory, anodyne, carminative, diuretic, expectorant, stimulant, tonic

RANGE: *P. balsamifera* native across Canada to boreal zone; *P. trichocarpa* native to British Columbia, southwest Yukon, and western Alberta

These native deciduous trees from the Willow family are very highly valued by many Indigenous Peoples across North America. Balsam Poplar and Black Cottonwood are usually found near damp areas and have very similar properties and uses, but only the latter grows exclusively in temperate climates of western Canada and US, and tends to be quite a bit taller, often up to 35 m. The resinous, fragrant leaf buds are the parts most used for medicine and are usually gathered in late winter or early spring. The leaves that emerge in spring are dark green on top, light blue-grey underneath, ovate, and finely serrated, the Black Cottonwood leaf tending to be flatter at the base. Flowers are either male or female, and only one sex is found on a single tree. In the spring, they emerge as greenish or reddish catkins, which then produce globular fruit that split open, turning to a cottony fluff that blows off in the wind, spreading the seeds. Harvest buds early, preferably from fallen branches, as the buds are larger higher up on the tree and it's a more sustainable way to collect them. Inner bark can be taken from these branches as well, and twigs may simply be chopped into smaller pieces. It is recommended that you wear gloves while gathering the buds as the resin can be difficult to remove if it gets on your hands.

MEDICINAL USES:

Upper respiratory tract infections, fevers, skin problems, rheumatism, muscle pain

- Resin from the buds can stimulate lungs to expel mucous and heal infection, particularly in cases of dry asthma and when cough is longstanding and unproductive.
- Buds and inner bark contain salicin, from which aspirin is derived, helping to reduce fevers and pain from sore muscles, rheumatism, or menstrual pain.
- Oil made from the bud resin can be used as is or in a salve for mild burns or sunburn, to soothe skin inflammation, disinfect, and ease the pain of arthritic joints, sprains, carpal tunnel, and sore muscles. New research suggests it may be effective in treating psoriasis. It reduces swelling and inflammation and prevents infection. Oil and salve will last for many years due to natural preservatives.
- Inner bark is anti-inflammatory and anodyne. It can be eaten fresh off the tree or dried and ground to use as a thickener for soups or added to bread.
- A few drops of tincture in water aids digestion, can be gargled for sore throats, or to heal mouth or gum infections.

OTHER USES:

- An extract made from the shoots can be used as a rooting hormone for cuttings. Soak the shoots in cold water for 24 hours.
- Indigenous Peoples have traditionally used the resin to waterproof the seams of canoes or burned it to repel mosquitoes.
- Due to its antimicrobial properties, a few drops added to other oils or salves help to preserve them longer.

TINCTURE: Pack a mason jar ¼ full with fresh buds (dried for a few days), 1:2 in 75% alcohol. Allow it to sit for 4–6 weeks, shaking often. Strain and bottle. Use diluted in water, 15–30 drops up to 4 times a day.

OIL: Put 1 cup fresh buds into a quart mason jar, fill with olive oil. Cover and keep in a warm place for 4–6 weeks. Strain and bottle. Use as a chest rub for respiratory infections, sprains, sore muscles, arthritis. May be combined with St. John's Wort and/or Wild Bergamot oil for burns.

CAUTION: Avoid use internally if sensitive to aspirin. Avoid if pregnant or breastfeeding.

BARBERRY

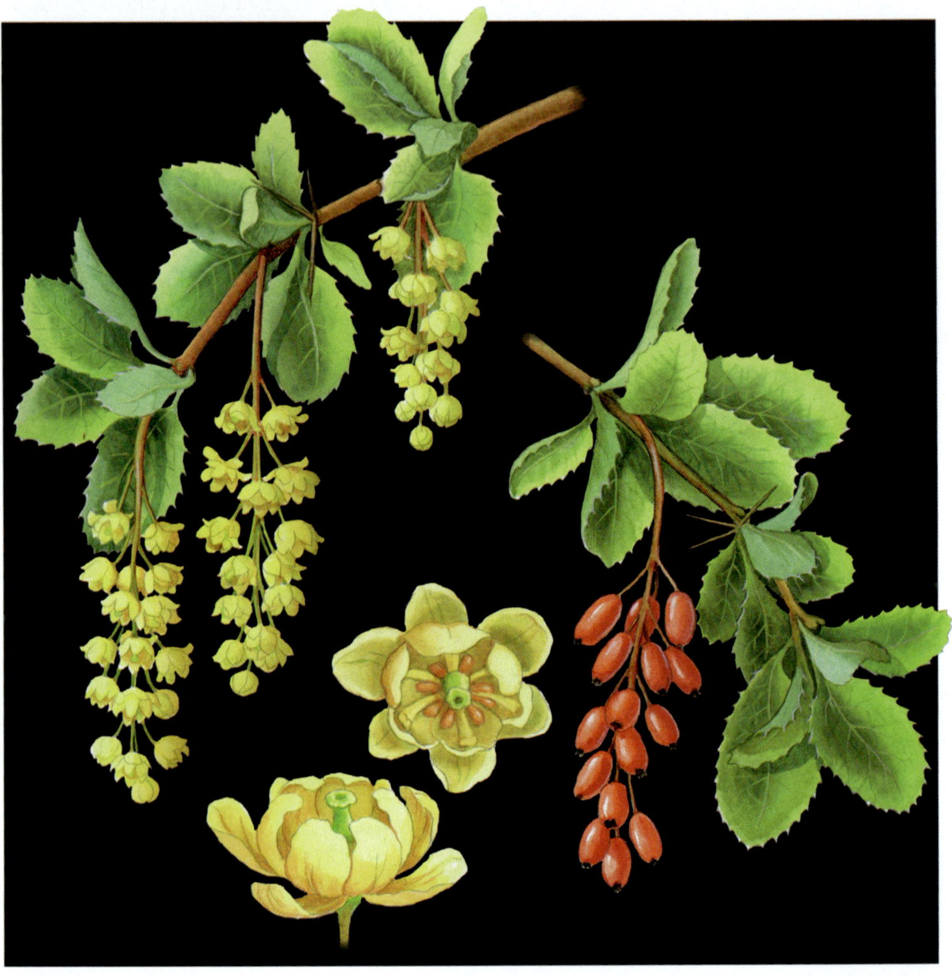

Berberis vulgaris

FAMILY: Berberidaceae

OTHER NAMES: Common Barberry, European Barberry, Jaundice Berry, *Fr.* Épine-vinette, Berbéris

PARTS USED: Bark of root (most concentrated) or stem, berries

CHARACTERISTICS: Cool, drying, bitter, astringent, sour

ACTIONS: Cholagogue, alterative, anti-inflammatory, antiemetic, laxative, hepatic tonic, antibacterial, purgative, antioxidant, sedative

RANGE: Introduced from British Columbia to Maritimes

Barberry is native to Europe but grows throughout northeastern Canada. It is a bushy, deciduous shrub, about 2.5 m. high with woody smooth stems, grey bark, three-pronged spines, and yellow roots. Leaves are alternate or in rosettes, and spoon-shaped with spiny notches and prominent veins on the underside. Flowers bloom between May and June and are small, pale yellow, and grow in pendulous clusters at the tip of the branches. The red, oblong berries appear in the fall, about 1 cm. in length. It can be found along field fences and in pastures. Harvest berries and root bark in the early fall; pare off the bark and dry roots in the shade before using.

MEDICINAL USES:

Liver and gallbladder problems, fevers, diarrhea, urinary tract infections, arthritis

- Roots, stems, and root bark are high in berberine, making it effective at fighting infection, increasing immunity, and improving the health and function of the liver and gallbladder. Used as a liver tonic, it stimulates bile production and treats inflammation of the gallbladder, stones, hepatitis, and jaundice.
- Astringency and antibacterial qualities make it an effective immune stimulant for treating diarrhea, dysentery, cholera, and giardiasis. Root bark decoction can reduce fevers. Alterative, it can help improve chronic illnesses characterized by congestion and tiredness.
- Tea made from the root bark and stems can improve stomach ulcers and indigestion.
- Supports the urinary system and relieves urinary tract infections and stones. Eases inflammation, infection, and discomfort.
- May lessen the symptoms of arthritis, rheumatism, and sciatica.
- Infusion can be used externally as an eyewash for infections or as a gargle to treat gingivitis or sore throat. Berries are astringent and rich in vitamin C, and a juice made into a syrup can help ease a sore throat and gingivitis.

OTHER USES:

- Indigenous Peoples used (and continue to use) the bark and stems to dye animal skins and fabrics.
- Berries are pleasantly acidic and can be eaten raw, or cooked in jams or jellies.

DECOCTION: Put ½ tsp. bark into 1 cup of cold water; bring to a boil. Simmer 10–15 minutes. Let steep 5 minutes. Add honey, as it is quite bitter. Drink 1–3 ounces, up to 3 times a day.

COMBINATIONS: With Dandelion Root or Burdock for cleansing the liver and bowel. With Red Clover and Bedstraw to cleanse the lymphatic system and relieve swelling.

RESEARCH: Recent studies have shown berberine and specifically Barberry may be effective at lowering blood pressure and LDL cholesterol, reducing the risk of cardiovascular problems like congestive heart failure, cardiac hypertrophy, and arrhythmia. It may also be promising at increasing insulin sensitivity and act as an anti-obesity and hypoglycemic agent in cases of diabetes. It can be considered a possible candidate for further research into these diseases, as well as thyroid and liver disorders.

CAUTION: Avoid use during pregnancy or breastfeeding. Not for children under two years of age. May be harmful in large doses, so do not use for more than 7 days at a time, and wait at least a week before using again. Large doses may cause nausea and vomiting. May temporarily decrease blood pressure and heart rate and cause lethargy. May interfere with some medications, check with healthcare provider before using.

BAYBERRY

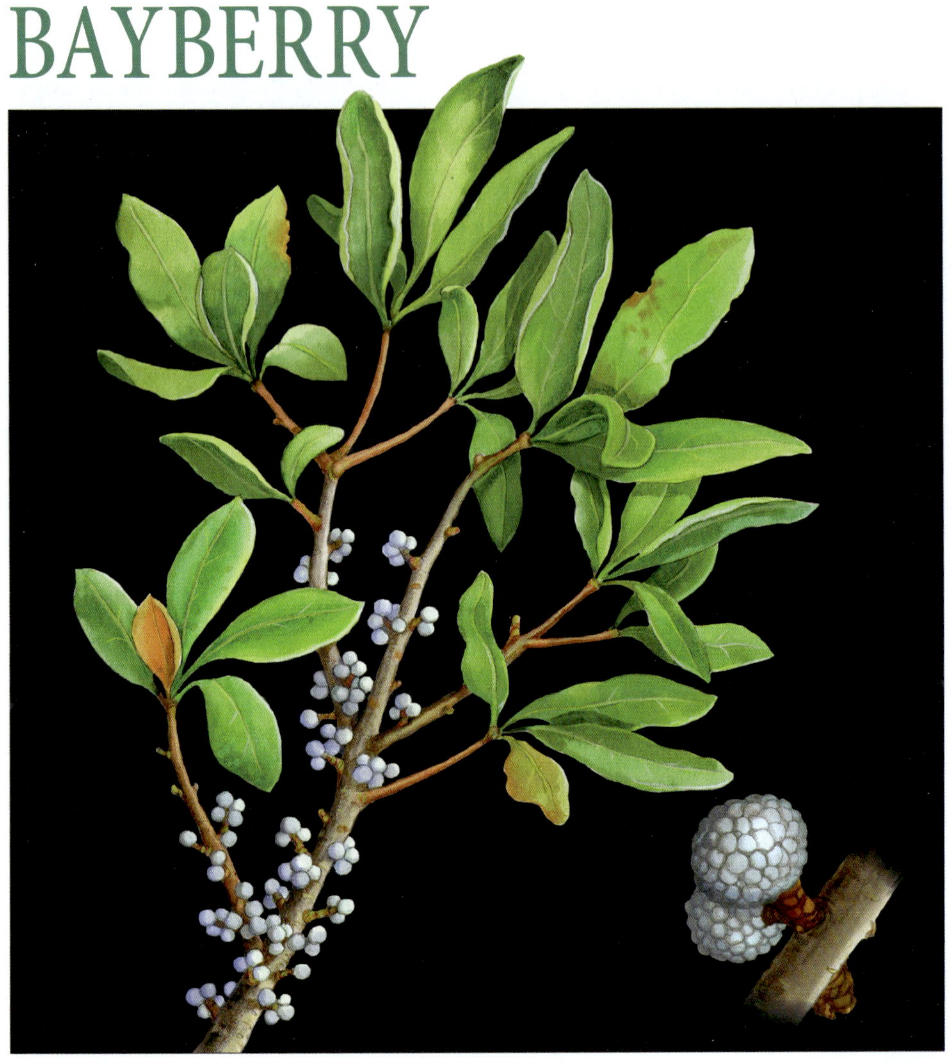

Morella (Myrica) pensylvanica

FAMILY: Myricaceae

OTHER NAMES: Wax myrtle, Candleberry, Waxberry, Northern Bayberry, Candlewood, *Fr.* Myrique cirier, Arbre à suif, Cirier de Pennsylvanie

PARTS USED: Bark and root bark, leaves

CHARACTERISTICS: Spicy, warm, astringent

ACTIONS: Circulatory stimulant, astringent, alterative, anti-inflammatory, antibiotic, analgesic, antibacterial, antipyretic, expectorant, diaphoretic, tonic, vermifuge

RANGE: Native from Ontario to Newfoundland and Labrador

Bayberry is a perennial native bush that grows abundantly along shorelines and near swamps and marshes, helping to control erosion along shorelines and preserving sand dunes. Usually 1–2 m. tall, it has alternate, lance-shaped leaves which are shiny, resinous, and fragrant when rubbed. The flowers are inconspicuous clusters of yellow-green catkins that appear from April to May. The fruit are small light-grey berries that grow along the stems and are covered in an aromatic waxy substance that is often used in candle-making. The root should be harvested in spring or fall, the bark removed and dried before using, then pulverized and stored in a dark container.

MEDICINAL USES:

Colds, flus, fevers, astringent for hemorrhoids, circulatory stimulant, gargle for sore throats, inflamed gums

- Has been used for centuries as an alterative to rally the body's defences against infectious diseases, especially to reduce congestion and mucus, to promote sweating where there is fever, improve circulation, and tone the tissues. One of the active components in the root bark is myricetin, which reduces inflammation and is antimicrobial and antioxidant.
- Effective against colds and flu, congested sinuses and fevers.
- Astringent effects help with diarrhea, mucous colitis, and dysentery, or when there are chronic digestive disorders with looseness in the bowel and inflammation. Small amounts stimulate digestion and bile production.
- Useful when women experience uterine prolapse or heavy periods. Infusion may be used as a douche for leukorrhea.
- Infusion can also be used as a gargle for sore throats or as a rinse for gingivitis or cankers. Some Indigenous people crush the root bark to a powder and use it as a poultice for skin ulcers or wounds or as snuff for headaches or nose polyps.
- The leaves are also used as a poultice for hemorrhoids or varicose veins.

OTHER USES: Berries can be boiled in water to separate the waxy coating, which can then be used to make fragrant candles. However, it takes literally a bucketful of berries to make a couple of small candles.

DECOCTION: Steep 1 tsp. of root bark in 2 cups of boiling water for 30 minutes. Add honey if desired. Will induce perspiration and improve circulation. Do not exceed 2 cups per day.

TINCTURE: Fresh bark 1:2, dried bark 1:5, 60% alcohol. Start with 2–5 drops, as it may cause nausea. Do not exceed 1–2 ml. per day. Best when combined with other herbs as it increases their effectiveness.

INFUSION: Steep 1 tsp. powder in 2 cups boiling water for 30 minutes. Add honey if desired. Will induce perspiration and improve circulation. Sip slowly, do not exceed 2 cups per day.

CAUTION: Emetic if taken in large doses. Start with a small dose. Avoid if pregnant or breastfeeding, or if you have a history of stomach or colon cancer, kidney disease, or high blood pressure.

BEARBERRY

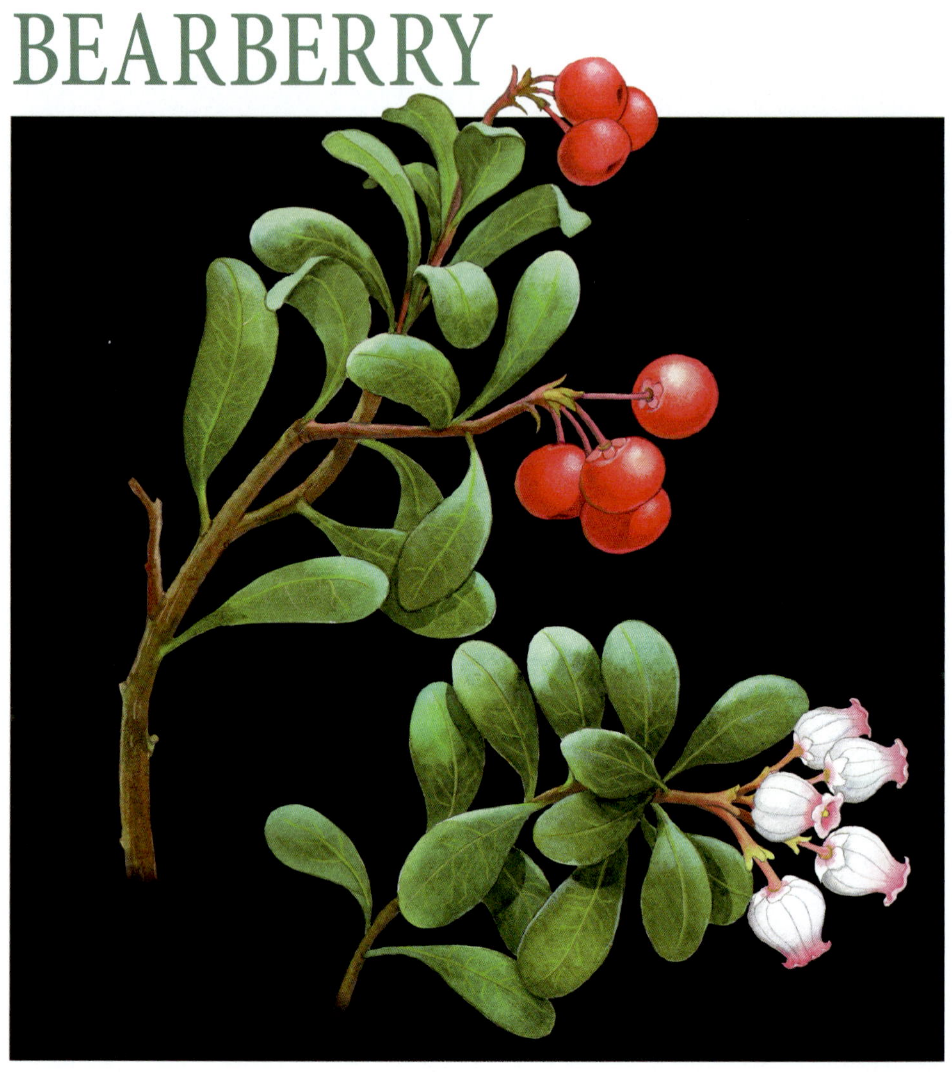

Arctostaphylos uva-ursi

FAMILY: Ericaceae

OTHER NAMES: Uva ursi, Mealberry, Sandberry, Foxberry, Hog Cranberry, Kinnikinnick, *Fr.* Raisin d'ours

PARTS USED: Leaves, stems, fruit

CHARACTERISTICS: Bitter, astringent, cool

ACTIONS: Anti-inflammatory, antiseptic, astringent, diuretic, urinary antiseptic, tonic, antibacterial, antiviral, antifungal, mild tonic

RANGE: Native across Canada

This low-growing evergreen shrub probably earned its name, *uva-ursi*, which means "bear's grape," because bears find the berries tasty—whereas people consider the flavour unpleasant. Growing to a height of about 20 cm., its trailing branches are short and woody, covered in a pale brown bark. The shoots are slightly hairy and rise upward from the stems. The leaves are alternate, leathery, and spoon-shaped, dark green on top and paler underneath with a coarse network of veins. The flowers appear in drooping clusters in June, each one urn-shaped, usually white, sometimes with a reddish lip. The berries that appear in the fall are edible and resemble a small red currant, however they are dry and mealy. It grows in dry, open woods, in gravelly or sandy soils. Collect leaves in September or October, only in fine, dry weather when the dew has evaporated, taking only green, unblemished leaves. Dry in the sun or a warm, dry, well-ventilated shed.

MEDICINAL USES:

Cystitis, urinary tract infections, diarrhea, leukorrhea

- Primarily used by herbalists as a diuretic and treatment for uncomplicated bladder and urinary tract infections, painful urination, stones, and other inflammatory diseases of the urinary tract. Its natural antibiotic effect works best if the patient is on a vegetable-based diet where the urine is alkaline; acid can neutralize the effect. Also a powerful astringent that soothes and tonifies the entire urinary system.
- Antibacterial and astringent properties help treat intestinal infections, diarrhea, and dysentery. Aids sluggish digestion.
- Tones and reduces discharge in leukorrhea and STDs. Tones the uterus in cases of prolapse and helps prostatitis.
- Has been used in folk medicine for years as a headache remedy. The leaves are dried and smoked, producing a mild narcotic effect.
- Salve made from the fruit can speed healing when applied to wounds.

OTHER USES: Used by many Indigenous Peoples to make "kinnikinnik," a herbal mixture used as a smudge or smoked in the sacred pipe during ceremonies.

INFUSION: Dried herb up to 2 tsp. per dose, don't exceed 7 days. You can take ½–1 tsp. baking soda in water to increase alkalinity if taking for UTIs. Herb may be taken every 3–4 hours throughout the day until resolved. Do not take vitamin C or acidic juices or fruit while taken treatment. If condition worsens, or if there is fever or kidney pain, contact your doctor.

TINCTURE: Dried herb 1:5 in 50% alcohol, 1–4 ml. in water 2–3 times a day.

COMBINATIONS: Used with Dandelion root and leaf to prevent recurring UTIs, with Marshmallow root to relieve burning, Echinacea to help infection, and Licorice root for inflammation. Goldenseal helps with chronic diarrhea and dysentery.

RESEARCH: Based on only a few definitive trials, this herb shows great promise at reducing cystitis and UTI infections. Contains a high concentration of arbutin, which converts in the urine into hydroquinone, a highly potent antibacterial. It also contains other components like ursolic acid and allantolin, which together soothe irritation, reduce inflammation, help promote growth of new cells, and shrink, tighten, and heal mucous membranes.

CAUTION: Overuse can cause nausea, vomiting, and liver damage. Avoid if pregnant or breastfeeding, and do not give to children under twelve. Avoid if you have high blood pressure or Crohn's disease, digestive problems, ulcers, or kidney or liver disease. May affect certain medications like lithium, diuretics, or iron supplements.

BLACKBERRY

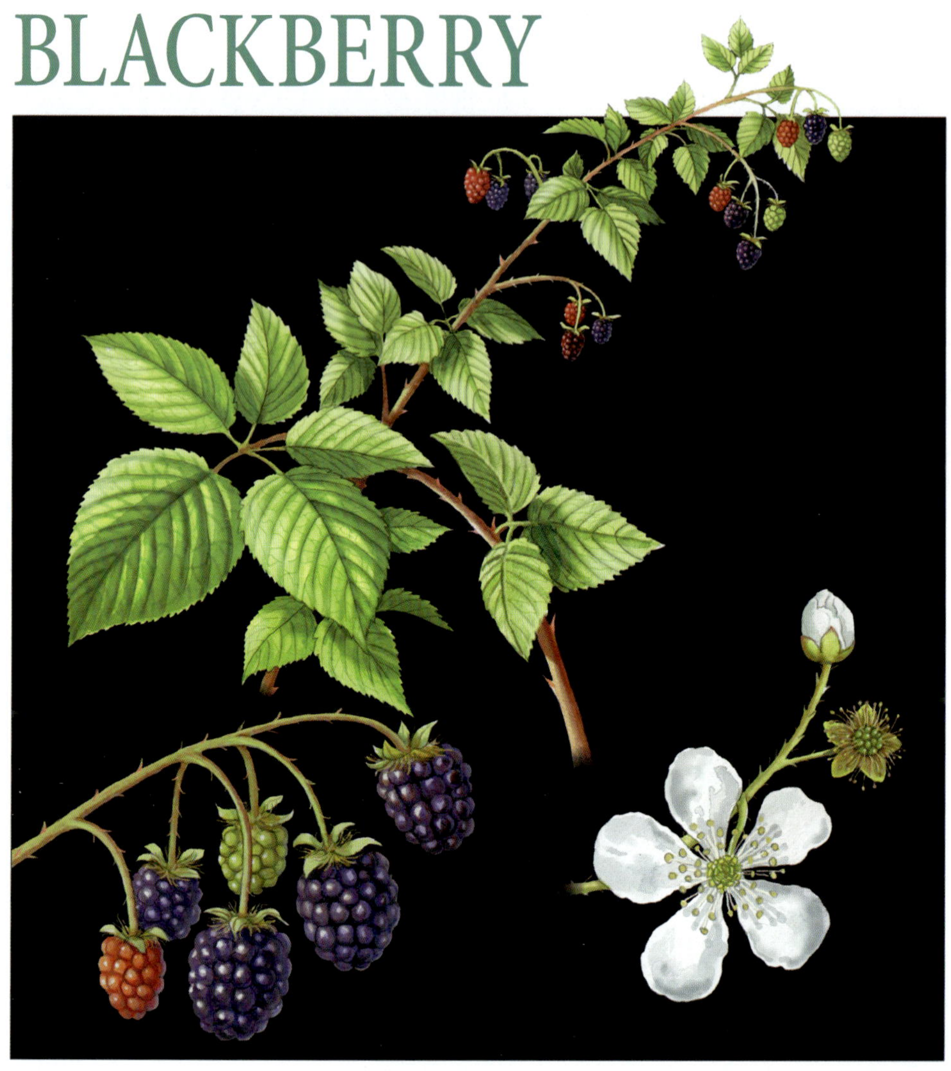

Rubus canadensis (Canadian Blackberry)
R. ursinus (Trailing Blackberry)

FAMILY: Rosaceae

OTHER NAMES: *Fr.* Mûrier

PARTS USED: Leaves, fruit, root bark

CHARACTERISTICS: Berries sweet, leaves and root bark astringent, cool

ACTIONS: Astringent, antiseptic, antioxidant, anti-inflammatory, diuretic, antispasmodic, tonic

RANGE: *R. canadensis:* introduced in British Columbia, native southern Ontario to Maritimes; *R. ursinus* native to southern British Columbia

Many different varieties of Blackberry grow throughout Canada, their invasive nature annoying those who are oblivious to their many attributes. *R. canadensis* is a perennial shrub with mostly smooth arching reddish stems and can grow 2–5 m. tall. Its toothed compound leaves grow in groups of 3 or 5 arranged alternately up the stem. Clusters of white or pinkish 5-petalled flowers appear in early summer and turn into green fruit in August as the flowers die back. These ripen to red, and then turn dark purple or black as they become succulent, sweet, juicy berries that can be eaten by the handful. You can tell the difference between raspberries and blackberries by the core: a raspberry's core is hollow, whereas a blackberry's core is solid when picked. The leaves can be harvested during flowering and thoroughly dried for later use; the roots may be dug up at any time, the bark peeled off and dried in the oven. Be aware of spraying notices and avoid plants with disfigured leaves or flowers as this may indicate contamination. Also, black bears love these berries and may be present.

MEDICINAL USES:

Diarrhea, heavy menstruation, urinary tract infections, mouth infections, hemorrhoids

- Leaves and root bark contain tannins which are astringent and help dry and tighten tissues, resolve mucus, and control bleeding. Root contains higher concentrations. The berries have many important vitamins and minerals and contain polyphenols which are highly antioxidant, destroying free radicals and fighting stress and inflammation.
- Reduces inflammation in the intestinal tract. Relieves diarrhea and dysentery, especially in children. Restores tone in the digestive system and reduces hyperpermeability in the gut. Helps prevent stomach ulcers and combats Helicobacter pylori bacteria. Cream or ointment can be used to treat hemorrhoids.
- Infusion of leaves or decoction of root bark makes a good mouthwash for spongy gums, thrush, mouth ulcers, toothaches.
- Leaves and root bark, along with juice of the berries, have traditionally been used to treat anemia, menorrhagia, and leukorrhea. Leaf extract has been shown to have hypoglycemic properties.
- Poultice can stop minor bleeding and help heal skin ulcers, bruises, psoriasis.
- Decoction of root bark is diuretic and helps with urinary problems.
- Berries are highly nutritious, containing vitamins C and K, manganese, and fibre. They are known for their anticancerous properties, as they are rich in antioxidants that destroy free radicals and strengthen immunity.

OTHER USES:

- Plump berries make a tasty jam, especially when mixed with Blackcurrants.
- May be used to make wine or added to brandy or other sweetened alcohol to make liqueurs.

INFUSION: 2 tbsp. dried leaves in 2 cups of water. Cool and drink ½ cup every couple of hours for diarrhea.

DECOCTION: 1 ounce of root bark boiled in 3½ cups water. Reduce to 2½ cups. Take ½ cup every 2 hours.

TINCTURE: Dried herb, 1:5 in 40% alcohol, 1–4 ml. up to 3 times a day.

CAUTION: Wilted leaves may be toxic. Use either fresh or fully dried. Do not exceed recommended dosage.

BLACK COHOSH

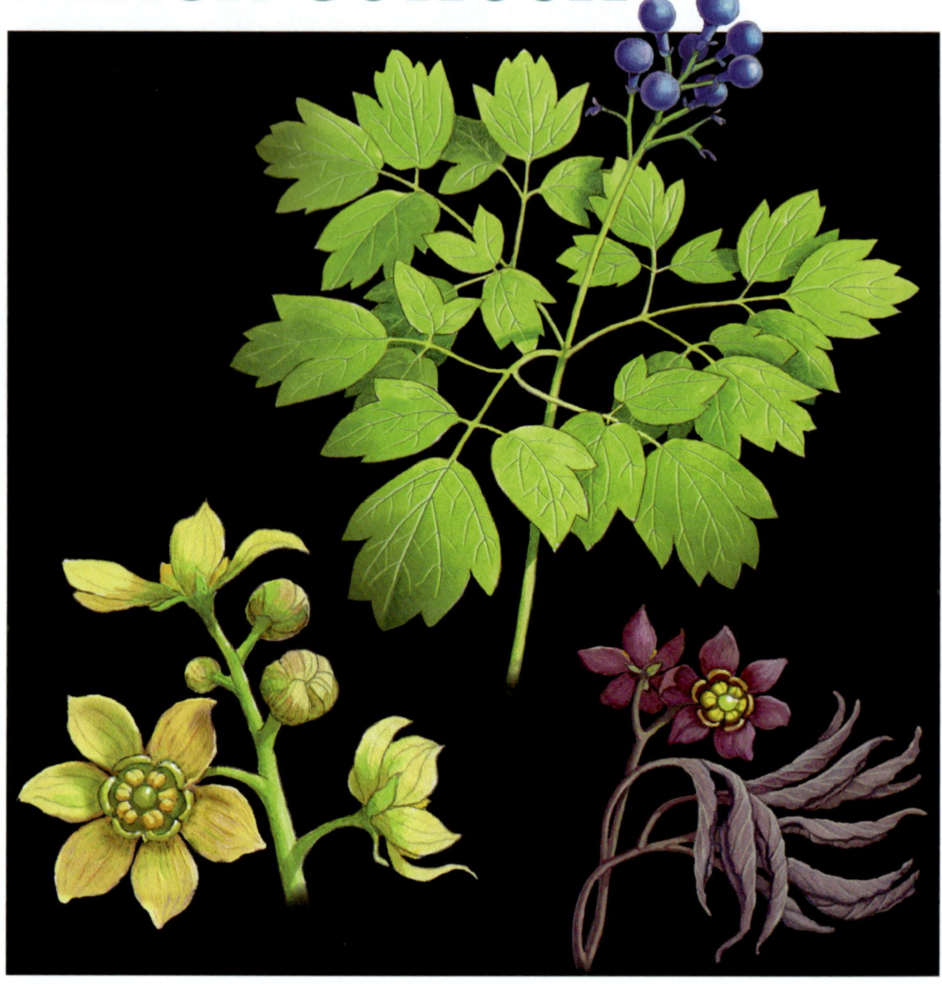

Actaea (Cimicifuga) racemosa

FAMILY: Ranunculaceae

OTHER NAMES: Black Snakeroot, Rattle Root, Black Bugbane, Fairy Candle, *Fr.* Actée à grappes noires, Cimicaire à grappes

PARTS USED: Root

CHARACTERISTICS: Sweet, pungent, slightly bitter, cool

ACTIONS: Alterative, anodyne, antispasmodic, antidepressant, antirheumatic, antivenomous, anti-inflammatory, slightly astringent, cardiotonic, diuretic, diaphoretic, emmenogogue, hypotensive, expectorant, relaxant

RANGE: Native to Ontario, introduced in Quebec

This plant's roots have a long history of use as a traditional remedy by Indigenous Peoples, and this knowledge was passed down to the first settlers, primarily as a women's medicine, but also in the treatment of other diseases, including rheumatism. It lost popularity in North America in the early 1900s, but later in the 1950s the Germans began to research its effectiveness for menopause, and it is still widely used today throughout Europe and North America. This native perennial grows in shaded woods, but is commonly grown in gardens. Its fragrant white bottlebrush-like flowers, which reportedly repel bugs, grow on tall, arching racemes reaching up to 1.5 m. high in midsummer. Its basal leaves are sharp and irregularly toothed, compound, and alternate with 2–5 leaflets, terminating in a 3-lobed leaflet. Its black, gnarled roots are harvested in early fall after the flowers have faded and leaves have died back. They can be cut into pieces and dried or tinctured fresh for future use.

MEDICINAL USES:

Menopause, irregular periods, cramps, PMS, rheumatism, coughs, nerve pain

- One of the most important herbs for female problems, although it is not exclusively for women. Treats scanty periods, irregular menses, delayed or absent periods, cramps, spasms, low back pain, fluid retention, mood changes, and PMS.
- Reduces perimenopause and menopausal symptoms: hot flashes, mood swings, anxiety, insomnia, night sweats, depression (especially when combined with St. John's Wort).
- Eases discomfort from rheumatism caused by dampness, arthritis, neuralgia, sciatica, neck and lower back pain, inflammation, any pain that is heavy, achy, shifting, and comes and goes.
- Antispasmodic actions relieve symptoms of bronchitis, asthma, whooping cough, pneumonia, respiratory conditions associated with cold and dampness. Use a decoction of the root combined with honey as a cough syrup.

OTHER USES: Fresh or dried plant repels bugs.

DECOCTION: ½–1 tsp. in 1 cup water, simmer 10–15 minutes. Drink 2–3 cups per day.

TINCTURE: Best fresh in brandy or vodka. 1:2 in 50% alcohol. Start with 2–4 ml. 1–3 times a day. Increase gradually if needed. Continue for at least 8 weeks. If headache occurs, reduce dosage.

COMBINATIONS: For menopause with Red Clover, St. John's Wort, Chasteberry, or Dong Quai (*Angelica sinensis*). For arthritis with Willow Bark, Sarsaparilla, or Poplar Bark.

RESEARCH: Since the active ingredients in Black Cohosh are unknown and it is unclear how they exert their influence on the body or what dosage is effective, any studies that have been conducted on its efficacy have been inconclusive. Some have found it to be ineffective at reducing menopausal symptoms, while other studies have concluded there was sufficient evidence that it reduced symptoms, and in 2017 it was approved in Europe as an effective treatment for menopause.

CAUTION: Not for use during pregnancy, except during labour. Large doses may cause headaches, dizziness, nausea. Avoid use if taking Tamoxifen, as it augments the effects of the drug. No studies have yet been done to prove safety after 12 months of use. Use only products from a reputable dealer, as some products contain unlisted ingredients.

BLACK WALNUT, BUTTERNUT

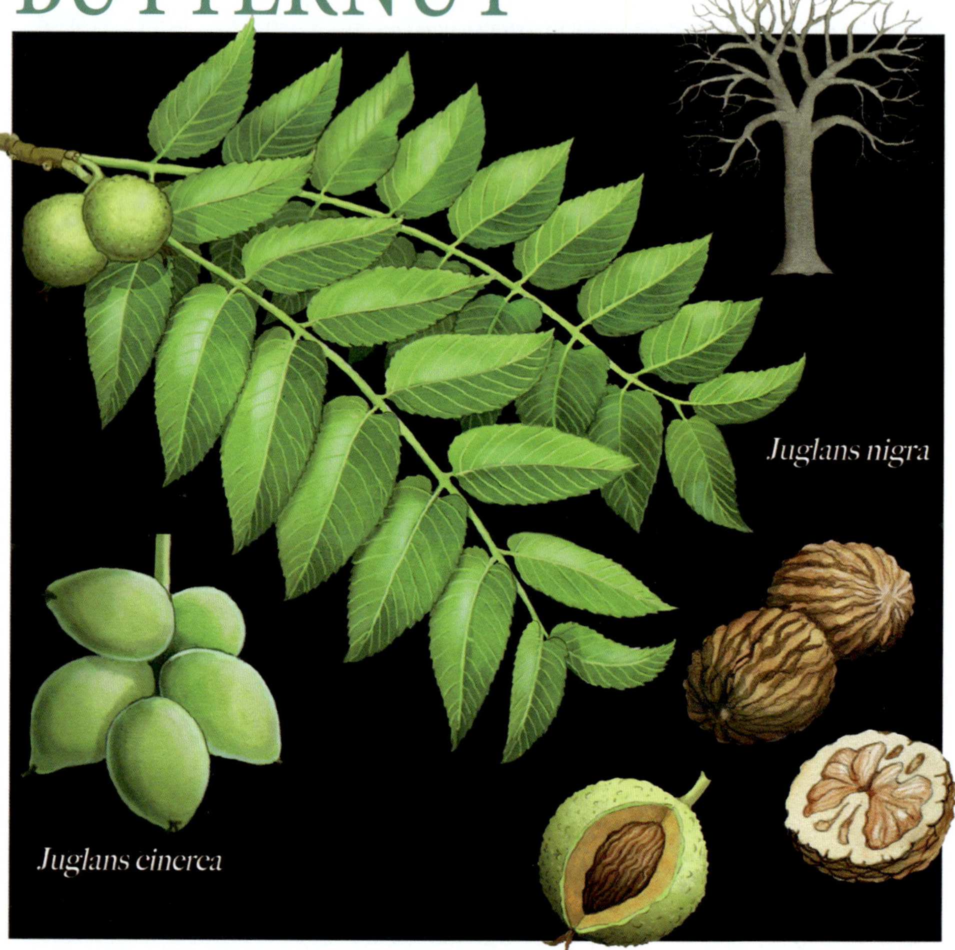

***Juglans nigra* (Black Walnut), *Juglans cinerea* (Butternut)**

FAMILY: Juglandaceae

OTHER NAMES: *J. nigra:* Eastern Black Walnut, *Fr.* Noyer noir; *J. cinerea:* Butternut, White Walnut, *Fr.* Noyer cendré, Noix longues

PARTS USED: Fruit, inner bark, leaf, hull, roots

CHARACTERISTICS: Slightly warming, drying, bitter

ACTIONS: Alterative, anodyne, anti-inflammatory, antifungal, antioxidant, anticancer, astringent, tonic, laxative, vermifuge, antiparasitic, antibacterial

RANGE: *J. nigra*: Native to Ontario, Quebec, New Brunswick; *J. cinerea*: Native to Southern Ontario, Quebec, New Brunswick, introduced in Manitoba, Prince Edward Island

Black Walnut trees, found throughout most of Eastern and Central Canada, have a long history both as a food and a herbal medicine among Indigenous Peoples and settlers. Another tree, Butternut (*J. cinerea*), can easily be mistaken for Black Walnut. Both have edible nuts and have very similar medicinal uses; however, the Butternut has more elongated, sticky fruit in clusters of 2 to 5 or more and usually has 11–17 leaflets on a hairy stalk. Black Walnut is usually taller, reaching up to 30 m., with 15–23 leaflets and round fruit in groups of up to three. Its roots and leaves secrete a substance called juglone which inhibits other types of plants or trees, and even its own seeds, from growing beneath it, protecting itself from competition. The fruit ripens and falls off the tree in September or October, so harvest soon after, picking nuts that are green and slightly soft. Remove hulls with gloves as the flesh stains hands and clothing. Discard the hulls that are black or wormy, then wash thoroughly in a bucket, being careful not to discard the water onto your plants. Leave out in the sun to dry for a couple of weeks before cracking. Bark should be dried for 1 year before using to prevent cramping.

MEDICINAL USES:

Chronic constipation, diarrhea, parasites, high blood pressure, cholesterol, fungal infections, skin problems, mouth infections

NUTS: Used as a nutritional food, walnuts are usually eaten raw or roasted or pressed for their oil. Higher in protein, phytosterols, omega-3 fatty acids, and tocopherols than most other popular nuts, it makes them beneficial in cancer prevention and heart disease. They lower blood pressure and reduce high cholesterol, purifiy the blood, and antioxidants scavenge for free radicals. The oil is extracted, warmed, and applied to the scalp for dandruff, or to ease muscular or joint pain. Eating a few walnuts a day boosts memory and learning ability and improves immunity.

HULLS: Traditionally the black, sticky part of the green hulls were usually used for gastrointestinal irritation, diarrhea and constipation. and as an antiparasitic, but it is also antifungal, and when dried and ground it is used to treat warts, cold sores, and athlete's foot. Hull extract may help ulcers, shingles, abscesses, cancers, boils, acne, eczema, and other types of skin itching and inflammation; however, be aware that it stains the skin. May be used on scalp to reduce hair loss. Decoction may be used as a gargle for mouth or throat infections, tonsillitis, bleeding gums, and thrush. Powder rubbed on teeth strengthens tooth enamel. Used traditionally for hypothyroidism and to improve digestion.

LEAVES: Used to treat diarrhea, colic, worms, sunburn, itching, dandruff, and externally to reduce fever and rheumatic joint pain. With hulls, they have a cleansing action on the digestive tract, relieving both constipation and diarrhea.

BARK: Root bark is used by the Cherokee in a decoction as a laxative, for toothache and decay, chewed and used as a toothbrush. Bark and leaves ground together as a paste is used as an antibacterial on wounds and to treat ringworm and athlete's foot. Inner bark is used in decoctions or tinctures for constipation, and to aid digestion, stimulate liver, and treat skin conditions.

OTHER USES:

- Brown, yellow, or orange dye can be made from the fresh hulls to dye clothing or hair.
- The tree itself is valued for its dark wood, which is prized by cabinet makers and is resistant to decay.
- The green, unripe walnuts are used to make a traditional Italian liqueur called Nocino by macerating them in alcohol, sugar, and spices.

SHELLED WALNUTS: Take 5–10 per day to improve blood pressure.

INFUSION: Put 2 tbsp. of bark or leaves in 1 cup boiling water, take 2–3 times a day.

TINCTURE: Use fresh hulls, fill a mason jar ⅓ full of vodka, fill jar with coarsely chopped hulls, and top up with more vodka to cover. Macerate about 6 weeks, strain. Take 5–20 drops 3–4 times a day, increasing slightly each day until it takes effect.

SALVE: Break up fresh green hulls into pieces and place in a mason jar to about half full (use gloves!). Fill the jar with oil (olive, almond, coconut, etc.). Place the opened jar in a pan with water and gently heat (do not boil) for 2–3 hours. Remove from heat, cover with a cloth, and let sit for a few days to further infuse. Discard hulls and use to make salves for skin problems.

COMBINATIONS: A tincture called Wormwood complex made from Black Walnut hulls, Wormwood, and Cloves is used as a remedy against parasitic infections.

RESEARCH:

- Studies conducted on the kernel extracts have concluded that it could be a promising remedy for inflammatory diseases such as rheumatoid arthritis and some skin disorders. Extracts have been found to contain twenty-six substances that have anti-inflammatory activity.
- A powerful antioxidant, it contains arginine, an amino acid that turns into nitric acid, which is a vasodilator that can lower blood pressure, and plant sterols and omega-3 fatty acids, which raise HDL (good cholesterol) and reduce plaque buildup in the arteries.
- Juglone is considered to be a significant anticancer compound that may be effective in treating many commonly occurring cancers.
- Black Walnut is one of the most important medicinal plants, with great potential for further research.

CAUTION: Bark is considered poisonous, use with caution. Eating more than a handful of nuts may cause an allergic reaction in some people. Do not use spoiled nuts. Leaves may cause allergic reactions in some people. Use with caution if you suffer from cirrhosis, stomach or intestinal ulcer, thrombophlebitis, gastritis, or are pregnant or lactating due to lack of research. Avoid taking at the same time as other medications.

BLOODROOT

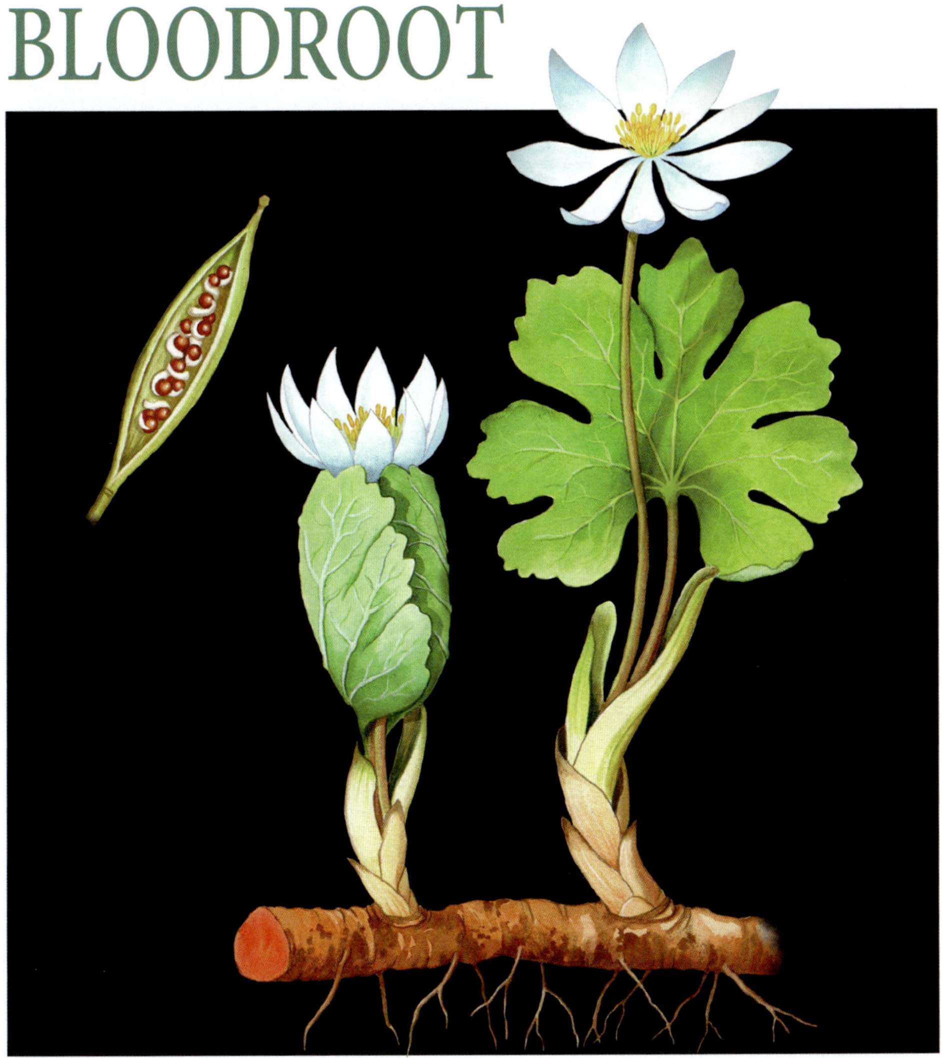

Sanguinaria canadensis

FAMILY: Papaveraceae

OTHER NAMES: Red root, Snakebite, Sweet Slumber, Bloodwort, Puccoon, Tetterwort, *Fr.* Sanguinaire

PARTS USED: Dried rhizome

CHARACTERISTICS: Bitter, acrid; in small amounts, drying and cooling; in large amounts, warm and stimulating

ACTIONS: Expectorant, stimulant, alterative, antibiotic, abortifacient, diuretic, emmenagogue, febrifuge, antispasmodic, diaphoretic, antioxidant, anticancer, emetic in large doses

RANGE: Native to Manitoba, Ontario, Quebec, New Brunswick, Nova Scotia

Bloodroot is a low-growing native perennial and a powerful medicinal herb that has been used by Indigenous Peoples for centuries—but it can be extremely poisonous if not used correctly. It's identified by its orangey-red rhizome, which is 2.5–10 cm. long with orangey-red rootlets, and oozes a red juice when cut open, hence its name.

Found in woods and clearings, it can grow up to 25 cm. tall, usually having only one large leaf with several lobes. In early spring, when the flower first sprouts from the rhizome, it is wrapped in a pale-green, lobed leaf. The leaf opens and a beautiful, waxy, white flower with golden stamens emerges, usually only lasting a day or two. The seedpod appears late in the summer and contains shiny bright-red seeds, which have a worm-like substance attached to each one. When the seeds are thrown out of the pod, this substance attracts ants. The ants then carry the seeds back to their nests, which are often far from the mother plant—the perfect place for a new plant to sprout up.

Please note: Bloodroot is endangered and should be cultivated, not collected in the wild. The root should be dug up in the fall after the leaves die off, then dried quickly or it will deteriorate.

MEDICINAL USES:

Bronchitis, pneumonia, skin cancer, heart palpitations

- Antimicrobial and expectorant, it eliminates phlegm, reduces inflammation in the lungs and relaxes the muscles to ease coughing. Used in formulas for swollen lymph nodes.
- Used by many Indigenous Peoples for a variety of ailments, including colds, coughs, diarrhea, general debility, poison ivy, snakebites, and as an emmenagogue and abortifacient.
- There is evidence that it reduces plaque and gingivitis in the mouth, but recent studies have shown a link between Bloodroot use and oral leukoplakia, or precancerous lesions in the mouth and gums.
- Highly antioxidant, it has been used on skin conditions like acne, psoriasis, eczema, warts, skin tags and moles. However, recently a product once sold as a veterinary medicine called black salve, which contains Bloodroot, activated charcoal, and zinc chloride (a corrosive), among other ingredients, has been marketed as a remedy for skin cancer or other skin conditions. Use of this product can have disastrous effects, including permanent disfigurement and recurring cancers. Clinical evidence shows Bloodroot could possibly one day be an effective treatment for skin cancer, but its misuse through self-treatment can be hazardous.

DECOCTION: ⅛ tsp. dry powdered root per 1 cup of boiling water.

TINCTURE: 1–2 drops topically or mixed with water as a mouthwash.

CAUTION: Bloodroot is not used much today due to its toxicity, although if taken orally in small doses for short periods of time it can be relatively safe. However, due to its unpredictable effects self-treatment is not recommended. Bloodroot is toxic in large doses or with prolonged use. May cause nausea and vomiting, burns to the skin and stomach, vertigo, tunnel vision, or glaucoma. Do not use if pregnant or breastfeeding. Use only with extreme caution.

BLUE COHOSH

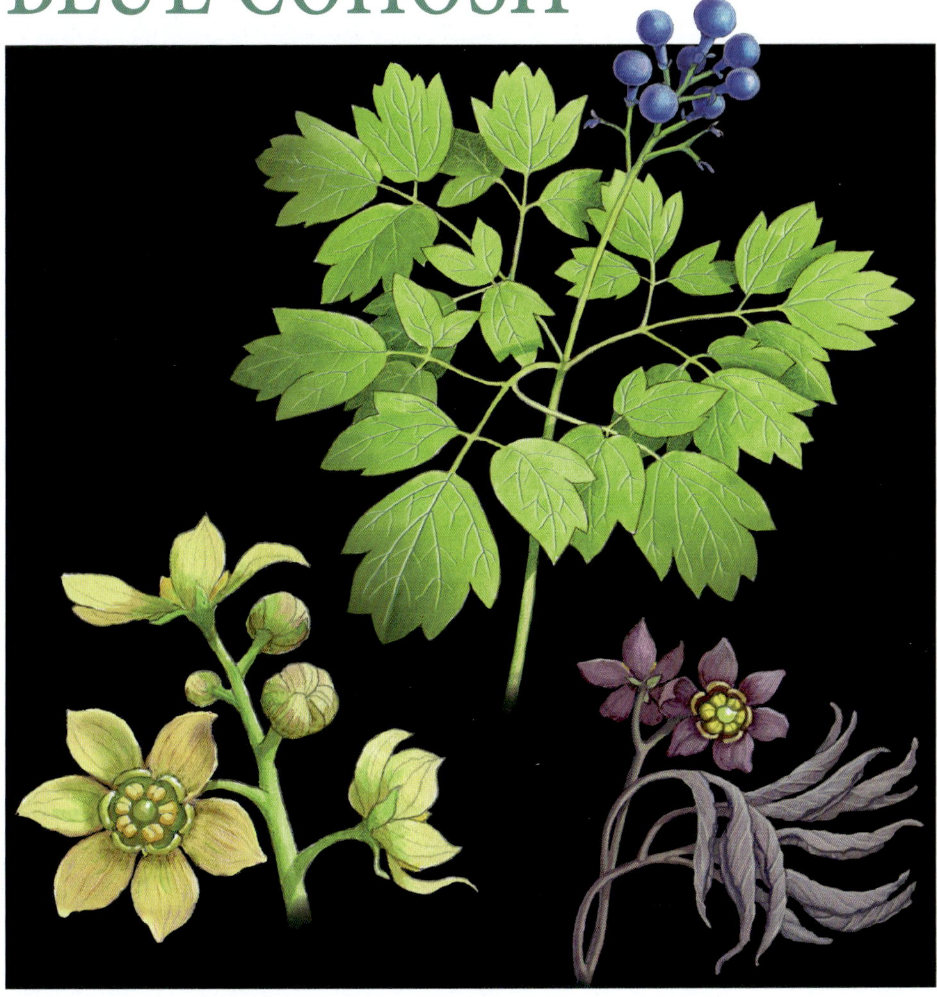

Caulophyllum thalictroides

FAMILY: Berberidaceae

OTHER NAMES: Papoose Root, Blueberry Root, *Fr.* Cohosh Bleu, Léontice faux-pigamon

PARTS USED: Root, rhizome

CHARACTERISTICS: Warming, relaxing, drying, acrid, bitter

ACTIONS: Antispasmodic, anti-inflammatory, emmenagogue, relaxing nervine, uterine tonic, abortifacient, diuretic, diaphoretic, emetic

RANGE: Native from Manitoba to Nova Scotia

Blue Cohosh is another herb traditionally labelled as a women's herb, as it was historically used by Indigenous Peoples and settlers for menstrual problems and during childbirth. The erect central stem of this woodland perennial grows 30–90 cm. tall, is smooth and light green to purplish in colour, and terminates in a panicle of small flowers with 6 sepals that are greenish yellow or purplish, with insignificant yellow-green petals, 6 yellow stamens, and a round beak-like ovary. It blooms from mid to late spring before the leaves have fully developed, then the flowers are replaced by round green berries which eventually turn bright blue later in the summer. Roots should be collected in the fall and dried for later use in teas or tinctures. The berries and aerial parts are usually considered toxic.

MEDICINAL USES:

Childbirth, delayed menstruation, cramps, rheumatism, spasmodic coughing, anxiety

- Contains several active alkaloids, including methylcytisine, and saponins which have been proven to act on uterine muscles, resulting in an oxytocic response, increasing the strength of uterine contractions. Traditional use was to administer small doses (1–7 drops a day) over a week or two before childbirth to tone the uterus in cases of poor circulation or uterine weakness, or a slightly larger dose in cases of stalled labour. Often used by midwives to prepare a woman for childbirth in a formula called "Mother's Cordial," containing Partridgeberry, Raspberry leaf, Black Cohosh, and False Unicorn. It eases pain and strengthens contractions. Particularly useful if labour is slow and the mother is exhausted. Should only be used under supervision and in small doses.
- Contains caulosaponin, which encourages menstruation. Uterine tonic, for inflammation, cramps, delayed menstruation, dysmenorrhea, breast pain, leukorrhea, vaginitis.
- Can ease arthritis and rheumatic pain, neuralgia.
- May help with spasmodic asthma, whooping cough, bronchitis.
- In formulas for anxiety, often combined with Skullcap.
- Used externally for toothache and as a remedy for Poison Oak or Poison Ivy.

OTHER USES: Some claim the seeds can be roasted to use as a coffee substitute (the roasting process is supposed to remove the toxins). However, it is not recommended.

TINCTURE: 1:5 in 60% alcohol. Take 5 drops every 4 hours or as advised by a professional. Best if used in formulas.

COMBINATIONS: With False Unicorn, Raspberry leaf, Motherwort, and Yarrow where there is weakness or congestion in the uterine tissues.

RESEARCH: There are some safety concerns around the use of Blue Cohosh during childbirth because of a small number of reports of adverse reactions in the foetus, including congestive heart failure. Due to the heart-stimulating effects, it could be damaging to the baby's heart in certain cases, particularly if guidelines are not followed. It should be noted that in one or more of these cases a higher dose was used than is recommended, and quality and purity checks were not carried out, so the herb could have been contaminated.

CAUTION: Use only root, as aerial parts may be toxic. Not for use during pregnancy except in the last couple of weeks and only in small doses. May provoke uterine contractions and cause miscarriage. Excessive doses may cause high blood pressure, nausea, vomiting, headaches, and incoordination. Contraindicated for people with diabetes, angina, high blood pressure, or heart disease, as it may cause narrowing of blood vessels to the heart. Avoid in hyperglycemia as it raises blood sugar levels. Powdered root may cause irritation of the mucous membranes. Touching plant may cause irritation in some people. Use only under strict supervision by a herbal practitioner.

BLUE FLAG IRIS

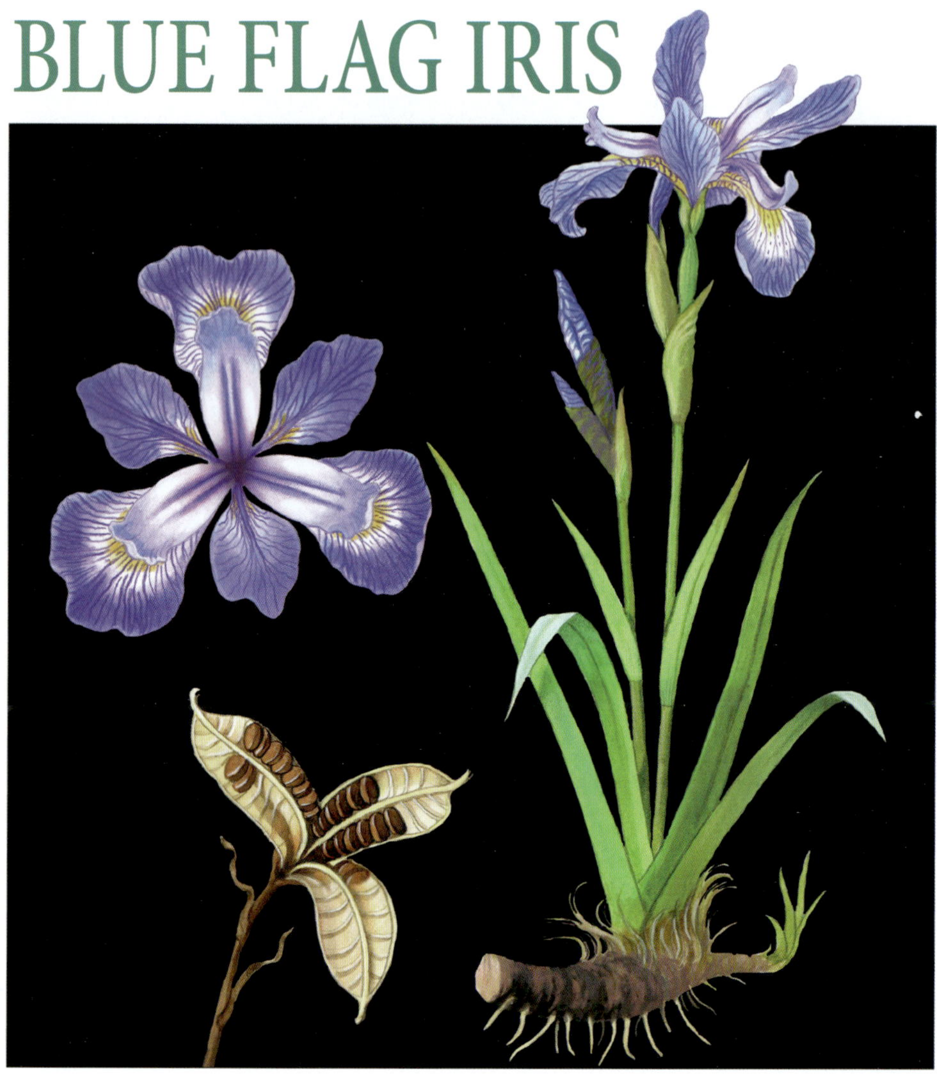

Iris versicolour

FAMILY: Iridaceae

OTHER NAMES: Flag Lily, Poison Flag, Wild Iris, *Fr.* Fleur-de-lis, Iris versicolore

PARTS USED: Rhizome, dried

CHARACTERISTICS: Bitter, acrid, cool, drying

ACTIONS: Alterative, anti-inflammatory, cathartic, diuretic, stimulant, emetic, laxative, lymphagogue, cholagogue, astringent, diaphoretic, hepatic

RANGE: Native to Nunavut, from Saskatchewan to Newfoundland and Labrador

This showy native perennial prefers damp areas like ditches, wetlands, or riverbanks, growing to a height of 50–90 cm. It has narrow sword-shaped leaves and pretty blue or purple flowers that bloom in June or July. There are often several flowers along its sturdy stem, each one with three colourful sepals streaked with violet, yellow, and green markings and three shorter violet-striped petals. The fleshy horizontal root has annual joints and a slight odor along with a pungent, acrid taste and should be a light pinkish-brown colour inside. Avoid using roots that are dark or reddish brown inside.

Dig up roots early in the fall, slice transversely, and dry for later use. Take care not to confuse Blue Flag with Sweet Flag, as they look very similar before the flower blooms.

MEDICINAL USES:

Liver congestion, glandular congestion, hepatitis, jaundice, various skin diseases

- Works primarily to correct problems associated with liver congestion, such as hepatitis, jaundice, constipation, indigestion, and skin problems. Stimulates bile production, and relieves stagnation in the liver and spleen. Helps treat hepatitis and jaundice. Use only in small doses as it will cause diarrhea and vomiting in large amounts and should not be used if the body is in a weakened state.
- In small doses and repeated at short intervals, it stimulates the glandular system and lymphatics where there is stagnation or enlargement. Used for enlarged thyroid, enlarged spleen, or swollen lymph nodes.
- Soothes chronic skin diseases like herpes, acne, psoriasis, eczema. Works through the liver to detoxify and purify the blood.
- Was used by Indigenous Peoples to induce vomiting in cases of food poisoning.
- Roots can be boiled in water and mashed to make a poultice to treat pain, cuts, burns, bruises, snakebites, and swelling, or to relieve arthritic joints.

OTHER USES:

- Flowers can be made into an infusion that can be used as a litmus test for acids and alkalis.
- Leaves can be dried and used to weave baskets or mats.
- Some Indigenous Peoples carried the root as protection against rattlesnakes.

TINCTURE: Dried root, 1:5, 50% alcohol. Take 5–10 drops up to 2 times a day.

CAUTION: Blue Flag's rhizomes are poisonous and excessive use can cause vomiting, diarrhea, fatigue, and dehydration. Fresh root is an irritant and can cause burning in the mouth and mucous membranes. Should only be used dried and only under supervision of a certified herbalist. Do not use if pregnant or breastfeeding.

BLUE VERVAIN

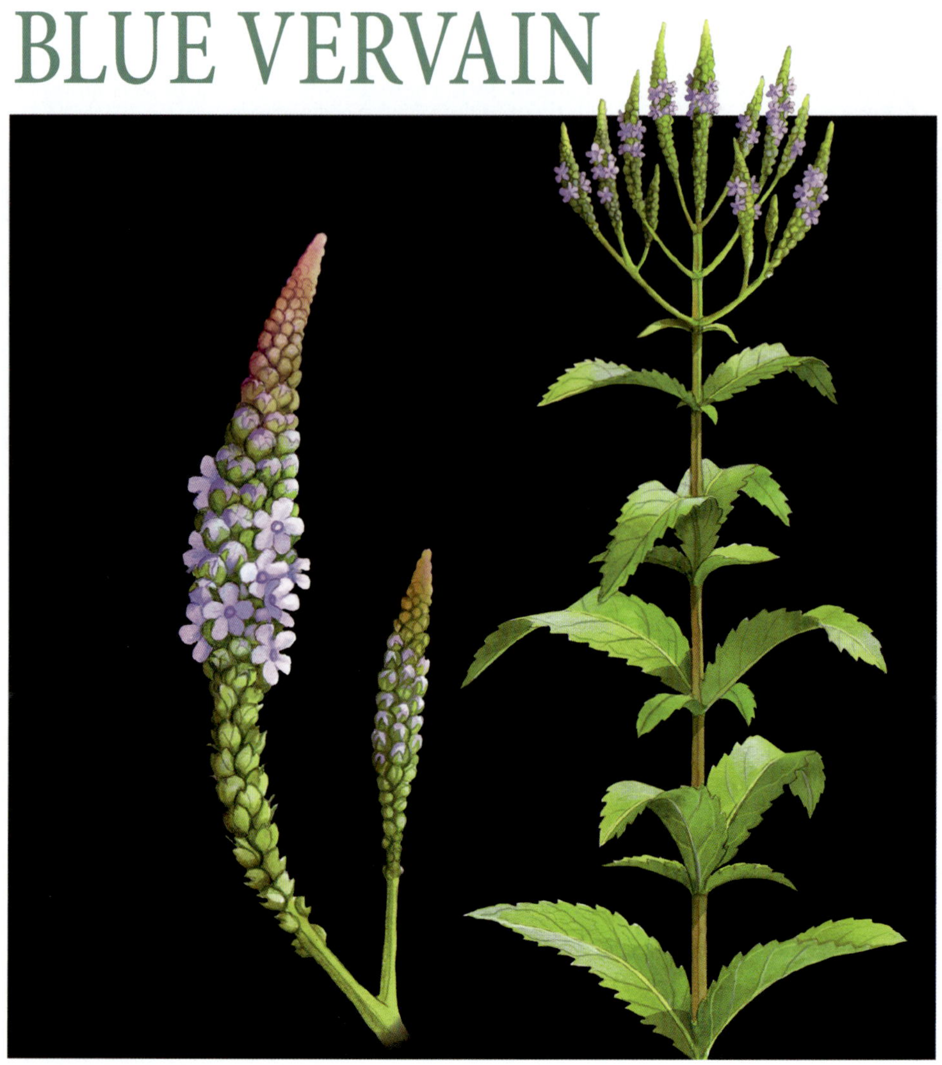

Verbena hastata

FAMILY: Verbenaceae

OTHER NAMES: Blue Verbena, Indian Hyssop, Swamp Verbena, Herba Sacra, *Fr.* Verveine bleue

PARTS USED: Whole plant

CHARACTERISTICS: Cold, bitter, drying; root astringent

ACTIONS: Astringent, antimicrobial, anti-inflammatory, antidepressant, antioxidant, antispasmodic, bitter tonic, diaphoretic, diuretic, emmenagogue, emetic (in large doses), nervine, febrifuge, galactagogue, vulnerary, tranquilizer

RANGE: Native to British Columbia, and from Saskatchewan to Maritimes

This common weed native to North America is similar in medicinal properties to the European variety *Verbena officinalis*, which has been revered as a sacred healing herb for centuries. It is a tall, erect, branching perennial that grows from 0.6 to 1.5 m. high with intense blue-violet flower spikes and a reddish square stem and opposite lanceolate leaves that are conspicuously veined and coarsely serrated. It blooms from mid to late summer, each flower spike being up to 13 cm. long, the individual flowers having 5 lobes and no noticeable scent. It grows in ditches and along roadsides and in pastures and wetlands throughout Canada, and makes a nice addition to gardens. Harvest when the plants come into bloom, tincture fresh or dry quickly in a cool, dark place for later use in teas.

MEDICINAL USES:

Anxiety, stress, insomnia, fever, gingivitis, indigestion, PMS

- Primarily used as a nerve tonic, it is helpful in people who are anxious, stressed, or depressed, often with frayed nerves and burnout. It restores balance and calm, acting as a neuroprotective agent, sedative, and muscle relaxant. Helps those who have difficulty falling asleep due to an overactive mind or stomach tension. May be used over long periods of time to nourish the nervous system.
- Powerful diuretic and antimicrobial, it can be used at the beginning of a fever to stimulate perspiration and remove toxins. Also nourishes and strengthens during convalescence by improving liver function.
- Its bitter qualities stimulate the liver and help treat a number of chronic liver problems such as cirrhosis and jaundice. Calms the digestive system and relieves nervous stomach indigestion.
- Gentle astringent, soothes inflamed gums and treats gingivitis. Helps teething babies. May be used externally for minor wounds and sores.
- Used as a uterine tonic to relieve cramps, pain, and headaches due to PMS.

FOLKLORE: Once believed to have magical properties. Druids and sorcerers used the European variety in their rites and incantations; it was used in love charms, as it was said to have aphrodisiac qualities. Called Herba Sacra, priests used it in rituals as it was supposedly used to staunch the wounds of Jesus. It was often worn around the neck for good luck and to ward off headaches.

INFUSION: 2 tbsp. dried herb in 2 cups boiling water. Steep 10 minutes, strain. Best if combined with other herbs due to its bitter taste.

TINCTURE: Fresh 1:2, dry 1:4, in 40% alcohol. Take 1–2 ml., 2–4 times a day.

COMBINATIONS: With Motherwort, Skullcap, Rose, Tulsi for anxiety, stress. With Peppermint and Elder flower for fevers. With Milk Thistle, Dandelion root, and Burdock root for liver support and digestive health. With Hops and Valerian for sleep problems. With Goldenrod flowers and Mullein for headaches.

CAUTION: Not recommended during pregnancy due to danger of miscarriage in large doses. Otherwise no known safety concerns.

BOGBEAN

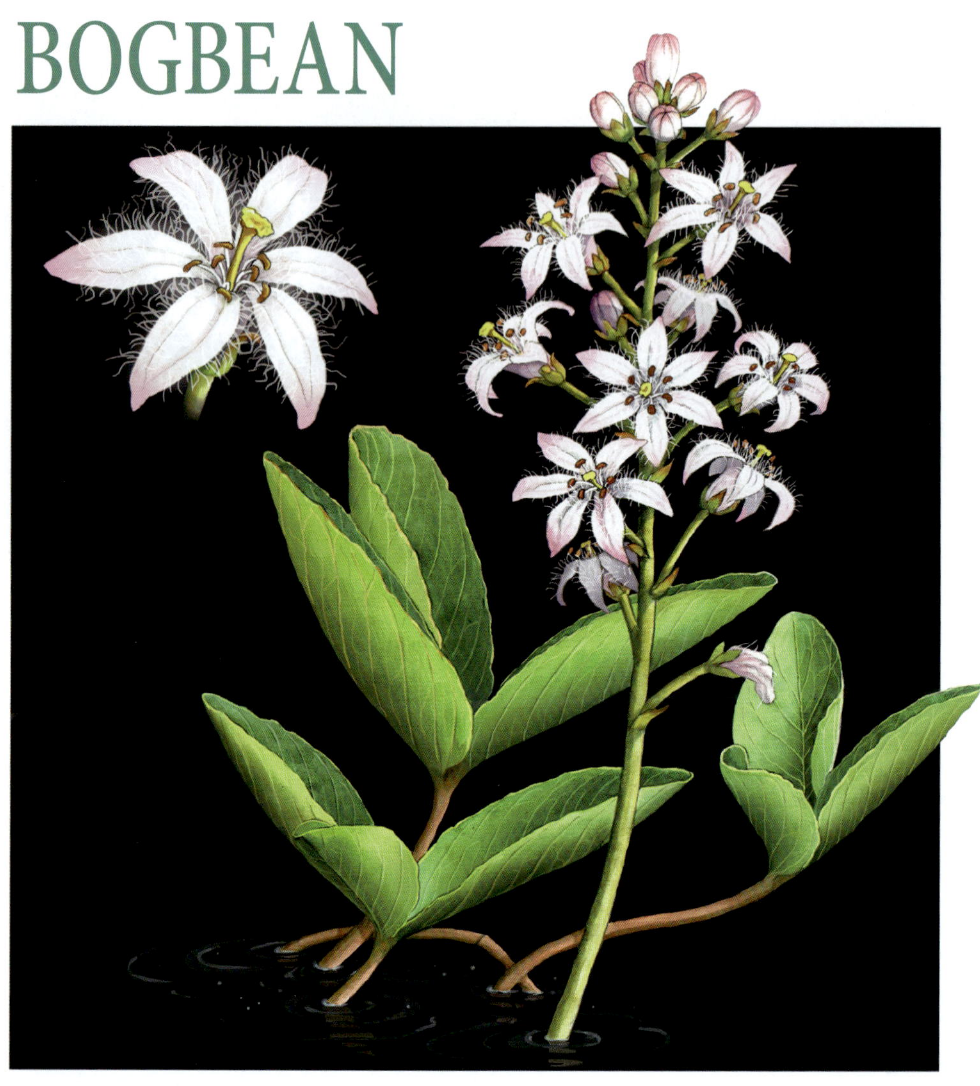

Menyanthes trifoliata

FAMILY: Menyanthaceae

OTHER NAMES: Buckbean, Marsh Trefoil, *Fr.* Trèfle d'eau, Herbe à canards

PARTS USED: Whole plant, mostly leaf

CHARACTERISTICS: Cool, very bitter

ACTIONS: Bitter tonic, anti-inflammatory, antirheumatic, antimicrobial, cathartic, antioxidant, astringent, carminative, diuretic, emetic, emmenagogue, febrifuge, stomachic

RANGE: Native across Canada

As its name suggests, this native plant grows in wetlands, ponds, bogs, swamps, and marshes. It has been used for centuries in both Europe and North America as a digestive tonic and to relieve joint pain. The stalk is usually up to 30 cm. high, rising above the water and topped with 3 smooth, oval leaflets with smooth or toothed edges. Flower stalks produce clusters of rank-smelling white or pinkish star-shaped flowers, each about 1.3 cm. wide with 5 or 6 pointed lobes covered in white hairs. They bloom from late May into June. The fruit are oval capsules containing tiny yellowish seeds that float on the water when released. Gather the leaves in late spring to early summer, when the plants come into bloom, leaving the roots intact, and dry before using as the fresh leaves may cause vomiting. The root is edible but its acrid taste may be removed by dehydrating, pulverizing to a powder, and rinsing with water; however, this removes some of the minerals and active ingredients.

MEDICINAL USES:

Digestive and liver disorders, arthritic and rheumatic conditions, chronic infections, exhaustion and debility

- Very bitter digestive tonic, relieves digestive disturbances due to sluggishness and liver disorders, tonifies the digestive tract and increases flow of saliva and digestive juices. Relieves chronic diarrhea and stimulates bile production. Helps indigestion, hypoacidosis, bloating, and flatulence.
- May help with minor arthritic pain, gout or rheumatism, muscular pain, weakness, exhaustion, fibromyalgia and debility. Can assist with anorexia, or where there is a problem gaining weight, with lack of appetite and low vitality. Use in small doses.
- Infusion can be taken internally or used as a poultice for muscle pain and arthritis. Pounded roots or salves can be used for inflammatory skin conditions.

OTHER USES: Leaves were once used as a substitute for hops in beer-making. Powdered roots can be mixed with flour for making bread.

INFUSION: For a digestive tonic, add 1 tsp. herb to 1 cup boiling water, cover and simmer for 10 minutes. Take ½ cup 20 minutes before meals. Good for those with food sensitivities, bloating, or slow digestion.

TINCTURE: Fresh 1:2, dry 1:5, in 50% alcohol. Take 10–30 drops, 3 times a day.

COMBINATIONS: Usually combined with other digestive herbs such as Celery seed, Gentian, Calamus, and White Willow.

RESEARCH: In-vitro studies have observed the root extract can protect cells from DNA damage and moderately affects growth of certain bacterial and fungal pathogen strains. Could possibly play an important role in treating disease in future research.

CAUTION: Avoid in large doses. May irritate the digestive tract, especially if there is gastric inflammation, ulcers, diarrhea, colitis, or infection, as it stimulates production of hydrochloric acid. May cause vomiting or have a laxative effect. Avoid use if pregnant due to lack of studies.

BONESET

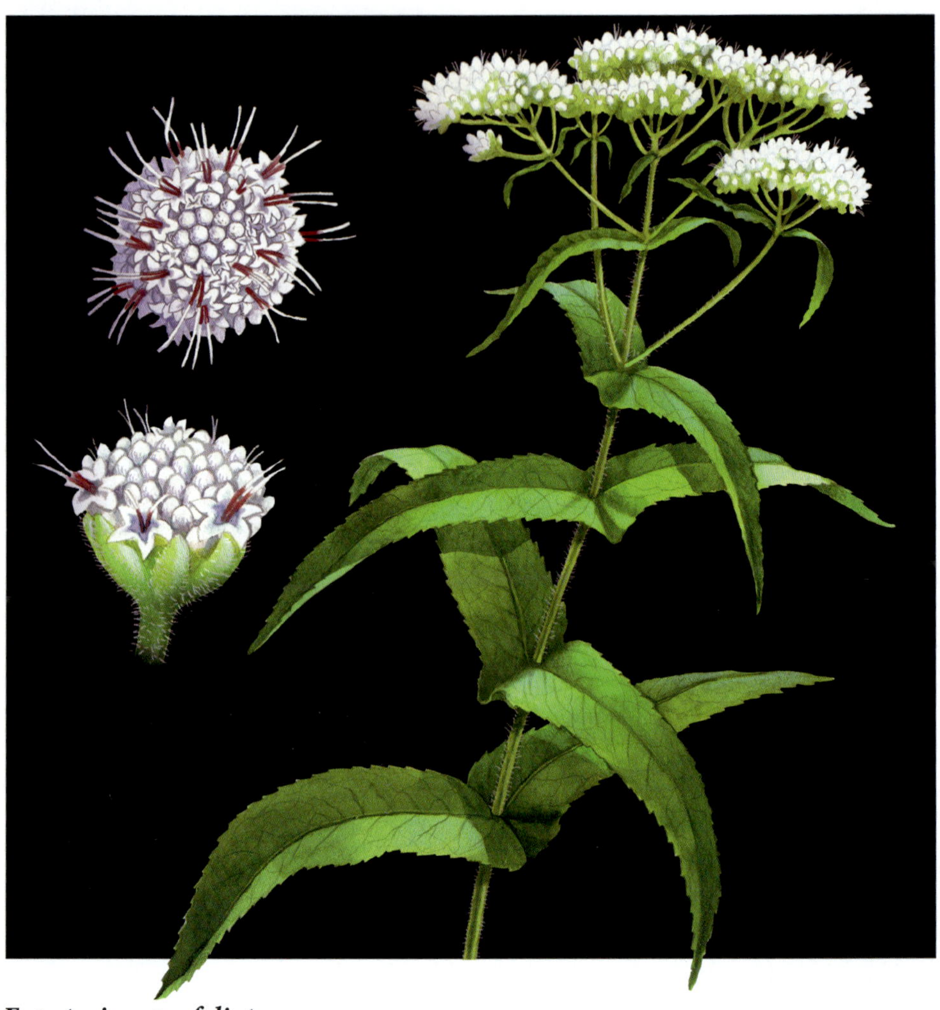

Eupatorium perfoliatum

FAMILY: Asteraceae

OTHER NAMES: Feverwort, Thoroughwort, Ague-weed, Indian sage, *Fr.* Eupatoire

PARTS USED: Aerial, dried

CHARACTERISTICS: Cool, bitter, pungent, drying

ACTIONS: Febrifuge, diaphoretic, expectorant, laxative, anticatarrhal, anti-spasmodic, tonic, diuretic, emetic, anti-inflammatory, antibacterial

RANGE: Native from Manitoba to the Maritimes

Boneset is native perennial that has always been popular in North America, both among Indigenous Peoples and European settlers, as a remedy for that deep-seated ache in one's bones at the onset of a flu or cold. It was used extensively during the pandemic of 1918–1919 to prevent infection, relieve the muscle aches and pains associated with the disease, and speed up recovery time. It has an erect, hollow, bristly stem 0.6–1.2 m. high, branched at the top with large, opposite leaves at right angles to the ones below, which are united at the base and appear to be pierced through by the stem. They are lance-shaped and tapered to a point, the edges finely toothed with fine hairs on the underside. The slightly aromatic flowerheads consist of 10–20 white, hairy-looking florets that bloom from July through September. It can be harvested after the flowers open, but because the fresh herb contains a toxic chemical called tremerol, it should always be dried for use in infusions, as this neutralizes the toxin. It is usually found along streams and marshes and prefers wet ground.

MEDICINAL USES:

Aches from colds and flu, congestion, intermittent fever, nervous stomach, rheumatism, arthritis

- Used primarily in viral and bacterial infections, it aids the immune system by stimulating white blood cells to fight the infection, treats high fever and chills by promoting sweating, clears mucus congestion, reduces inflammation, and loosens phlegm. Best when taken in a hot infusion; however, it is intensely bitter, so should be used with caution, as it can cause vomiting if used in large doses.
- Good for any damp congestion in the body, such as chronic sinus congestion. Loosens phlegm and reduces inflammation in the respiratory tract.
- Low doses in a cold infusion soothes and relaxes the stomach and relieves bloating and indigestion of nervous origin. A mild laxative, it improves appetite, aids in recuperation, and promotes sleep.
- Relieves aches and pains of rheumatism and arthritis. May be applied as a poultice.
- Named in the nineteenth century as a cure for dengue fever (or "breakbone fever"), which caused intense muscle pains. It was once used to treat malaria, typhoid, and snakebites.

TINCTURE: Dried flowering herb 1:5, 60% alcohol. Take 10–30 drops every 1–2 hours in hot water at first for fevers, increase gradually if necessary.

INFUSION: For fevers, add ½–1 tsp. dried herb to 1 cup of hot water, infuse 10–15 minutes. Add honey if desired. Drink every 1–2 hours until sweating occurs, dose may be increased, but if you start to feel nauseous, stop. It's your body's way of telling you it's enough.

COMBINATIONS: Mix with Echinacea, Elder flower and berry, Licorice root, and Yarrow for an effective cold and flu remedy.

RESEARCH: There has been limited research done on humans, but the information that does exist supports the traditional use in treating malaria, combatting colds and influenza, supporting the immune system, and fighting inflammation. This is attributed to its polysaccharide content and polyphenolic compounds, which inhibit viral attachment to the host cells.

CAUTION: Avoid taking in large doses or over a long period of time. May cause vomiting. Do not use if you are pregnant or breastfeeding. Not recommended for people with liver disease or stomach ulcers.

BORAGE

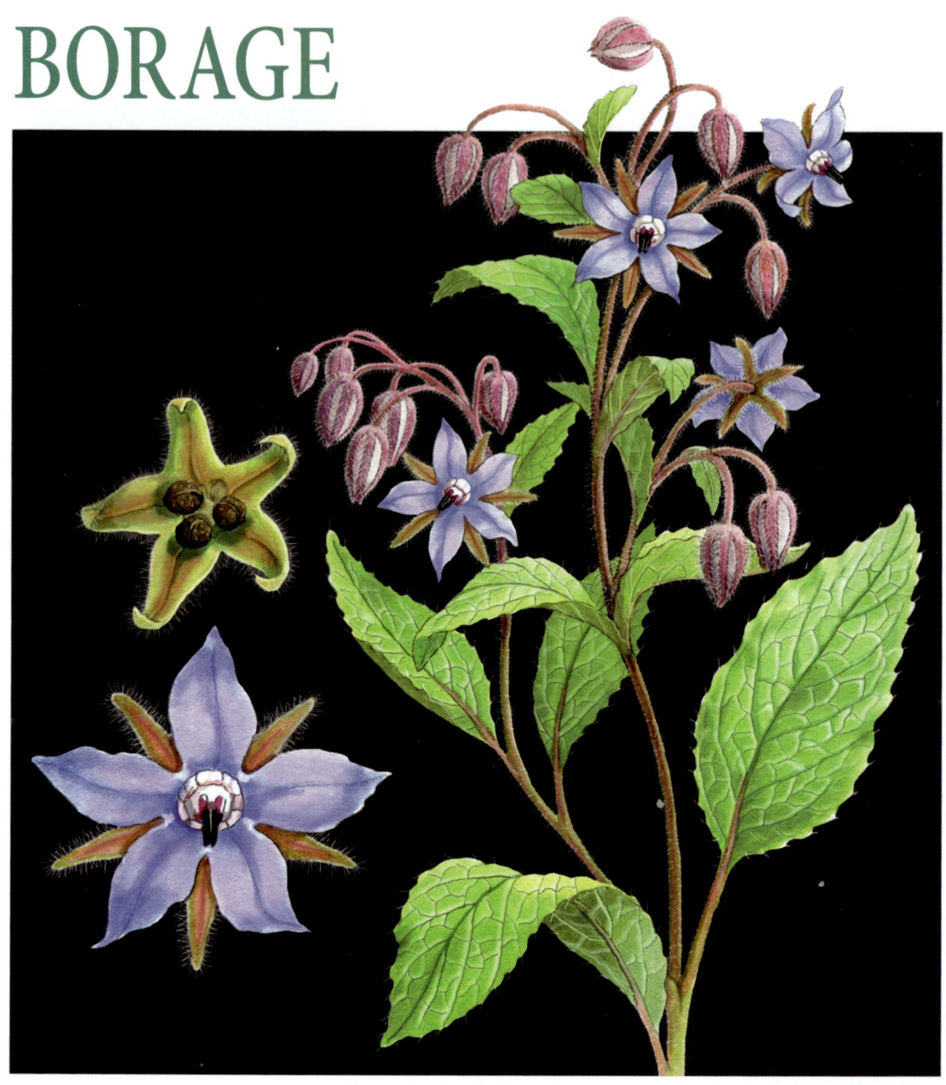

Borago officinalis

FAMILY: Boraginaceae

OTHER NAMES: Starflower, Beeplant, Beebush, *Fr.* Bourrache

PARTS USED: Flowers, leaves, seeds

CHARACTERISTICS: Cooling, moistening, slightly sweet

ACTIONS: Aperient, diuretic, diaphoretic, demulcent, febrifuge, emollient, anti-inflammatory, expectorant, galactagogue, adrenal tonic, antidepressant

RANGE: Introduced, British Columbia to Manitoba

This pretty blue annual flower, traditionally served in wine before going off to battle, was once known for its ability to instill bravery and banish melancholy. Whether it was the wine or the flowers that gave soldiers courage, we can't be sure, but it continued to be used up until the last century and is still prescribed by some herbalists for depression and other ailments. It is believed to have originated in Syria and spread throughout southern Europe and North Africa, eventually becoming naturalized and cultivated by colonists in North America. A robust annual with hollow reddish or green stems and thick, wrinkled leaves, it is almost entirely covered in hairs, except for the striking blue flowers, which bloom from June to October. The plant grows 60–90 cm. in height, has alternate oval leaves, and has flowers with 5 petals in the form of a star, 5 hairy sepals, and prominent black anthers, which are replaced by 3–4 brown nutlets. It is widely cultivated for its seed oil, which is rich in a fatty acid used to fight inflammation. Leaves should be picked on a sunny day before the flowers have opened, are best when young and not too hairy, and preferably used fresh, although the leaves may be dried for later use. Flowers can be picked right after blooming and may be dried, candied, or frozen into ice cubes. Keep from direct light and use within 3 months.

MEDICINAL USES:

Asthma, arthritis, skin conditions, cerebral arteriosclerosis, lung infections, urinary disorders

- Seed oil is the richest plant source of gamma-linolenic acid (GLA), an unsaturated fatty acid (omega-6) that is anti-inflammatory and boosts immunity. May lessen symptoms in people with rheumatoid arthritis, memory loss, heart conditions, menopause, gingivitis, diabetes, PMS, breast pain, asthma, and some autoimmune disorders, however there needs to be more research done to verify these claims.
- Used as a poultice or infused oil, it can help chronic inflammatory skin diseases like eczema, dermatitis, and psoriasis, reduces itch; and treats insect bites, rashes, sores, ringworm. Hydrating, soothes dry, irritated skin.
- Natural sedative, adrenal tonic, causes a significant reduction in anxiety and restores balance to the nervous system. Specific for neurasthenia, added to formulas for depression. Can help with hyperthyroidism, and reduce stress and tension.
- Reduces inflammation of arthritis, lessens swelling and pain. May take up to a month to take effect.
- Increases effectiveness of other medications used for urinary and respiratory disorders, arthritis and skin diseases.

OTHER USES:

- Flowers are added to salads, drinks or confections, young leaves have a cucumber-like flavour, may also be used in salads or teas.
- Beneficial for gardens as it is rich in nitrogen and other plant nutrients, it attracts bees, and also aphids, which can keep them off other plants.

INFUSION: 1–2 tsp. in 1 cup boiling water, taken up to 3 times a day.

TINCTURE: Dried herb 1:5 in 50% alcohol, take 1–3 drops 3 times a day.

CAUTION: Plant contains pyrrolizidine alkaloids, which can be toxic to the liver and aggravate cirrhosis, hepatitis, and other liver ailments. Only use seed oil that is labelled as non-hepatotoxic or PA free. Avoid if pregnant, lactating, or taking anti-coagulants. May cause bloating, nausea, or headache in some people. Not for children under twelve. Avoid long-term use, preferably no longer than 2 months at a time, and large doses. Contact with leaves may cause dermatitis in a small number of people.

BUGLEWEED

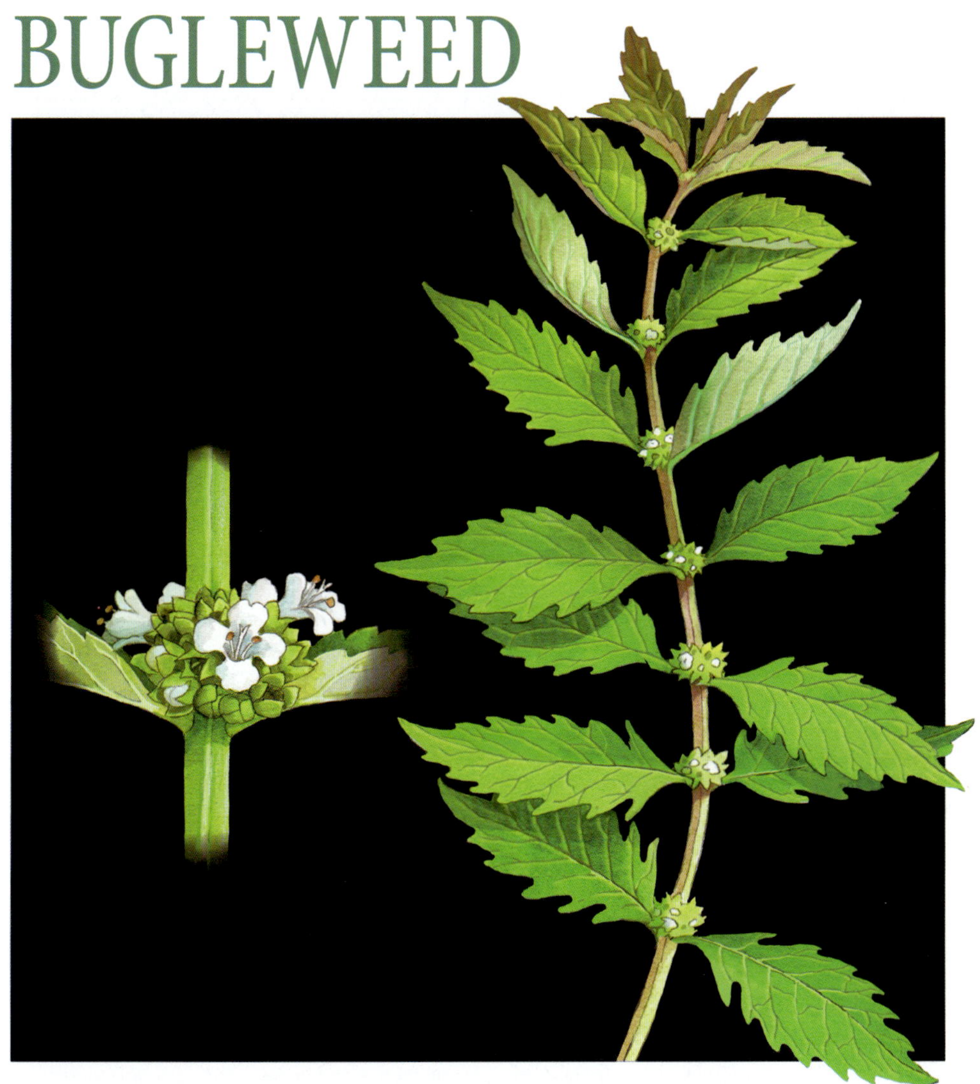

Lycopus virginicus*; *Lycopus americanus*; *Lycopus europaeus

FAMILY: Lamiaceae

OTHER NAMES: *L. virginicus:* Virginia Water Horehound; *L. americanus:* American Water Horehound, *L. europaeus:* European Bugleweed, Gypsywort, *Fr.* Lycope

PARTS USED: Whole plant

CHARACTERISTICS: Bitter, cooling, aromatic

ACTIONS: Antioxidant, anti-inflammatory, antitussive, astringent, cardiac tonic, mildly narcotic, sedative

RANGE: *L. virginicus* native to Ontario and Quebec; *L. americanus* native across all provinces; *L. europaeus:* introduced in British Columbia, Ontario, Quebec, Nova Scotia

Bugleweed, a native perennial and member of the Mint family, would easily be confused with Mint if not for the lack of the distinctive aroma. Although *L. virginicus* is most often used medicinally, *L. americanus* is quite similar and interchangeable medicinally, along with its European relative, *L. europaeus.* They should not be confused with a plant that is often called Bugleweed or Common Bugle, *Ajuga reptans*, which belongs to another family of herbs. *L. americanus* and *L. virginicus* grow up to a height of around 60 cm. Its usually unbranched stem is sometimes covered in fine hairs and is squarish with opposite, lance-shaped, hairless leaves that are narrowly lobed toward the base but more coarsely toothed at the top. Often the central vein has fine hairs on the underside. The tiny flowers grow in clusters in the leaf axils, the calyx forming a tube with 4 broad teeth. The flower is also in the form of a tube with 4 fused petals and may be white or pinkish with tiny pink spots, replaced by 4 small square-shaped nutlets in late summer. Usually found in low, wet places, the whole plant can be gathered during the summer and dried for future use.

MEDICINAL USES:

Hyperactive thyroid, Graves' disease, tachycardia, anxiety, coughs, pulmonary bleeding

- This herb is a specific for overactive or hyperthyroid conditions that may include rapid, thin pulse, palpitations, anxiety, and insomnia, and is usually taken as a tincture or infusion. However, these issues dealing with the thyroid or heart can be complex, so should be treated under the supervision of a medical practitioner.
- Relaxing, bronchodilating and expectorant. Useful for dry, chronic coughs, especially if accompanied by a fever, and for mild asthma.
- Mild sedative. Traditionally used by Cherokee people to calm the heart and promote sleep by chewing the roots, and to treat snakebites by chewing the root and swallowing half, applying the rest to the wound. Often fed to children to give "eloquence of speech."
- Heart tonic, where there is tachycardia or rapid heartbeat with weak circulation. Slows and strengthens the heart, reduces inflammation, and relieves anxiety and insomnia, particularly when recovering from debilitating diseases where heartbeat affects the sleep.
- Mild gastric tonic, improves digestion, calms upset stomach.
- Eases excessive menstrual bleeding.

TINCTURE: Fresh 1:2 or dried 1:5 in 50% alcohol. Take 1–2 ml. 3 times a day.

INFUSION: 2 tbsp. dried herb to 2 cups of boiling water. Take 1 cup 3 times a day.

COMBINATIONS: May be used with Hawthorn, Motherwort, or Lemon Balm (cardiotonic and nervine herbs) for hyperthyroid conditions. Combines well with Elecampane or Pleurisy root for dry coughs.

RESEARCH:

- Studies done using *L. europaeus* show promise in the treatment of hyperthyroidism and Graves' disease. One of the main constituents, rosmarinic acid, has been shown to decrease thyroid hormones and improve heart-related symptoms, almost as much as beta-blocker medications. Low doses were found to have more cardiac effects, reducing heart-rate and blood pressure, whereas larger doses tended to be more effective at reducing thyroid hormones.
- It was also found to have a significant effect as a cough suppressant and sedative. When tested against several strains of *Staphylococcus aureus*, which have become highly resistant to antibiotics, the herb showed no significant antibacterial action, but when taken along with tetracycline and erythromycin, the herb multiplied the efficacy of the antibiotics.

CAUTION: Avoid during pregnancy or breastfeeding, or if taking thyroid or heart medications. Long-term use should be monitored by a healthcare professional.

BURDOCK

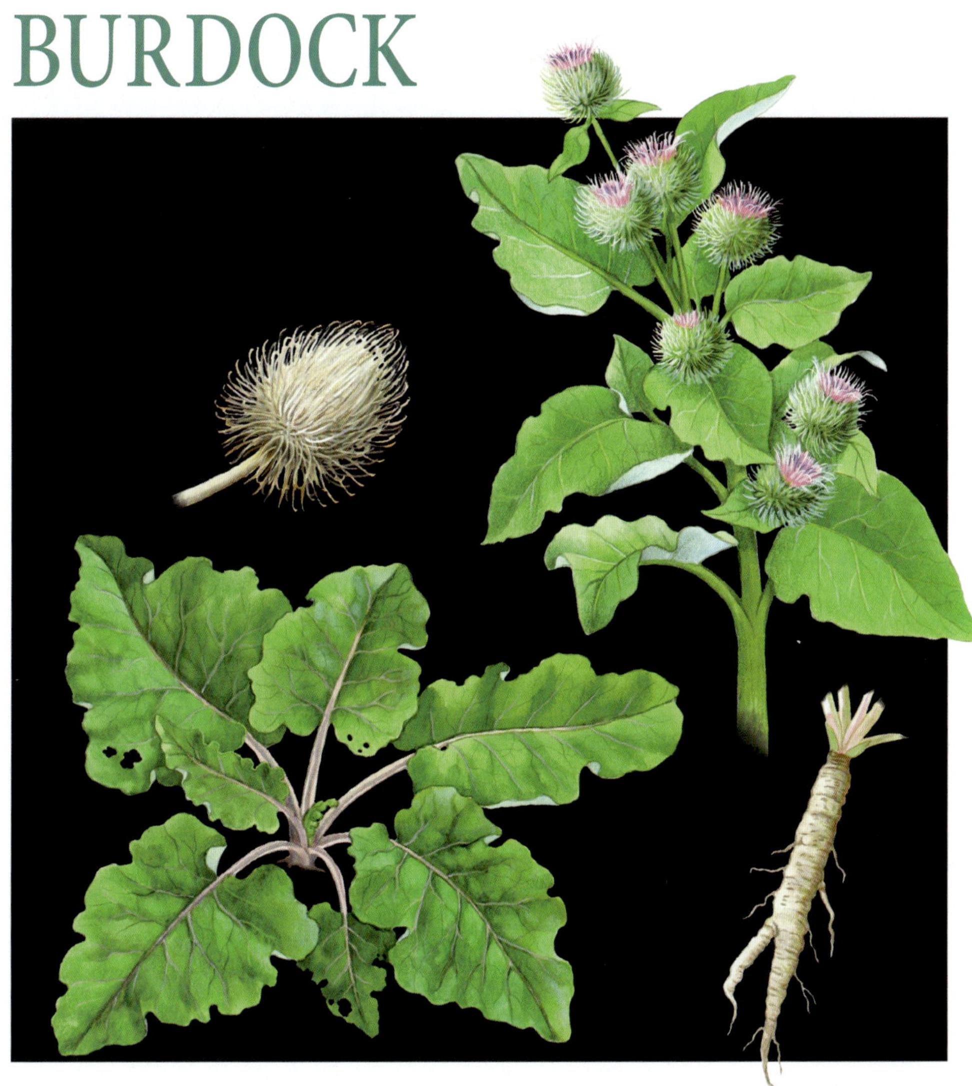

Arctium lappa

FAMILY: Asteraceae

OTHER NAMES: Greater Burdock, *Fr.* Grande bardane

PARTS USED: Root (chronic conditions), seeds (acute disorders) and leaves

CHARACTERISTICS: Bitter, slightly sweet, cool, drying

ACTIONS: Alterative, diuretic, diaphoretic, nutritive, mild laxative, tonic, vulnerary, relaxant, antibacterial, antifungal, carminative, demulcent, antioxidant, anti-inflammatory, hepatoprotective, anticancer, cholagogue

RANGE: Introduced in all provinces and Northwest Territories

Burdock is another one of those pesky weeds people hate having on their property, mainly because of its burrs that will attach to just about anything, particularly house pets. However, it's one of the best detoxifying herbs. It grows mainly in waste places, meadows, and woods and can grow up to 1.8 metres tall. The lower leaves are large, wavy, and heart-shaped, covered with fine hairs, and light grey on the underside. The upper leaves are smaller and oval-shaped with less of the downy covering. The flowerheads are purple and enclosed in a round spiny shell with prickles that hook on to everything that passes by. The long taproot is collected after the first year of growth in early spring, sliced and dried quickly for later use, or eaten fresh as a vegetable. Do not confuse with Rhubarb leaves, which are toxic.

MEDICINAL USES:

Skin diseases, blood purification, urinary problems, arthritis, PMS

- Contains many minerals, especially iron, that make it valuable for the blood. Beneficial as a detoxifier and blood and liver tonic, as it promotes sweating and detoxifies the epidermal tissues, assists in absorption of nutrients, aids digestion, and improves lymphatic function, relieving bloating and water retention. It works best if used in moderate doses over a long period of time. The seed is said to be better used for acute illnesses, whereas the root is more beneficial for chronic problems of the kidneys, bladder, skin, and bowel, and is more permanent.
- Alleviates the pain of arthritis, rheumatism, sciatica, and lumbago by its diuretic action, which increases the removal of urine and toxic substances.
- Due to its ability to increase circulation to the skin and its mucilaginous, demulcent nature, it helps chronic skin eruptions like acne, psoriasis, eczema, boils, and herpes. It can be taken internally in an infusion and/or used externally as a wash or poultice. Crushed seed can be poulticed on bruises, and the leaves can be used on burns, ulcers, or sores, on the forehead to relieve headache, or on the scalp to relieve itchiness or dandruff. Studies have shown it may even inhibit cancer growth.
- Digestive herb, the bitterness in the leaf can stimulate bile production, cleanse the liver, and repair the damaging effects of alcohol. The demulcent quality soothes the digestive tract and contains inulin, which feeds healthy bacteria.
- Relieves mild urinary tract infections, reduces congestion, and flushes harmful acids from the kidneys.
- Regulates the menstrual cycle, relieves mastitis and menopausal symptoms, eases swollen prostate glands.

OTHER USES:

- The stalk, when cut before the flower opens, peeled, and boiled, makes a tasty vegetable.
- The young leaves can be eaten in salads, but are slightly laxative.
- The root may be boiled and eaten like carrots.

DECOCTION: 2 tsp. dried root in 2 cups boiling water, soak overnight, boil again and simmer 5–10 minutes. Drink 3 times a day.

TINCTURE: Fresh root 1:2, dried 1:5, in 60% alcohol. Take 30–90 drops 3 times a day.

COMBINATIONS: Burdock and Red Clover make a good blood tonic. Burdock can be combined with Yellow Dock or Dandelion root to detoxify and stimulate digestion. Burdock may exacerbate skin conditions temporarily, so it may be combined with other diuretic remedies like Dandelion, Cleavers, Violet, Red Clover, or Yellow Dock. Start with a low dose.

RESEARCH: Contains phenolic acids quercetin and luteolin, which are powerful antioxidants. The seeds possess some anti-inflammatory and inhibitory effects on the growth of tumours such as pancreatic carcinoma. The leaf extract has been found to inhibit growth of microorganisms in the mouth, and daily consumption of the infusion could be effective at preventing and reducing recurrence of acute colonic diverticulitis. One study showed significantly lower levels of inflammation in people with bilateral knee osteoarthritis after taking daily doses of Burdock root tea for 6 weeks, as well as an improvement in blood lipids and blood pressure. There is much potential for further research into this amazing plant.

CAUTION: May interact with some medications, particularly blood thinners and diabetes medications. When gathering seeds, be careful to remove the splinters clinging to them, use a mask and gloves as they can be extremely irritant.

CALENDULA

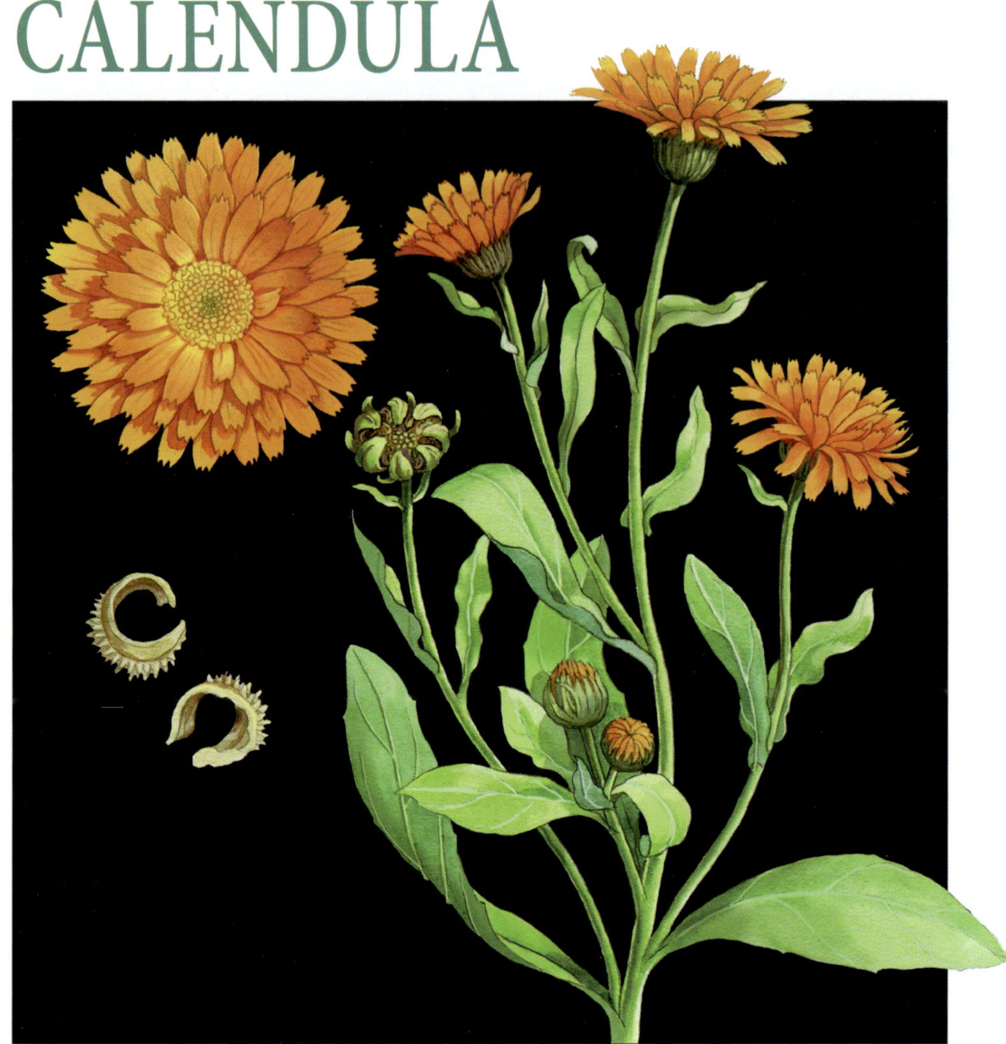

Calendula officinalis

FAMILY: Asteraceae

OTHER NAMES: Marigold, Pot Marigold, *Fr.* Souci des jardins, Souci officinal

PARTS USED: Flowerheads, leaves

CHARACTERISTICS: Slightly bitter, salty, warm, drying

ACTIONS: Antibacterial, anti-inflammatory, antifungal, astringent, antioxidant, antiviral, hepatoprotective, cholagogue, diaphoretic, emmenagogue, lymphagogue, slightly stimulant, vulnerary

RANGE: Introduced and cultivated across southern Canada

This common annual garden herb is a native of Southern Europe and Asia which was brought to America by settlers for its pretty blooms and valuable medicinal qualities. It has a branching, slightly hairy stem about 30 cm. high, with alternate lance-shaped leaves and a large solitary terminal flowerhead on each stem. The 3-toothed petals are actually ray florets, or individual flowers grouped together, and range in colour from bright yellow and orange to russet red. Do not confuse Calendula with Garden Marigolds of the genus *Tagetes*, which are often planted in gardens to repel pests due to their unpleasant smell.

Pick the entire flowerhead for medicines, as many of the medicinal constituents are found in the green bases or calyxes; however, only the petals should be used if eating them raw in salads, as the small hairs on the calyx can be irritating. They should be picked often to encourage new growth, and only after the dew has evaporated, then dried on screens out of the sun for 7–10 days.

MEDICINAL USES:

Skin problems, wounds, varicose veins, digestive problems, swollen lymph nodes, periodontal disease

- Used medicinally since the twelfth century for its wound-healing properties, it is known for its anti-inflammatory and antioxidant effect on many types of skin conditions as well as a variety of internal complaints where there is pain, irritation, and swelling. It increases the amount of blood and oxygen to the wound, hydrating and softening tissues.
- Compresses soaked in diluted tincture or infusion help heal abscesses, scalds, ulcers, cracked nipples, stings, sprains, diaper rash, eczema, dermatitis, and minor wounds. It staunches bleeding, helps prevent infection, gangrene, and pus formation, relieves swelling and redness, and speeds healing. Infusion is good for cleaning out wounds.
- Useful for healing varicose veins, both as a compress and internally to relieve swelling, pain, and inflammation.
- Effective internally for digestive issues such as GERD, peptic ulcers, Crohn's, colitis, and gastritis, relieves pain and heals mucous tissue in the digestive tract.
- Stimulates the lymphatic system; acute or chronic swelling of the lymph nodes from infections, helps build immunity.
- Used in a mouthwash for thrush, bleeding gums, periodontal disease.
- Crushed calyx and flower stems can be applied to skin and covered with a bandage to help dissolve warts and corns.
- Brings on suppressed menstruation and relieves premenstrual symptoms.

OTHER USES:

- A rinse adds golden highlights to hair.
- Boiled flowers create a yellow dye for fabrics.
- Cheap alternative for saffron in cooking.

TINCTURE: Dried flowers 1:5, 60% alcohol, take 1–3 ml. 3 times a day.

INFUSION: 1–2 tsp. dry herb in 1 cup boiling water. Take 3 times a day.

SALVE: Combine macerated oils of Calendula, Plantain, Chickweed, St. John's Wort, and Violet; heat gently, adding just enough beeswax to solidify the oils (usually 28 grams beeswax to 1 cup oil). When melted, remove from heat and add several drops of vitamin E and essential oil if desired. Pour into jars.

COMBINATIONS: Internally can be combined with Agrimony, Plantain, Yarrow, or Shepherd's Purse for digestive issues where tissue is sore and inflamed. For fatigue, lymphatic congestion, or swollen glands, add Red Clover or Cleavers. For external use combine with Plantain, St. John's Wort, Chickweed, or Violet.

CAUTION: Not recommended for internal use during pregnancy. May cause allergic reaction in sensitive individuals. Do not eat raw flower base (calyx) as it could be irritant to mouth and digestive tract.

CASCARA SAGRADA

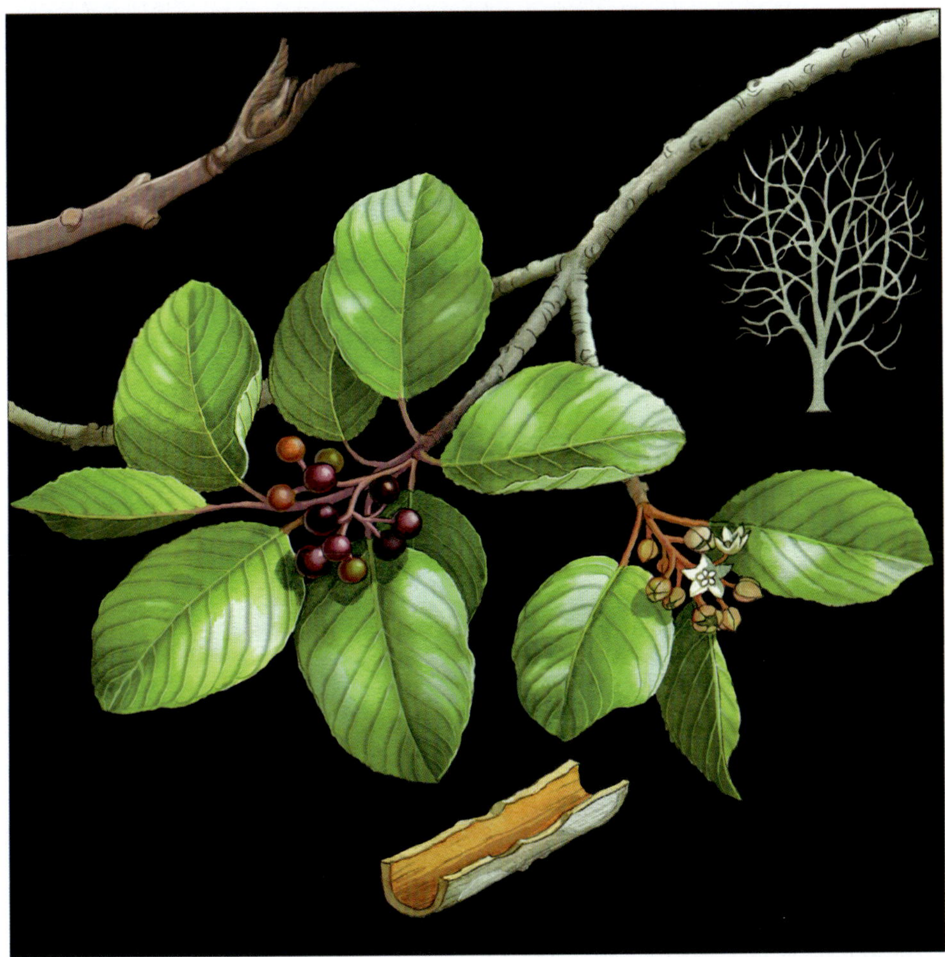

Frangula purshiana

FAMILY: Rhamnaceae

OTHER NAMES: Cascara Buckthorn, Chittam Bark, Sacred Bark, *Fr.* Nerprun cascara

PARTS USED: Aged bark

CHARACTERISTICS: Bitter, cooling

ACTIONS: Laxative, tonic, alterative, hepatic, stimulant, nervine

RANGE: Native to southern British Columbia

Cascara Sagrada, a deciduous shrub belonging to the Buckthorn family, has been used as a laxative for hundreds of years by Indigenous Peoples and Spanish settlers, who gave it the name Cascara Sagrada, Spanish for "sacred bark," because of its use as medicine. It usually grows only 5–10 m. tall; however, it has been known to reach 15 m. Its outer bark is light grey or brown and often spotted with lichens, the inner bark an orange-yellow, and it is usually found in wet, shady places, along streams or coastlines. In winter it grows small, hairy, rusty-brown buds resembling two angel wings, which in spring grow into shiny green, oval, alternate leaves which are sparsely serrated. The inconspicuous white flowers emerge in May or June, followed by green berries that turn red and eventually black. The best time to harvest is late spring to early summer. This shrub is endangered, so do not strip the bark from the trunk; instead, remove a branch about 1 cm. thick and strip the bark off as soon as possible. Use gloves, as the inner bark is extremely potent and can penetrate the skin. It should be left to dry in a paper bag for at least 1 year or up to 3 years before using, as it is too strong to consume fresh and will cause cramping, nausea, and diarrhea.

MEDICINAL USES:

Constipation, lack of appetite, digestive sluggishness, toxic liver, leaky gut

- Contains anthraquinone glycosides, which stimulate contractions in the intestinal wall, increasing peristalsis and strengthening the lower intestine to relieve acute or chronic constipation. Take before bed. It usually requires 6–8 hours to work.
- Smaller doses will tonify the colon and should be taken in combination with carminatives like fresh Ginger to reduce cramping, and/or Aniseed, Fennel, or Cardamom to ease nausea and mask the intense bitterness. People with chronic constipation need to modify their diet and eliminate processed and refined foods.
- Smaller doses taken 10–15 minutes before meals stimulate digestion and increase appetite, releasing enzymes from the pancreas, liver, and duodenum. Can prevent acid reflux, help detoxify the liver, and aid in repairing the intestinal wall where there is leaky gut syndrome. May relieve hemorrhoids caused by constipation and straining. Some herbalists claim that it will release stuck emotional issues as well.
- Rich in emodin, which is antifungal and antimicrobial, it expels a range of bad bacteria, fungi (such as candida), and some parasites. Possibly protects against osteoporosis and may have anticancer properties, but more study is needed.
- When combined with psyllium, relieves sluggishness and cleanses the colon.
- Unlike other products, Cascara Sagrada taken daily in small doses will not create a dependency, and is one of the safest laxatives. However, you should drink plenty of water while taking it, and don't use for more than 1 week as it may cause abdominal cramps and loss of electrolytes.

TINCTURE: As a laxative, take 1 tsp. before bed in a little water. To use as a bitter digestive tonic, take 1–5 drops, 10–15 minutes before meals. Combine with fresh Ginger, Aniseed, Licorice root, Fennel and/or Cardamom.

CAUTION: Not for use during pregnancy or breastfeeding. Fresh bark contains anthrone, which can cause intense cramping, diarrhea, and severe vomiting. Dry for 1–3 years before using. Long term use may result in loss of electrolytes, especially potassium, liver injury, and dependency. Avoid with inflammatory bowel disorders or obstructions.

CATNIP

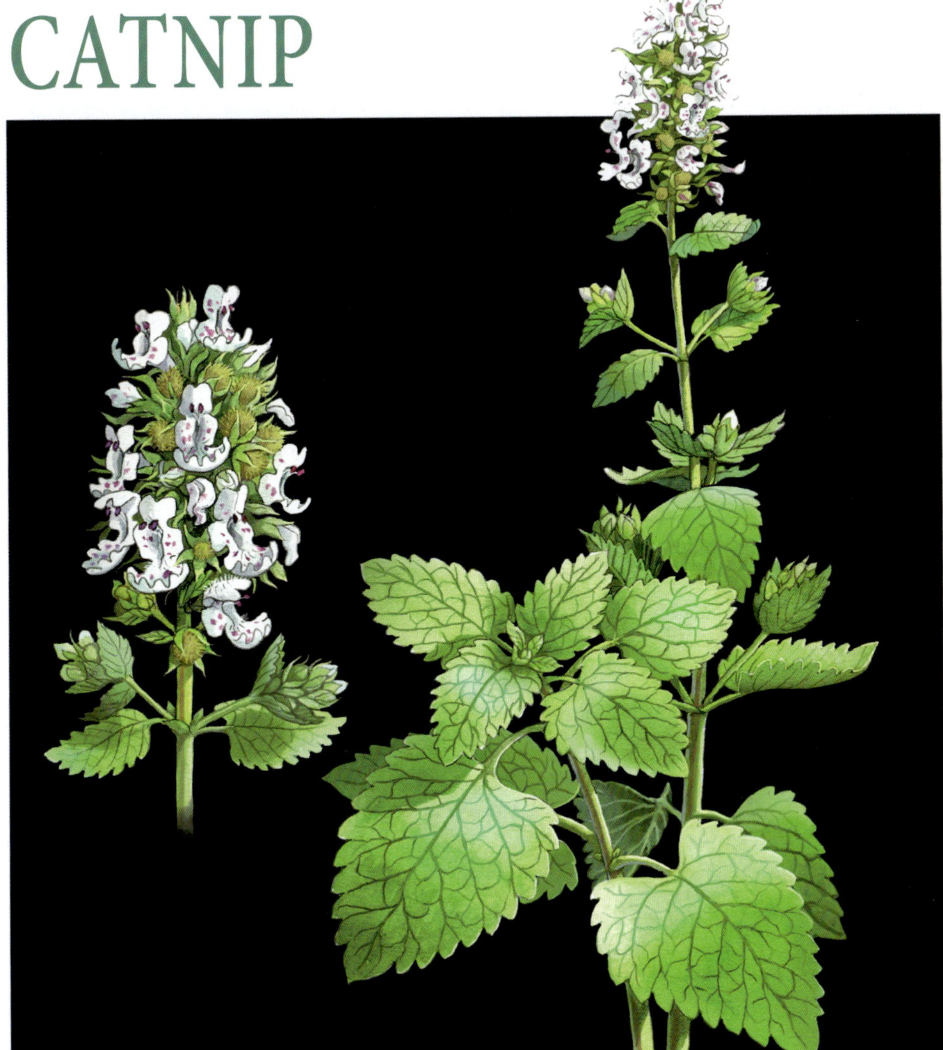

Nepeta cataria

FAMILY: Lamiaceae

OTHER NAMES: Catmint, *Fr.* Herbe à chat, Cataire, Chataire

PARTS USED: Flowers, leaves

CHARACTERISTICS: Cooling, drying, slightly bitter, astringent

ACTIONS: Antispasmodic, aromatic, carminative, diaphoretic, emmenagogue, nervine, sedative, tonic, febrifuge, anticatarrhal, anti-inflammatory, antimicrobial, antioxidant

RANGE: Introduced and cultivated across all provinces

Catnip is well-known for its ability to drive cats crazy. I've tried to grow Catnip for years, but all I succeed in doing is attracting all the felines in the neighbourhood to come over and roll in my garden in a drunken frenzy. I have stopped trying, although they say it's better to plant seeds; apparently as long as the plants aren't bruised, the essential oils that attract cats are not released, but I'm not convinced. Short of installing an iron cage around each plant and deep in the ground, I suspect the cats will get at them one way or another.

Most people have no idea this hardy perennial is also a medicinal plant, brought to America from Europe, Africa, and Asia as a garden plant. It has since escaped to the wild, and is found near roadsides, fields, and streams, but is easy to grow from seed if you can keep the cats away from it. It resembles Mint, belonging to the same family, only Catnip has more of a citrusy aroma. Leaves are opposite, toothed and heart-shaped, and the flowers, which grow from July often into October, are white, light blue, or purple, often with pink spots, and tubular. Harvest the flowering tops when in full bloom and dry for later use.

MEDICINAL USES:

Cold and flu, upset stomach, colic, cramps, nervousness and stress, amenorrhea and dysmenorrhea, toothache, skin irritation

- A relaxing, mild, aromatic herb that settles the stomach, calms nerves, and relieves gas pains, headache, motion sickness, vomiting, and trouble settling down to sleep.
- Diaphoretic, it promotes sweating, and can relieve colds, chills, fevers, congestion, and sore throat when ingested hot in infusion. When taken in cold infusion, it becomes tonic. The Ojibwa steep it with an equal amount of Tansy for fever.
- Antispasmodic, it relieves muscle pain, menstrual cramps, and gastrointestinal cramps or IBS. It is preferable to use fresh leaf tincture.
- Used by Indigenous Peoples in preparations, particularly for children, for colds, coughs, colic, stomach upsets, diarrhea, sore throat, fever, or bronchitis.
- Mildly anesthetic, the leaf chewed or rubbed on the gums relieves toothache pain and sore gums. Antimicrobial, infusion can be used as a gargle for sore throat.
- Used in a poultice for sore nipples, bruises, hives, swellings, and boils, it is a mild antibiotic and antifungal.

OTHER USES:

- Makes an effective mosquito repellant. Crush leaves and soak in vodka. Strain and put into a spray bottle.
- Young leaves are edible and can be added to salads.

TINCTURE: Fresh leaves 1:2, dried 1:5, in 50% alcohol. Take ¼–1 tsp. up to 4 times a day.

INFUSION: 1–2 tsp. in 1 cup water steeped for 10 minutes. Drink up to 3 times a day.

GASTRITIS INFUSION: Combine 2 parts Catnip, 2 parts Fennel seed, and 1 part Licorice root. Use 1–2 tsp. in 1 cup boiling water, infuse covered for 10–15 minutes.

COMBINATIONS: Often combined with Yarrow, Elder flower, Chamomile, Lemon Balm, Mint, or Boneset for colds, flu, and fevers. For stomach upsets, add Fennel, Chamomile, or Spearmint.

CAUTION: Not for use during pregnancy. Very large doses may induce vomiting and dizziness.

CELANDINE

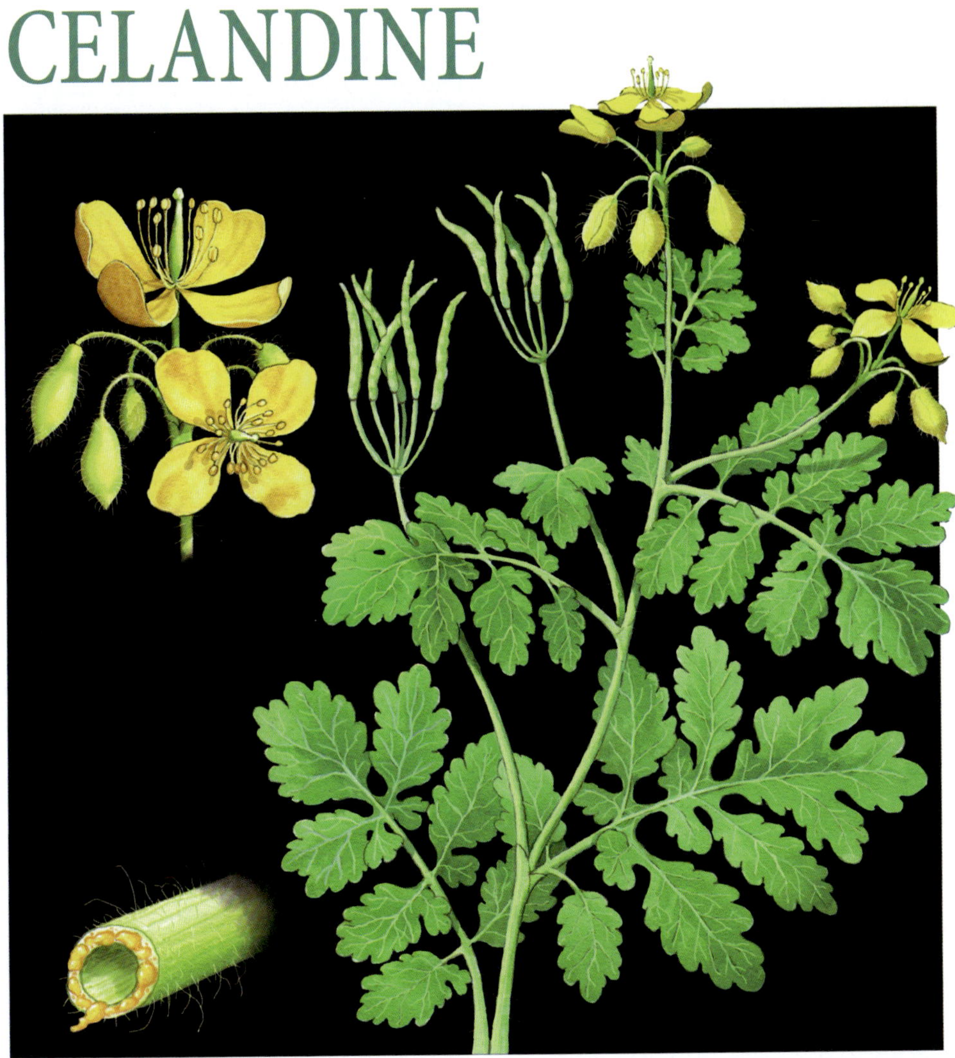

Chelidonium majus

FAMILY: Papaveraceae

OTHER NAMES: Greater Celandine, Nipplewort, Swallow Wort, Tetterwort, *Fr.* Grande chélidoine

PARTS USED: Whole plant

CHARACTERISTICS: Bitter, acrid, warm

ACTIONS: Antimicrobial, antiviral, antifungal, anti-inflammatory, antispasmodic, hepatic, gastric, anticancer, mild sedative, diaphoretic, diuretic, cholagogue

RANGE: Introduced in southwest British Columbia, Manitoba to Nova Scotia

Celandine is a biennial that is originally a native of Europe, Asia, and North Africa and has a long history as a herbal medicine both there and in North America. Its name derives from the Greek word *chelidon*, meaning "swallow," a bird that, according to folklore, arrived every year just as the flower began to bloom and fed it to their nestlings to improve their sight. It is very similar to our native Celandine Poppy (*Stylophorum diphyllum*), which has larger and showier flowers but no known medicinal use. Celandine grows at the edge of forests, in lowlands, foothills, and along roadsides, often reaching a metre in height. Its leaves are compound, alternate, lobed, and toothed, with a cluster of 2 to 6 bright yellow 4-petalled flowers at the end of a branched, sparsely hairy stem. When broken, the stems exude a yellow-orange latex sap rich in alkaloids and proteins that can be irritating to some people. The above-ground parts can be picked during the flowering season and used fresh or dried quickly in an oven. Roots may be dug in the fall and used fresh or recently dried.

MEDICINAL USES:

Liver congestion, indigestion, gallbladder complaints, toothache, eye inflammation, warts, corns

- Used for centuries in Europe for liver sluggishness, indigestion, gallbladder inflammation and stones, hepatitis, and jaundice, characterized by pain and tenderness in the upper abdomen, dull pain beneath the right shoulder blade, and a yellow tinge to the skin. It thins the bile and increases secretion, as well as reducing intestinal spasms, making it easier to expel stones and prevent their formation. However, recent testing has concluded that caution is necessary due to possible liver toxicity with this herb. It should only be used under supervision by a professional and in the proper doses. It is considered safe for short-term use to treat flatulence and dyspepsia. A careful diet is necessary when taking any liver-cleansing herb; avoid junk food, alcohol, excess sugar, and unhealthy fats.
- Typically the juice and yellow latex were used in folk medicine for eye inflammation, getting rid of warts, corns and calluses, eczema, boils, and rashes. The root was often chewed to relieve toothache. Skin ulcers and scabs on the scalp were treated with a salve made of powdered root mixed with pork fat and vinegar.
- Anecdotal evidence suggests that taking a decoction of Celandine for 2 weeks may cause significant reduction of cancer tissue in squamous cell carcinoma of the esophagus, and possibly stomach cancer, but more research needs to be done.
- May be effective used as an antispasmodic in a syrup in cases of chronic bronchitis and whooping cough.

TINCTURE: Dried herb, 1:2 in 50% alcohol, 1–2 ml. 3 times a day.

INFUSION: ½–1 tsp. dried herb in 1 cup boiling water, drink ½ cup at a time, up to 3 times a day.

JUICE: For warts or corns, dab with fresh juice 2 or 3 times a day. Avoid dabbing on the surrounding skin.

COMBINATIONS: Barberry, Dandelion root, and Burdock for liver congestion.

RESEARCH: Extracts have been shown to have antibacterial and antifungal properties, the root containing higher levels of isoquinoline alkaloids and showing a stronger effect. Tested using *Staphylococcus aureus* and *Pseudomonas aeruginosa*, two bacterial strains notorious for their drug-resistance and responsible for many hospital infections. Also the aerial parts of *C. majus* had a significant effect on *Candida albicans*. Other research on the isolated isoquinones shows it has anticancer activity in vitro and suggests it could be promising in cancer therapy.

CAUTION: Not for use during pregnancy or lactation. May cause liver toxicity, especially if taking other pharmaceuticals or liver medications or if taking alcohol; discontinue use if symptoms worsen. Sap can be irritant, use gloves when handling. Can stimulate an immune response so may decrease effectiveness of immunosuppressants. Not recommended for very young children or the elderly. Use only under supervision of a healthcare professional and for a short term only.

CENTAURY

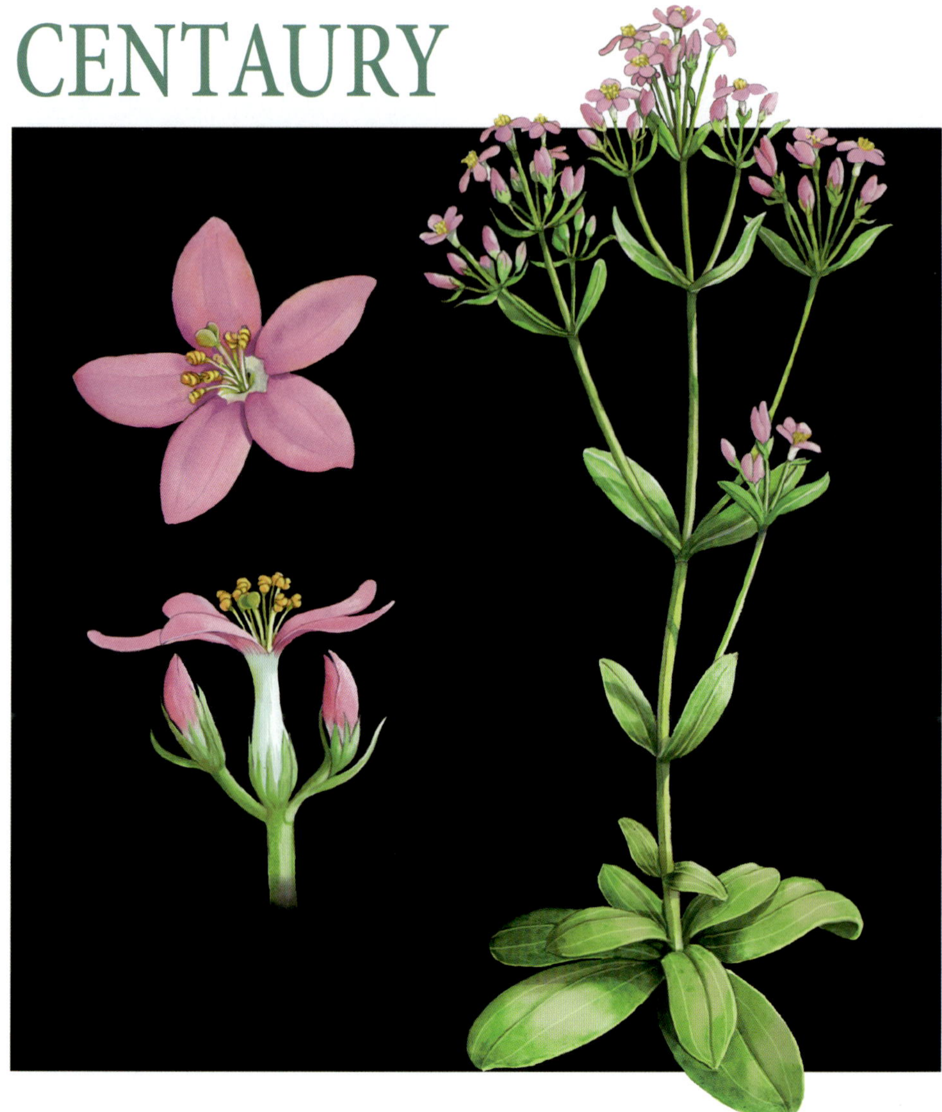

Centaurium erythraea (umbellatum)

FAMILY: Gentianaceae

OTHER NAMES: Filwort, Bitter herb, European Centaury, Common Centaury, *Fr.* Petite centaurée

PARTS USED: Aerial

CHARACTERISTICS: Bitter, cold

ACTIONS: Antioxidant, antidiabetic, aromatic, cholagogue, diaphoretic, digestive, emetic, hepatic, sedative, tonic

RANGE: Introduced in British Columbia, Ontario, Quebec, Nova Scotia

Centaury is an erect biennial (occasionally annual) in the Gentian family that originated in Europe and East Asia and has spread over fields, boggy meadows, and ditches throughout Eastern and Central Canada and US. Named after the centaur and renowned healer Chiron from Greek mythology, Centaury has earned the reputation of being one of the most useful bitter herbs, particularly in regards to digestive problems. Its stem grows up to 50 cm. high from a basal rosette and may or may not be branched, topped with pink, red, or lavender flowers growing parallel to the stem, and bright yellow anthers. Aerial parts can be harvested while still flowering and dried for later use.

MEDICINAL USES:

Anorexia, indigestion, jaundice, diabetes

- Primarily used as a bitter digestive tonic, where there is bloating, heartburn, and gas. It cleanses the liver, stimulates the bile flow from the gallbladder, and is mildly laxative. It improves the appetite and is useful in anorexia. Best taken before eating unless there is stomach inflammation or bloating, in which cases a few drops of tincture during or after meals is preferable. Long-term use protects against stomach ulcers and aids digestion. Effective for jaundice and hepatitis.
- May be effective at preventing arteriosclerosis and thickening of blood vessels due to injury or stents; however, there is no research to support this.
- Diaphoretic, it can be useful in fevers, as it induces sweating, which cools the skin.
- Tea has been used traditionally against worms, snakebites, insect stings, and other poisonings, as well as externally for lice and to clean and disinfect sores and wounds.
- May hold promise in treatment of type 2 diabetes, as it increases insulin levels and normalizes glucose levels.

OTHER USES:
- Flavouring in bitter herbal liqueurs and vermouth.
- May help fade freckles.

TINCTURE: Fresh herb 1:2 in 40% alcohol, a few drops on the tongue before meals for indigestion.

INFUSION: Steep ½–1 tsp. in ⅔ cup boiling water. Sip slowly, ½ hour before meals.

COMBINATIONS: With Barberry bark and Dandelion root for liver problems, with Senna for constipation, with Chamomile, Meadowsweet, or Marshmallow to soothe inflammation.

RESEARCH: Because of its longstanding use in traditional medicine, its bitter properties have been proven effective in cases of indigestion and other digestive disorders and loss of appetite. However, there is little evidence from clinical trials.

CAUTION: Avoid with GERD, stomach ulcers, high stomach acidity, inflammatory diseases of the digestive tract, and diarrhea. Do not give to children. Do not take while pregnant or breastfeeding.

CHAMOMILE

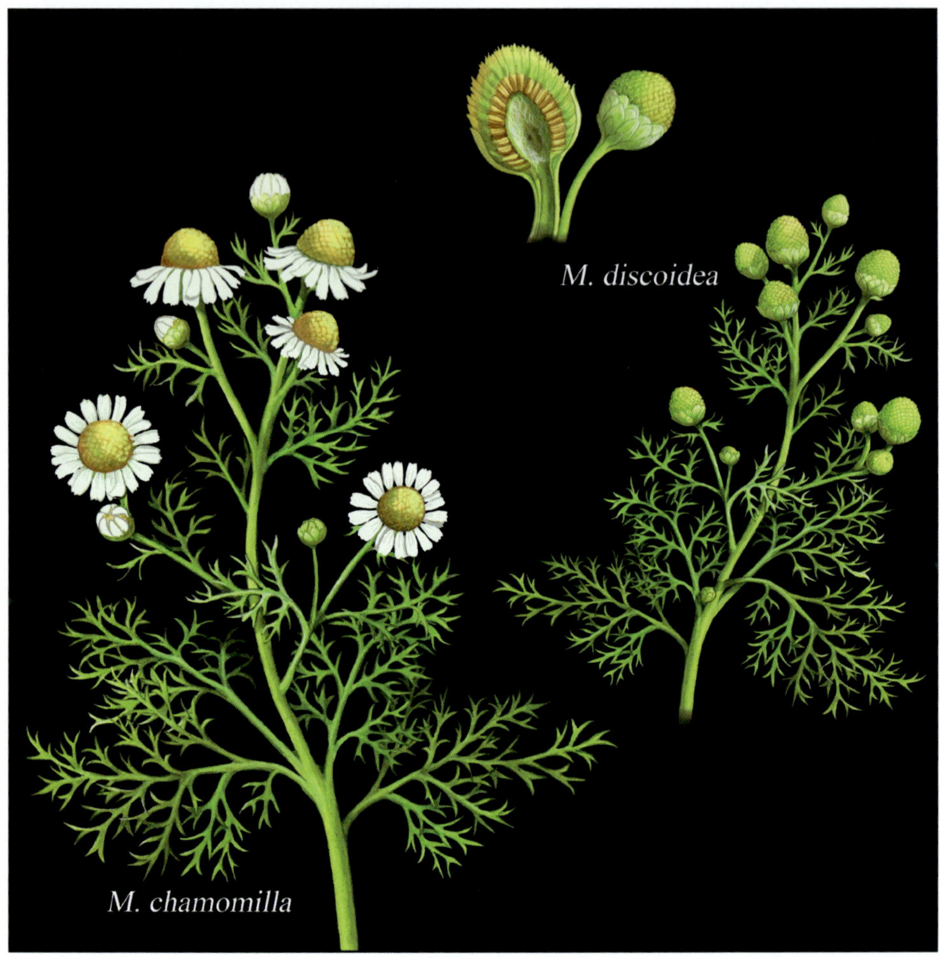

***Matricaria chamomilla*; *Matricaria discoidea* (Pineapple Weed)**

FAMILY: Asteracerae

OTHER NAMES: *M. chamomilla:* Wild Chamomile, German Chamomile, Scented Mayweed, *Fr.* Petite chamomille, Chamomille allemandy; *M. discoidea:* Rayless Mayweed, *Fr.* Matricaire odorante

PARTS USED: Flowers

CHARACTERISTICS: Aromatic, bitter, moist, cool

ACTIONS: Antiseptic, carminative, diaphoretic, sedative, antispasmodic, analgesic, anti-inflammatory, antimicrobial, nervine, stomachic

RANGE: *M. chamomilla:* Introduced British Columbia to Newfoundland and Labrador, except Prince Edward Island and New Brunswick; *M. discoidea:* Native to British Columbia, introduced in the Yukon, Northwest Territories, Alberta to Newfoundland and Labrador

There are several types of Chamomile, but these two varieties seem to be the most common in Canada. Both have similar properties, although German Chamomile, which originates in Europe, is most often used medicinally. They are small annuals, growing from 10 to 80 cm. tall, with feathery leaves and yellow cone-shaped flowerheads. German Chamomile has numerous short white ray petals surrounding the flowerheads, whereas Pineapple Weed has no ray petals, is usually somewhat shorter and close to the ground, and smells like pineapple. The flowers are picked in early summer and are more potent if used fresh, but can be dried for later use.

MEDICINAL USES:

Insomnia, indigestion, colic, fevers, colds, skin inflammations, anxiety, irritability

- Flavonoids and essential oils give chamomile its anti-inflammatory and sedative properties, making it an ideal remedy for problems related to tension, irritation, and anxiety. It relaxes the muscles, tendons, and digestive tract, soothes irritability, cools inflammation, and eases pain, making it easier to relax and sleep.
- A strong, hot infusion relieves digestive issues like bloating, indigestion, nervous stomach, and intestinal spasms. A few teaspoons of warm tea can ease colic in irritable children, relieve teething pain, and help them sleep.
- Helps ease PMS symptoms and relieve cramps and irritability.
- Can ease anxiety, calm the nerves, and improve sleep quality.
- Breathing the vapour can help congested sinuses or asthma, and taking the infusion internally helps clear mucus, reduce inflammation, and ease aching and muscular tension. Infusion may be used as a gargle or mouthwash for sore throats or mouth sores or to help gingivitis.
- A compress made from a strong infusion helps sore muscles or arthritic pain, and heals inflammation on the skin such as acne, rashes, eczema, psoriasis, or minor burns. A sterile cloth soaked in cooled tea and placed over the eyes can relieve an eye infection.
- Flowers macerated in oil can be massaged into arthritic joints.

TINCTURE: Dried flower, 1–4 ml. (10–20 drops for children) up to 3 times a day.

INFUSION: 2–3 heaped tsp. dried, in 1 cup boiling water, steep covered 10 minutes. Add honey if desired.

COMBINATIONS: With Fennel or Peppermint for indigestion, with Cramp Bark for menstrual pain or cramping, with Lemon Balm for children, and with Skullcap or Hops for insomnia.

CAUTION: Generally considered safe; however, some people may have allergies to plants in this family. May interact with blood thinners.

CHICKWEED

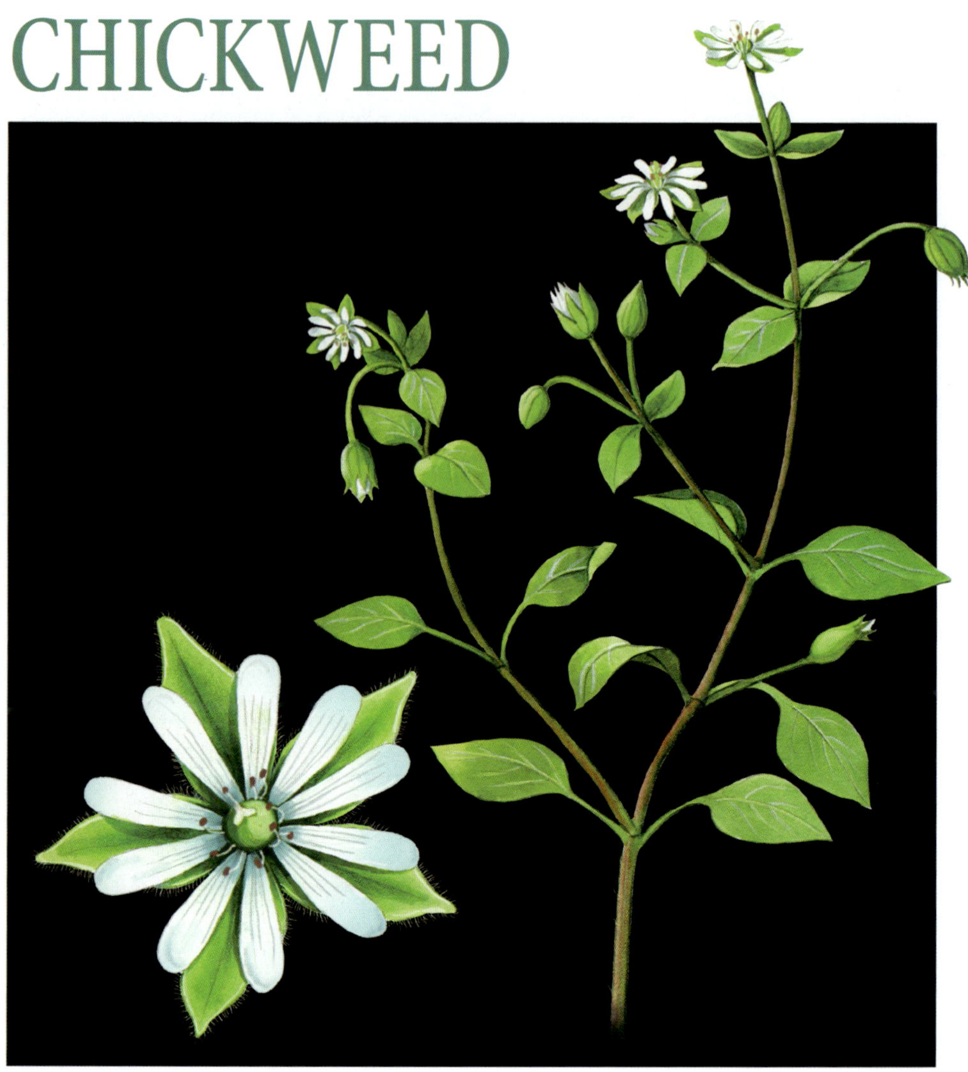

Stellaria media

FAMILY: Caryophyllaceae

OTHER NAMES: Starweed, Starwort, *Fr.* Stellaire, Mouron des oiseaux

PARTS USED: Aerial

CHARACTERISTICS: Sweet, mildly bitter, cool

ACTIONS: Anti-inflammatory, antioxidant, demulcent, emollient, expectorant, antitussive, antipyretic, alterative, astringent, vulnerary, diuretic, laxative, stomachic, antimicrobial, anti-obesity

RANGE: Introduced across Canada except Nunavut

Chickweed is a small, creeping plant, growing up to 30 cm. high with weak, many-branched stems that trail along the ground. Its name, *Stellaria media*, means "little stars," which perfectly describes its flowers. It is identified by a line of hairs running up one side of the stem then continuing along the opposite side when it reaches a pair of leaves. The opposite leaves are succulent, smooth, oval, and pointed. The small white flowers have 5 petals that are deeply divided, seeming like there are 10 petals, and are only open for 12 hours, on fine days. In the rain they droop, and at night the leaves fold over the delicate flowers and protect the tip of the shoot. They begin blooming in early spring and continue through till the fall. The seedpod is a small capsule with teeth that, once ripe, shake the seeds when the wind blows. It grows in fields and waste areas and should be collected between May and July. It is often mistaken for Grass-leaved Stitchwort (*Stellaria graminea*), which is hairless and has grass-shaped leaves, and Mouse-eared Chickweed (*Cerastium spp.*), which has densely hairy leaves. Neither has the same medicinal properties as *Stellaria media*.

MEDICINAL USES:

Skin irritations, weight loss, sore throat, respiratory infections, fever, inflammation

- The whole plant is edible, nutritious, and high in vitamins and minerals. Contains saponins, which improve absorption of minerals, and flavonoids, which contribute to its anti-inflammatory effect. It is mildly diuretic and laxative, works well as a cleansing herb and spring tonic, and helps in weight loss.
- In the form of an ointment or poultice it has a cooling, drying, and anti-inflammatory effect on skin irritations, itches, rashes, wounds, ulcers, boils, eczema, and psoriasis. A fresh poultice will actually heat up as it draws out infection from the body. Its emollient properties make it very soothing. As a decoction it can be used to treat rheumatic pain, wounds, or ulcers. It may also be added to bathwater to soothe inflammation, sunburn, or hemorrhoids. Tincture of the fresh herb has been used successfully to dissolve cysts and benign tumors.
- Treats fevers, inflammation, and other hot diseases. Soothes sore throat and reduces swelling and irritation in the sinuses as well as easing respiratory tract and reproductive inflammations.
- Has been found to have an effect on hepatitis B virus in vitro, but more research is needed.

POULTICE: Apply fresh chopped herb directly onto sores or wounds, cover with a clean towel, and leave for up to 3 hours. Replace if poultice begins to feel warm. If using older plants, cook in water and cool before applying.

INFUSION: 1–4 tbsp. fresh herb in 2½ cups boiling water. Infuse 10 minutes, strain, drink throughout the day.

TINCTURE: Fresh herb, 1:2 in 50% alcohol, take 1–2 ml. 3 times a day.

OIL: Macerate fresh or dried herb in olive oil for 4 days, then squeeze through cheesecloth. Combines well with Yarrow or St. John's Wort oils.

COMBINATIONS: With Calendula, Plantain, Chamomile, Lavender, Yarrow, or St. John's Wort in oils or salves for dry, itchy skin.

CAUTION: Contains saponins, avoid consuming in large quantities as it may cause vomiting or diarrhea. Generally safe.

CHICORY

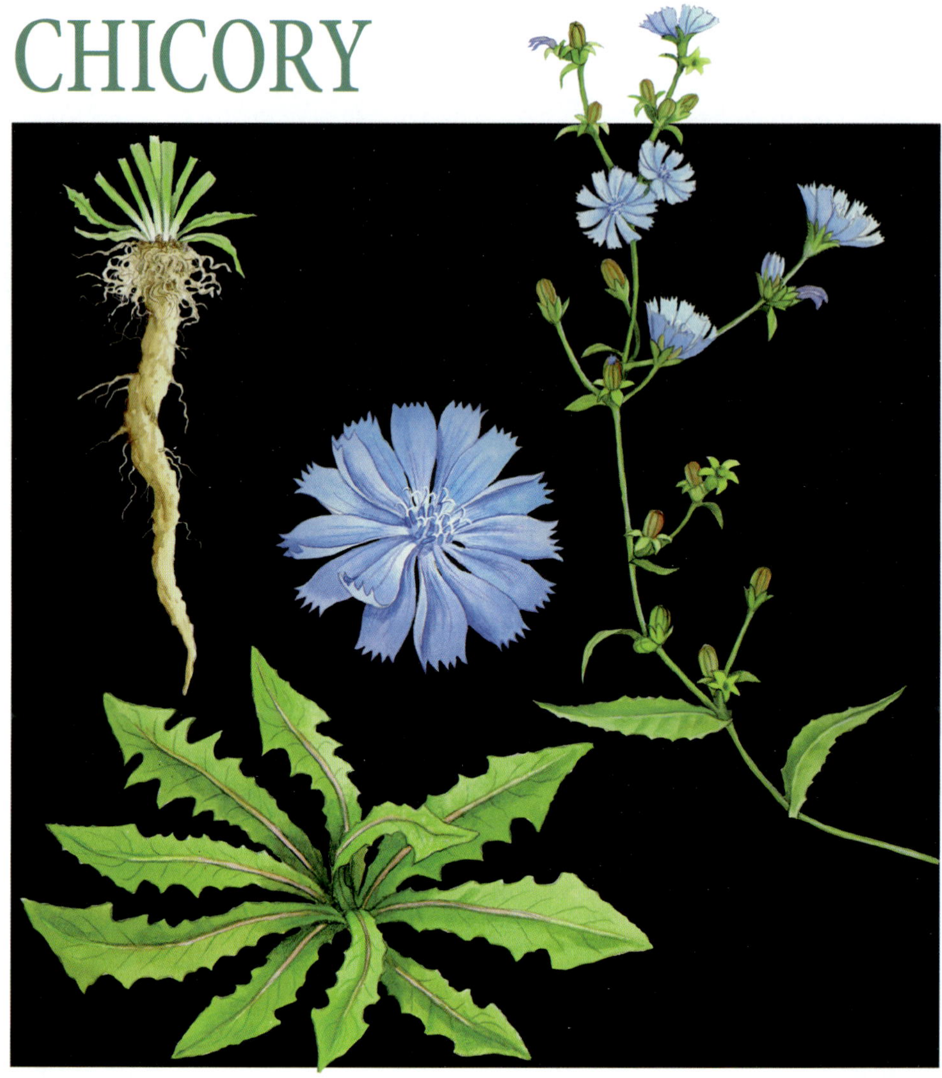

Cichorium intybus

FAMILY: Asteraceae

OTHER NAMES: Blue sailors, Coffeeweed, Succory, *Fr.* Chicorée sauvage

PARTS USED: Whole plant

CHARACTERISTICS: Cooling, slightly bitter, astringent, aromatic

ACTIONS: Stomachic, antibacterial, antifungal, anthelmintic, tonic, mild diuretic, sedative, mild laxative, anti-inflammatory, antipyretic, astringent, cholagogue, hepatoprotective, antioxidant

RANGE: Introduced across all provinces

Chicory is a hardy biennial or perennial originating from Europe and Asia, and has a long history of use in these countries as a medicinal plant. It grows almost a metre tall and can be found along roadsides and in fields from early summer right through to the fall. The stems branch out of a hairy rosette similar to Dandelion, and stretch in all directions looking somewhat angular and sparsely clothed with small leaves. Like Dandelion, Chicory also oozes a milky sap when cut. The delicate blue-mauve flowers appear in clusters of 2 or 3 and close up early in the afternoon. It has a large taproot, which is woody in the wild but when cultivated is large and fleshy and may be roasted and ground as a coffee substitute.

MEDICINAL USES:

Liver ailments, gallstones, digestive problems, swelling, and inflammation

- Benefits the liver; helps to treat jaundice, gallstones. The root contains inulin, which has little impact on blood sugar, making it suitable for diabetics. The juice of the leaves or a tea made from the flowering plant promote the production of bile and is useful for treating gastritis, flatulence, slow digestion, and chronic constipation. A decoction of the root can be laxative or diuretic, it cools heat, is used as a mild digestive tonic, regulates appetite, curbs sugar cravings, and tones the intestines.
- Romans macerated the root in honey wine to alleviate painful urination, jaundice, and kidney stones. Before the wars in Afghanistan, a decoction of the roots was used to fight malaria.
- Some research has been done on its effect on the heart, as it appears to slow a rapid heart rate, reduce lipid levels in the blood, and lower blood pressure.
- Poultices made from bruised Chicory leaves may reduce swelling, inflammation, and arthritic pain.
- Reduces anxiety and stress, mild sedative; when mixed with coffee it nullifies the effects of caffeine.
- Antibacterial and anti-fungal properties. Decreases biofilm formation and adhesion of bacteria to cells in cases of candida, streptococcus, and other pathogenic organisms.

OTHER USES:

- Root can be roasted and ground up as a coffee substitute.
- Used as feed for animals to remove parasites.
- Young leaves can be eaten fresh in salads; older leaves and stems can be boiled and eaten as a vegetable.

DECOCTION: 1 tbsp. dried herb or roasted root in 1 cup water, bring to a boil and simmer 10–5 minutes. Strain and drink 1–2 cups a day.

CAUTION: Do not use while pregnant or breastfeeding. Use in moderation over a short period of time. Avoid if taking anti-coagulant medications. May lower blood sugar levels.

CHOKECHERRY

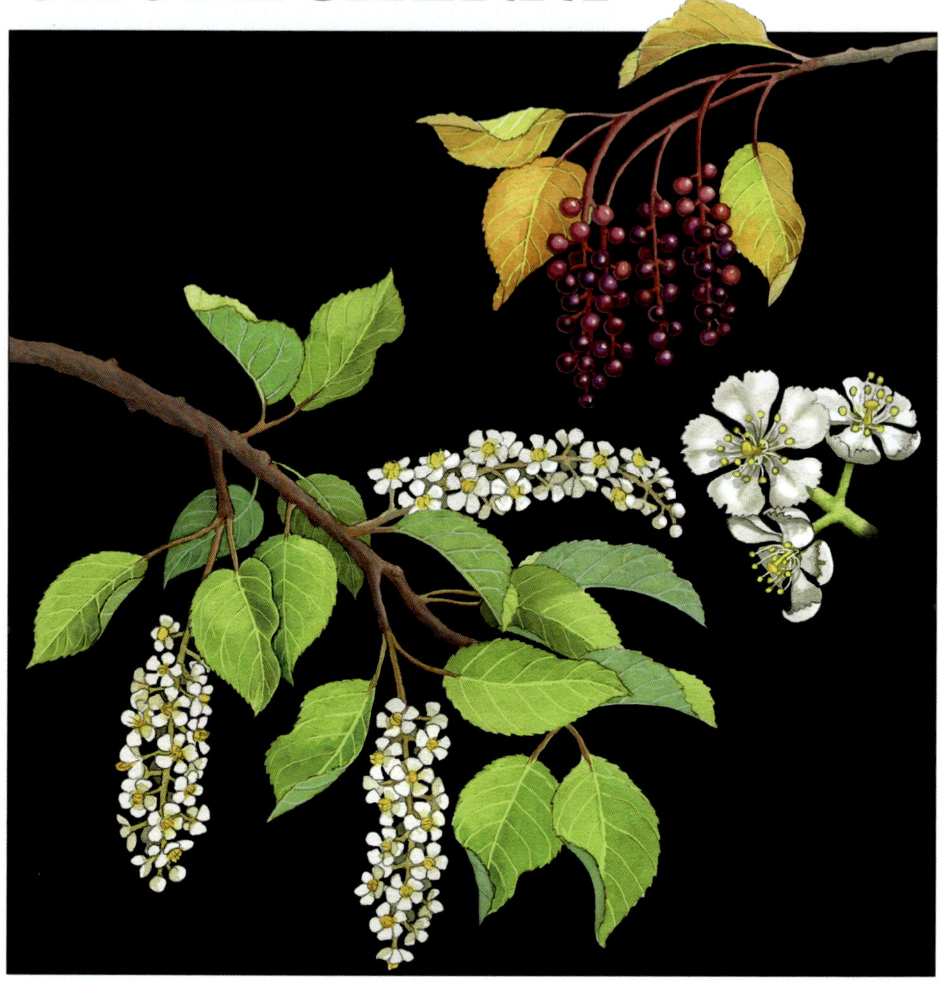

Prunus virginiana

FAMILY: Rosaceae

OTHER NAMES: Black Chokecherry, Bitterberry, *Fr.* Cerisier de Virginie

PARTS USED: Inner bark, berries

CHARACTERISTICS: Sour, astringent, cooling

ACTIONS: Astringent, blood tonic, sedative, appetite stimulant, pectoral, antioxidant, anti-inflammatory

RANGE: Native across all provinces and Northwest Territories

As you might expect, Chokecherry gets its name from its bitter, sour taste, which will make your mouth pucker from its astringency, particularly when eaten raw. But despite its reputation, it has been used by Indigenous Peoples for hundreds of years, both as a food and a medicine. It grows as a shrub or small tree, usually 6 to 9 metres tall, has oval, finely toothed leaves, and is easily identified by its flowers, which grow in racemes of up to 10 cm. long late in the spring. The red berries hang in drupes, turning to black as they mature. Each berry contains a single seed, which is considered toxic not only to humans but particularly to livestock, which may eat them and the leaves in large quantities, often causing sickness and death. Avoid confusing Chokecherry with Chokeberry from the *Aronia* genus; the latter grows in short bunches, a berry contains several seeds, and its leaves are more oblong. Bark and berries of the Chokecherry should be dried or cooked before using, and berries should be fully ripe.

MEDICINAL USES:

Respiratory tract infections, fever, childbirth, stomach upset, diarrhea, skin sores

- Seeds, leaves, and bark contain amygdalin, which hydrolyzes into hydrocyanic acid, which in small quantities can stimulate respiration and improve digestion; however, in excess it can cause respiratory failure and even death. Its healing and nutritive properties are well-known by Indigenous Peoples, who add the dried berries to their pemmican, consisting of dried meat (usually bison), bone marrow, and lard ground together, dried into cakes, and stored over the winter. Boiling or drying the berries or bark neutralizes the toxins.
- Some Indigenous Peoples also use the bark and berry juice during childbirth as a sedative to relieve labour pains and ease anxiety, and the astringency reduces the chance of hemorrhaging.
- Used as a digestive tonic, the bark and berries increase appetite and tone the circulation during convalescence, and relieve dyspepsia, ulcers, bleeding in the bowel, and diarrhea. The seeds have been found to contain some anticancer properties, although very little research has been done. Often combined with other digestive herbs such as Licorice, Ginseng, and Anise in tinctures to relieve digestive weakness.
- Strongly anti-inflammatory, may help reduce the development of diabetic microvascular complications.
- Excellent remedy for irritating spasmodic coughs and colds, bronchitis, persistent fevers, sore throat, and headache. Often the berries are used to make cough syrup.
- Powder or infusion of the black bark can be used for burns, sores, and ulcers.

OTHER USES:
- Green dye made from leaves and inner bark, purple dye from the fruit.
- Berries used to make jams, jellies, pies, syrup, and wine.
- Wood used in construction, to make arrows, or for carving pipe stems.

TINCTURE: Bark 1:5 with 60% alcohol, 30–90 drops up to 3 times a day.

INFUSION: Standard infusion or decoction, ¼–½ cups up to 3 times a day.

CHOKECHERRY JELLY: Put about 8 cups cleaned Chokecherries with 1½ cups water in a pot. Boil and simmer until berries are soft and mushy. Mash, cool, and pour through a sieve or cheesecloth, squeezing as much as possible. Add 1 cup sugar for every cup of juice (about 4 cups) plus 1 tbsp. lemon juice. Boil about 30 minutes or until it reaches gel stage. Pour into sterilized jars.

CAUTION: Not for use during pregnancy or breastfeeding. Seeds, bark, and leaves contain amygdalin, which breaks down into hydrocyanic acid, a toxin to humans and livestock. Boil before using, and add sugar to lessen toxicity. Use with caution.

CINQUEFOIL

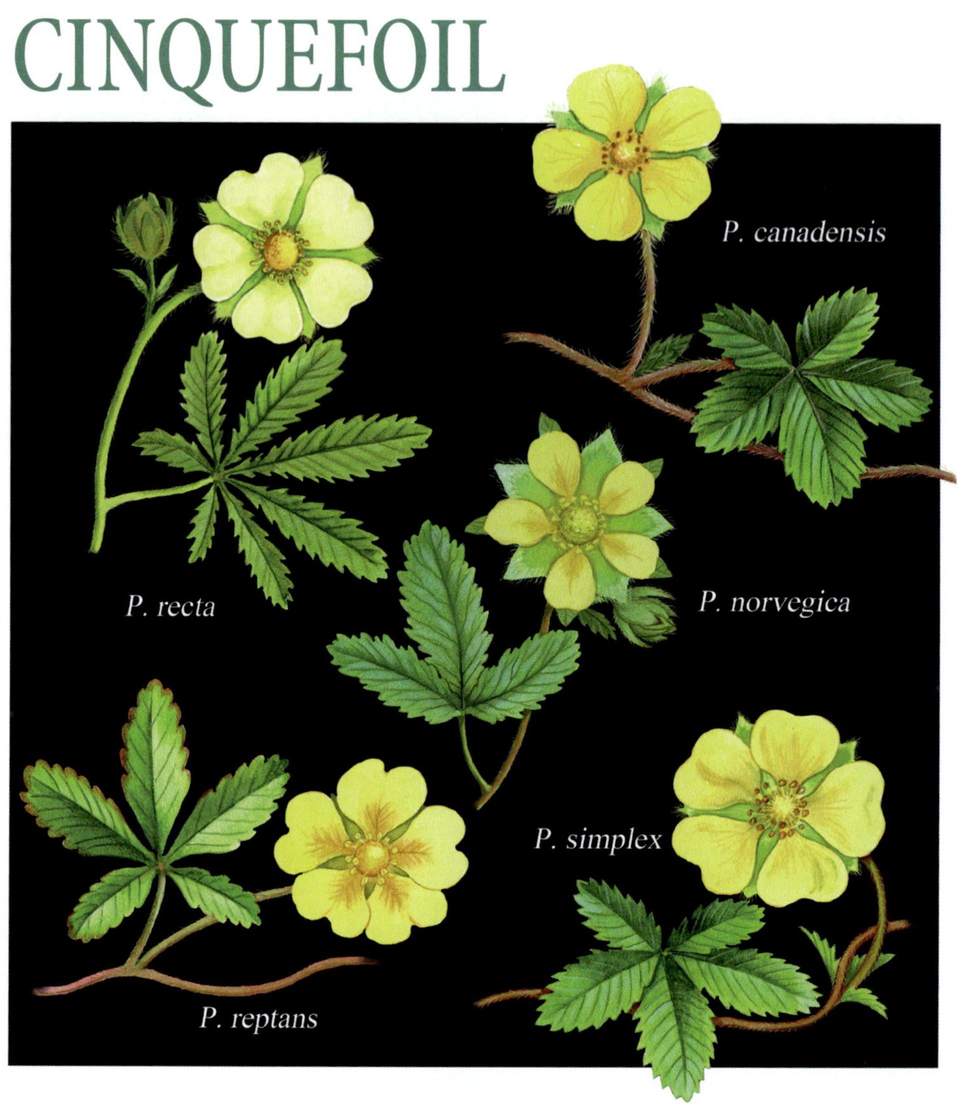

***Potentilla canadensis* (Dwarf Cinquefoil)**
***Potentilla norvegica* (Rough Cinquefoil)**
***Potentilla simplex* (Common Cinquefoil)**
***Potentilla recta* (Rough-fruited Cinquefoil)**
***Potentilla reptans* (Creeping Cinquefoil)**

FAMILY: Rosaceae

OTHER NAMES: Five fingers, Five Leaf, Tormentil, *Fr.* Potentille

PARTS USED: Herb, root

CHARACTERISTICS: Bitter, slightly sweet, cool, strongly astringent

ACTIONS: Astringent (especially the root), febrifuge, anti-inflammatory, disinfectant, antidiabetic, antidiarrhea, antiviral, anticancer, antioxidant, antibiotic, hemostatic, hypoglycemic, antispasmodic, tonic, vasoconstrictive

RANGE: Native and introduced across Canada

The Cinquefoil, or "five-leaf," is a small, hairy, native perennial. There are many different species growing in Canada, all of which are very similar physically as well as medicinally. Leaves are compound divided into 3, 5, or 7 sharply toothed, oblong leaflets, green on top and silvery underneath. The yellow flowers grow on long leafless stalks out of the axils of the leaves. They have 5 petals and bloom from June to September. The plant creeps along the ground, sending out hairy runners, similar to the strawberry plant. They may be gathered while in flower—preferably in June—and dried in the shade for later use. The root is best if dug up in April.

MEDICINAL USES:

Bleeding, diarrhea, fever, mouth infections, pain

- Cinquefoil has a long history of use as a folk remedy due to its high content of tannins, making it a powerful astringent.
- Decoction relieves pain from headaches, neuralgia, gout, arthritis pain, or premenstrual cramps, particularly if combined with Valerian root. May also be used as a compress.
- Stems bleeding, disinfects, soothes burns, sores, bruises, itching, shingles, or inflammation. Firms, tightens, and tones tissues.
- Cools intermittent fevers (hot and cold) and inflammation.
- Infusion used as a mouthwash can soothe a toothache, relieve mouth sores, bleeding gums, or infections. Juice or decoction mixed with honey can be used to treat hoarseness or cough.
- Relieves stomachaches, diarrhea, dysentery, IBS, colitis. Antispasmodic, eases cramps and pains in the digestive tract.

OTHER USES: Young leaves are good in salads.

FOLKLORE: This plant has been used for centuries as protection from witches and sorcery and was often hung over doors or windows to prevent disturbances. Images of the flower were carved into churches dating from the eleventh century. It was a symbol of strength and honour; the leaf was emblazoned on the shields of medieval knights to signify the five senses, or the power of self-mastery. Lovers used it in love potions and fishermen added it to their nets to increase catches.

INFUSION: 1 tbsp. dried root in 1 cup boiling water. Steep 30 minutes, drink lukewarm in small doses. Or use 2 tsp. dried herb and steep for 15 minutes.

COMPRESS: 1–2 tbsp. chopped fresh herb boiled in 2 cups water. Steep 20 minutes, strain, and cool. Soak compress in tea and apply to wounds or bruises.

COMBINATIONS: Add Plantain or Sorrel for wounds, use with Valerian for pain, headaches, or cramps.

CAUTION: Not recommended for use during pregnancy.

CLEAVERS

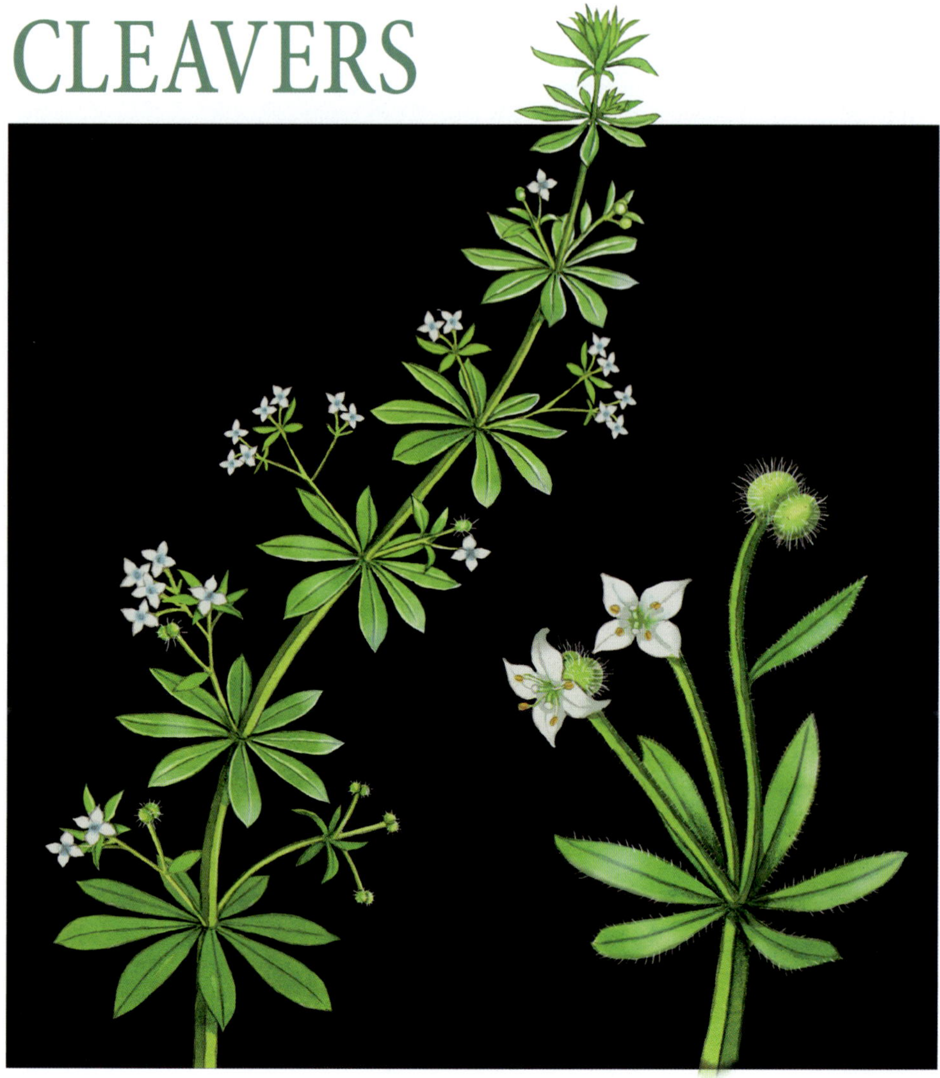

Galium aparine

FAMILY: Rubiaceae

OTHER NAMES: Goosegrass, Gripgrass, Catchweed, Catchweed Bedstraw, Sticky Willy, *Fr.* Gaillet gratteron, Gaillet jaune

PARTS USED: Aerial, fresh or dried

CHARACTERISTICS: Sweet, cool, salty

ACTIONS: Diuretic, adaptogen, lymphatic tonic, hypotensive, mild laxative, alterative, anti-inflammatory, aperient, mild astringent, febrifuge, tonic, vulnerary

RANGE: Native to British Columbia, Saskatchewan, Manitoba, Ontario, Northwest Territories; introduced in Alberta, Quebec, and the Maritimes

Plants in the genus *Galium* are found all over the world, and comprise over 3,000 species, many of them in Canada, but the one most often used for its medicinal properties is *G. aparine*, or Cleavers. These annual plants are slender, angular weeds with tiny lance-shaped or oval leaves arranged in whorls around the stem, and small flowers that are white, greenish, or yellow. They have weak stems so they grow in matted masses by attaching themselves to other plants and objects with their hooked bristles on the stalks and leaves. The flowers grow out of the axils of the leaves and are followed by little seedpods that are also covered in bristles and stick to anything that passes by, especially animal fur. Gather in May or June; may be hung in the shade to dry for later use, but best when the fresh herb is used, either in tinctures or infusions.

MEDICINAL USES:

Urinary infections, enlarged lymph glands, skin inflammations, insomnia, hypertension

- Juice from the fresh herb is rich in vitamin C and recommended as a diuretic for bladder infections where there is painful urination and helps prevent the build-up of minerals that can cause kidney stones. Calms, cools and soothes inflammation. Cleanses and decongests the lymphatic system, flushing out toxins and reducing swelling.
- Stimulates the lymphatic system, reduces swelling and heat, and drains the lymph glands. Removes waste products from the blood, keeping the immune system healthy. Reduces symptoms of tonsillitis, mumps, head colds, sinusitis, and swollen glands, soothing irritated tissues and inflammation.
- Crushed herb or fresh plant juice can be used as a poultice for hot, inflamed skin, sores, blisters, burns and scalds, psoriasis, ulcers, and insect bites.

OTHER USES:

- Can be used as a potherb when picked in the spring.
- Some use it as a hair tonic, claiming it makes it grow longer.
- A red dye can be obtained from the root.
- When juice is applied daily it may fade freckles.
- Roasted seed may be used as a coffee substitute.

COLD OR STANDARD INFUSION: 1 tsp. fresh herb, infuse 10–15 minutes, strain to remove bristles. Take 2–3 times a day.

TINCTURE: Fresh herb 1:2 in 40% alcohol, 2–4 ml. up to 3 times per day.

COMBINATIONS: With Echinacea, Red Clover, or Calendula for lymphatic cleansing, with Yellow Dock and Burdock for skin problems.

CAUTION: Juice may cause dermatitis in sensitive people. Filter to avoid throat irritation. Avoid ingestion if you have a tendency toward diabetes. Not recommended if pregnant or breastfeeding.

COLTSFOOT

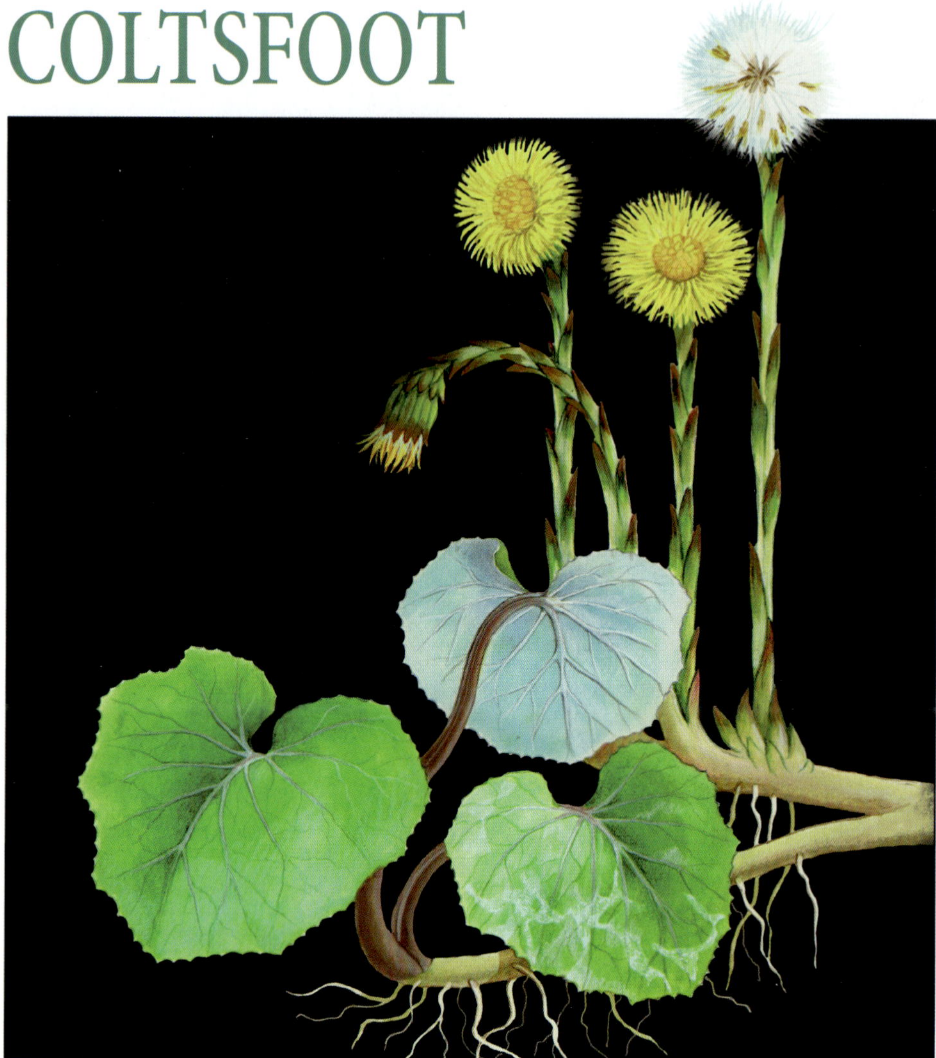

Tussilago farfara

FAMILY: Asteraceae

OTHER NAMES: Horsehoof, Coughwort, Son-before-the-father, *Fr.* Pas d'âne, Tussilage

PARTS USED: Dried leaves, roots, flower buds

CHARACTERISTICS: Bitter, salty, slightly sweet, astringent, cooling (fresh), warming (dried)

ACTIONS: Antitussive, expectorant, demulcent, anti-inflammatory, astringent, diuretic, emollient, antimicrobial, antispasmodic, antioxidant, relaxant, vulnerary, neuroprotective, antidiabetes, anticancer

RANGE: Introduced in British Columbia, Ontario to Newfoundland and Labrador

Native to Europe, Coltsfoot (or Tussilago, which means "cough dispeller") is one of the first wildflowers to bloom in early spring, but its leaves don't appear until long after the flowers have opened. The bright yellow flowers open in sunshine and close in cloudy weather, and are often mistaken for Dandelions. The difference is Coltsfoot's stem, which is covered in brown-tipped scales and grows upward from a creeping rhizome to between 7.5–30 cm. tall. Rosettes of the stalked leaves usually grow in after the flower has gone to seed. Each rosette is the shape of a horse's hoof, has irregular toothed edges, and is covered with a woolly coating, which becomes smooth and waxy on top as the leaf matures, with a grey woolly underside. The soft seed heads resemble those of the Dandelion and are used by birds to line their nests. Coltsfoot typically grows along cliffs, ditches, or riverbanks and tolerates wet areas. Flowers should be gathered before fully bloomed and dried in the shade; leaves should be harvested in early summer, and chopped and dried for later use.

MEDICINAL USES:

Dry coughs, bronchitis, asthma, sinus congestion, gastroenteritis

- Contains mucilage, which soothes mucous membranes and is useful for upper respiratory problems with a dry, unproductive cough that is chronic and persistent, as well as asthma, whooping cough, laryngitis, pharyngitis, and bronchitis. It can be used fresh in infusions, and has a licorice-like flavour. It can also be used dried in infusions, syrups, and cough drops, or it can be smoked.
- Crushed fresh leaves can be applied to burns and skin ailments, boils, insect bites, abscesses, or inflamed areas. A poultice of the flowers can be applied to the skin for inflammation, eczema, and insect bites.
- Indigenous Peoples and colonists once soaked blankets in hot infusion to wrap around a patient with whooping cough.
- Powdered leaves used as snuff for sneezing, sinus congestion, headache, or nasal obstruction.
- Soothes irritation in the gastrointestinal tract, treats inflammatory conditions where there is ulceration.

OTHER USES: Young leaves, flower buds may be added to salads or soups, but should be used sparingly due to toxicity.

TINCTURE: Dried herb 1:5, 45% alcohol, 2–5 ml. up to 3 times a day.

INFUSION: 1–2 tsp. dried leaves in 1 cup boiling water, drink up to 3 times a day.

COMBINATIONS: With Horehound, Marshmallow, Ground Ivy, Mullein, White Horehound, Plantain, or Licorice, for coughs. Avoid combining with St. John's Wort, Boneset, Borage, Comfrey, Gravel Root, or Tansy.

CAUTION: Contains pyrrolizidine alkaloids, which can be toxic to the liver. Do not exceed recommended doses or take for more than 2 weeks. Avoid if pregnant or breastfeeding and do not give to children under fifteen. Do not take if you have liver or heart disease, or high blood pressure.

COMFREY

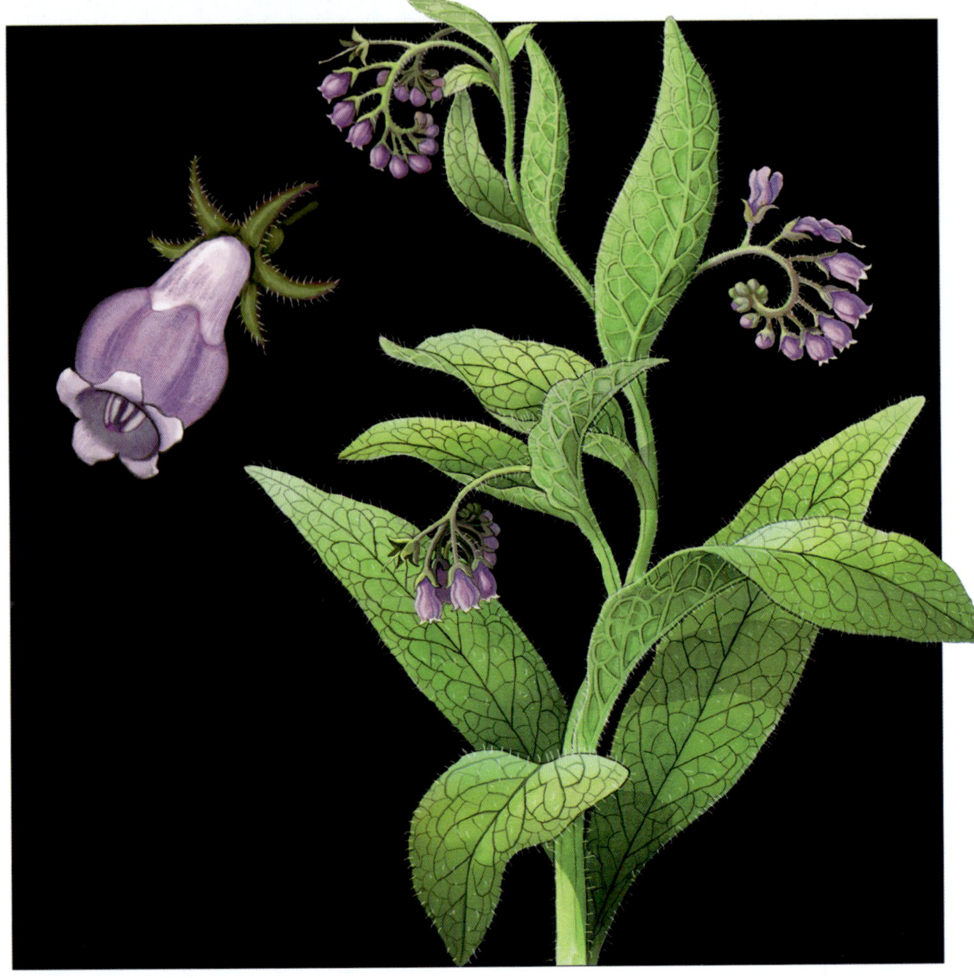

Symphytum officinale

FAMILY: Boraginaceae

OTHER NAMES: Common Comfrey, Boneset, Knitbone, *Fr.* Consoude officinale, Langue de vache

PARTS USED: Root, leaves

CHARACTERISTICS: Cooling, mucilaginous, slightly astringent, bitter, sweet

ACTIONS: Anti-inflammatory, tonic, demulcent, vulnerary, astringent, anodyne, analgesic, antioxidant, vulnerary

RANGE: Introduced across all provinces

This tenacious perennial, a member of the Borage family, is found across North America on moist grasslands, waste places, and old fields. Originally from Europe, it grows to a height of 30–90 cm. and spreads rapidly from even a small piece of the root, quickly taking over a garden. The stems and large alternate lance-shaped leaves are covered in coarse, bristly hairs, and produce a mucilaginous gel when broken. The bell-shaped flowers emerge in May and June and can vary widely in colour, from pink or purple to blue, white, and even yellow. The plant has a long history of use, both internally and externally; however, due to the presence of pyrrolizidine alkaloids, which can damage the liver, it is no longer recommended for internal use, but is highly valued and considered safe when used externally over a short period of time. The leaves are generally harvested during flowering and dried in bundles upside down out of the sun for later use. The roots may be dug up in the fall or early spring, cleaned, and cut into thin slices before drying.

MEDICINAL USES:

Broken bones, bruises, sprains, varicose veins, arthritis, sore muscles, skin ulcers

- The plant contains allantoin, a cell proliferant that speeds up the healing process and encourages new cell growth. Also contains rosmarinic acid, which is an anti-inflammatory, antiviral, and antibacterial, and tannins which help heal surface damage. Particularly useful in external treatment of cuts, bruises, sores, ulcers, eczema, and other skin conditions. Preparations include salves, ointments, and oils, but especially poultices and compresses from the decoction, as allantoin is more soluble in hot water.
- Helpful for osteoarthritis, swelling, and stiffness in the joints, acute myalgia, back pain, sprains, contusions, sports injuries. Compresses are indicated to be effective in healing bone fractures and injured tendons or ligaments more rapidly. However, bones need to be set properly before using Comfrey.
- The astringency of the root has been used internally throughout history in the form of decoctions or tinctures to stop hemorrhages and diarrhea, for broken bones, or as a demulcent to soothe coughs and lung problems with no ill effects if used for short periods. However, because of the presence of pyrrolizidine alkaloids, particularly in the roots, it is no longer recommended for internal use due to liver toxicity.
- A decoction of the root is used in a compress for mastitis, bleeding, and hemorrhoids.

OTHER USES: Leaves make an excellent compost, as they add many nutrients to the soil.

DECOCTION: Standard decoction of root used in compresses. Fresh leaves or crushed root may be applied to skin in the form of a poultice.

OIL: Macerate root and/or dried leaves in oil for 4 to 6 weeks. Filter out plant material and store out of sunlight.

COMBINATIONS: Calendula and Plantain to help healing; Marshmallow for dry, cracked skin.

RESEARCH: Clinical studies have confirmed its effectiveness; after 12 days of external treatment twice a day on patients with joint and back pain, swelling, myalgia, and sports injuries, most showed a marked improvement. Fresh abrasions healed 3 days faster and myalgia pain and sprained ankles improved significantly.

CAUTION: Contains pyrrolizidine alkaloids that may damage the liver and cause hepatic veno-occlusive disease, which creates obstructions in the veins surrounding the liver and could be life-threatening. Avoid internal use. Considered safe for use externally, but avoid using for more than 10 days at a time without guidance from a healthcare professional. Wounds should be cleaned and disinfected meticulously before using as it will seal quickly and could cause infection or debris to be trapped in the wound. Do not use where there is pus or infection already in the wound. Broken bones should be set properly before using. Not for use during pregnancy or breastfeeding, or for children under eighteen.

CRAMP BARK

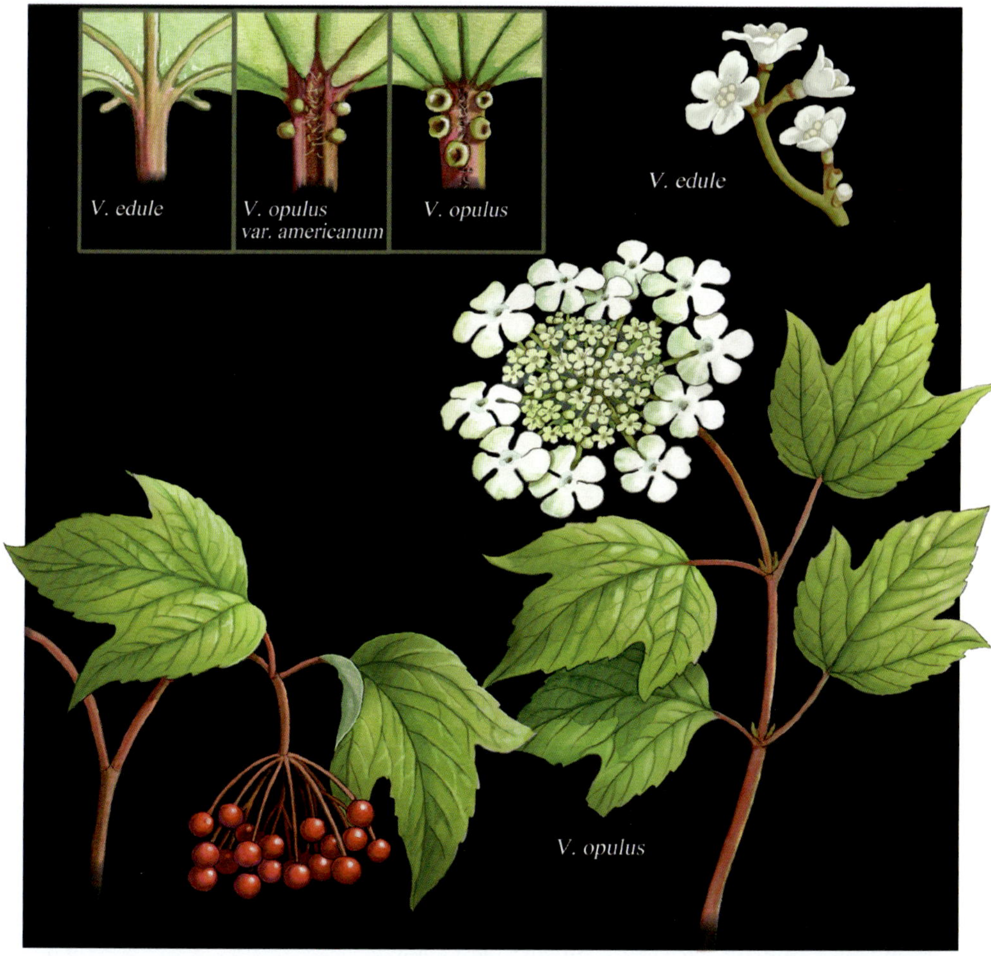

Viburnum opulus; Viburnum opulus var. americanum (trilobum); Viburnum edule

FAMILY: Adoxaceae (Caprifoliaceae, Viburnaceae)

OTHER NAMES: *V. opulus*: European Highbush Cranberry, Guelder Rose, American Bush Cranberry, *Fr.* Viorne obier; *V. edule*: Squashberry, Mooseberry, *Fr.* Viorne comestible; *V. opululus var. americanum:* American Bush Cranberry

PARTS USED: Bark, root bark, berries

CHARACTERISTICS: Bitter, sweet, astringent, warm, dry

ACTIONS: Anti-inflammatory, anti-abortive, antispasmodic, astringent, sedative, nervine, antioxidant, antimicrobial, vasodilator

RANGE: Native and introduced across Canada

The name Cramp Bark gives an indication of this deciduous shrub's usefulness as an antispasmodic in relieving cramps and muscle pains, but its history includes many other uses. It was originally native to Europe but eventually became naturalized, and now both the European and the American variant are found in abundance across Canada, along with its native cousin *V. edule*, which has similar properties but is not as strong medicinally. Cramp Bark grows up to 4 m. in height, the 3-lobed leaves are opposite and usually serrated with a rounded base. Flower clusters are comprised of an outer ring of larger white 5-petalled sterile flowers surrounding the centre of small fertile yellowish flowers, which eventually ripen into bright red drupes of bitter-tasting berries, which tend to smell like old socks, but when cooked into jellies with oranges or apples can be quite tasty. They are incidentally not related to the true cranberry, of the *Vaccinium* family. The *V. edule* variety has only one type of flower, and its berries do not hang in drupes. The best way to distinguish the varieties is by the glands at the base of the leaf. The bark is the part most commonly used for medicine, peeled from the root or branches. It should be collected in spring and summer when its properties are the strongest and dried for later use.

MEDICINAL USES:

Cramps, muscle spasms, menstrual cramps, irritable bowel, headaches, arthritis, high blood pressure, anxiety

- With its antispasmodic and sedative properties, it helps relieve all kinds of cramps and muscle spasms and the pain associated with them. The active components, particularly scopoletin and viburnin, interfere with calcium channels in muscle cells, which helps reduce contractions. Also, coumarin, a mild sedative, has a calming effect on the nervous system.
- Has a long history of use as a uterine tonic; eases bloating and PMS, relaxes menstrual cramps, and tones the uterine muscles. Can be used in cases of dysmenorrhea and endometriosis. Works best if you start taking it 1–2 days before menstruation. In pregnancy, it can stop uterine contractions that come too early, preventing miscarriage, improving muscle tone, and strengthening the uterus for labour. It also helps return the uterus to normal after the birth and helps prevent prolapse in later years.
- As a fomentation, liniment, or internally as a tincture, it relieves muscle spasms, backaches, chronic muscle tension, arthritic pain, restless legs, and headaches that start in the nape of the neck and radiate upward. Pain is often caused by tension due to emotional or physical causes, trauma, anxiety, or overexposure to stress hormones.
- Its cardiotonic effect dilates blood vessels, improves circulation, and lowers blood pressure. Relieves palpitations, angina, and with other herbs can work toward improving the health of the cardiovascular system. Eases anxiety and balances stress hormones.
- Can be used in formulas as an antispasmodic for chronic coughs, hiccups.
- Reduces tension in the gastrointestinal tract due to anxiety, indigestion, diarrhea. Nourishes and strengthens the mucosal lining.
- May be effective at helping expel kidney or ureteral stones.

OTHER USES:

- Berries are rich in vitamins C and K and can be used in jellies, syrups, and jams.
- A red dye can be made from the fruit.

DECOCTION: 2–3 tsp. dried bark in 1 cup water. Simmer 15–20 minutes, strain. Ginger or other spices may be added to mask the bitterness. Drink hot up to 3 times a day.

TINCTURE: Bark 1:5 with 50% alcohol, 20–50 drops 4 times a day or as needed.

COMBINATIONS: With Yarrow, Hawthorn, or Motherwort for cardiovascular problems. With Marshmallow or Mullein for coughs.

CAUTION: May be used during pregnancy under close supervision of a qualified herbalist if there is threat of miscarriage. Avoid with low blood pressure or if taking blood thinners. Raw berries may cause vomiting or diarrhea if eaten in large quantities. Avoid while breastfeeding.

CULVER'S ROOT

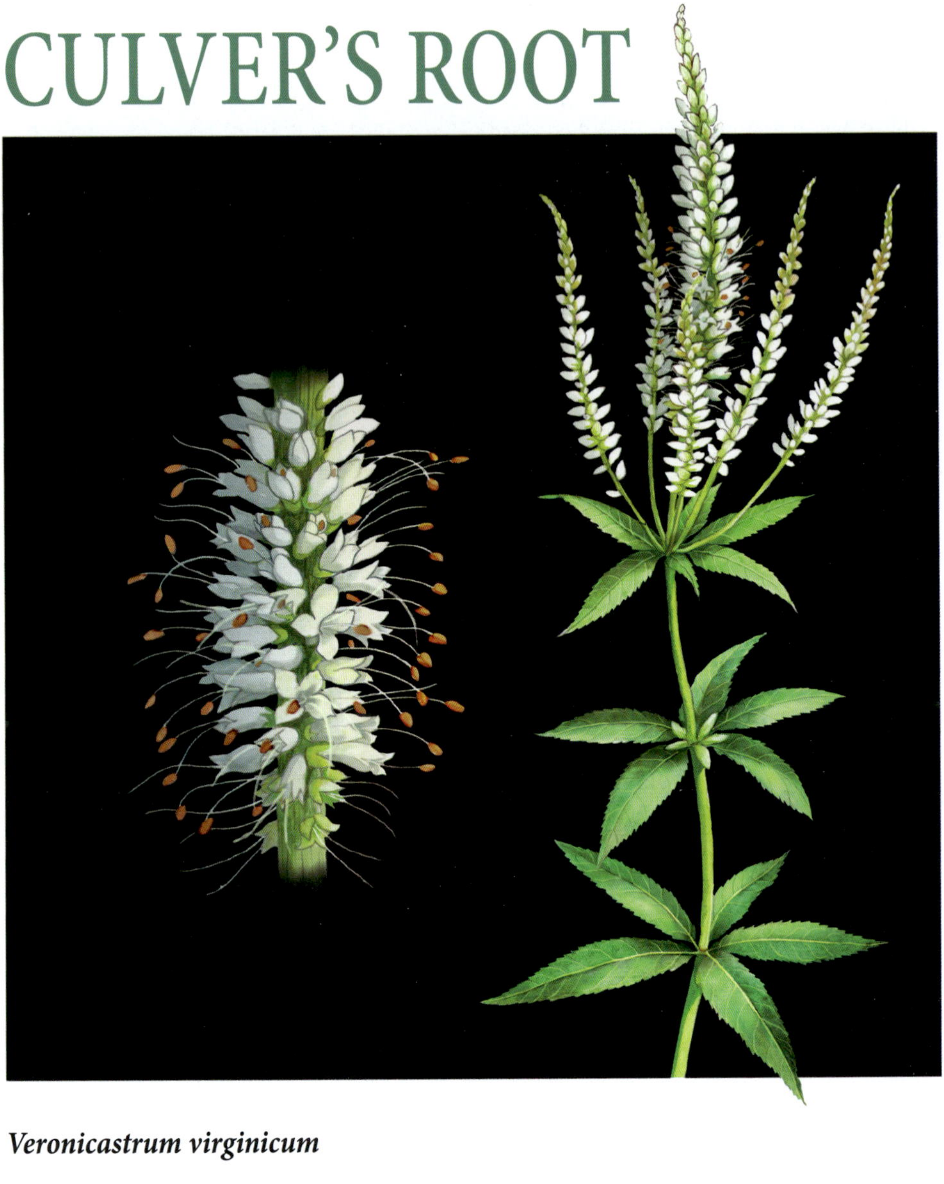

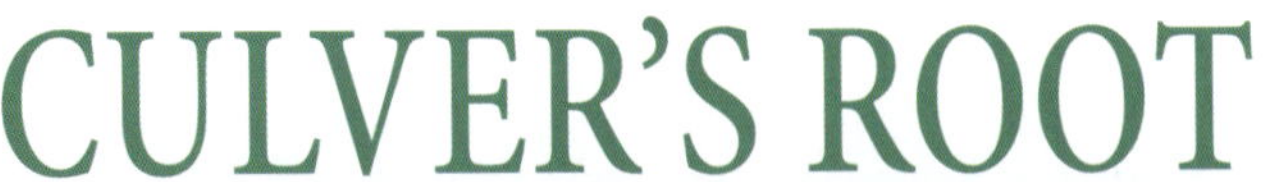

Veronicastrum virginicum

FAMILY: Plantaginaceae

OTHER NAMES: Black Root, Culver's Physic, Tall Speedwell, Bowman's Root, *Fr.* Véronique de Virginie

PARTS USED: Dried root, rhizome

CHARACTERISTICS: Bitter, astringent, cooling

ACTIONS: Diuretic, cholagogue, purgative, emetic, diaphoretic, antispasmodic, laxative, digestive, anodyne, cathartic, tonic, antioxidant, anti-inflammatory, aperient

RANGE: Native to Manitoba and Ontario

This bitter-tasting root typically grows in meadows and at the edge of damp forests of southeastern Canada. It has been used for many years by Indigenous Peoples and more recently was adopted by European settlers for its beneficial effect on sluggish digestion and to improve liver function. An erect perennial of about 1.8 m. tall, it has smooth stems covered in fine down and whorls of 3–7 slender, lance-shaped, finely toothed leaflets. The tall flower spikes are composed of numerous tiny white, pink, or blue tubular flowers that bloom from July to early fall. Roots are thin with a blackish bark, rhizomes grow horizontally up to 15 cm. Dig up in the fall, clean well, and dry for at least 1 year before using to lessen the emetic and laxative effect.

MEDICINAL USES:

Chronic constipation, sluggish digestion, liver disorders

- A digestive tonic, it stimulates the gallbladder, which increases the flow of bile and promotes motility in the digestive tract. Relieves chronic constipation and liver disorders, often accompanied by headaches, back pain, depression, bloating, cramps, pain around the liver, cold extremities, and loss of appetite, although these symptoms can be caused by other disorders. Strengthens and tonifies, benefits the immune system.
- The Seneca people used the fresh root to induce vomiting for purification rituals and to clean sores from tuberculosis; the Chippewa believed it cleansed the blood. The Cherokee people chewed the plant to relieve colic.
- Its effect on the liver often relieves chronic skin and joint problems. Infused oil can be applied topically to relieve inflammation.

DECOCTION: 1–2 tsp. (start with a low dose) dehydrated root to 1 cup cold water. Heat to a boil, simmer 10 minutes and strain. Drink 1 cup 2–3 times a day.

COMBINATIONS: Root powder extract mixed with dried Yarrow herb extract for acne (antimicrobial). With Dandelion root, Chicory root, or Barberry for liver stagnation. With Fennel seed, Peppermint, Ginger for indigestion, stomach cramps, bloating.

CAUTION: Use only dried, as the fresh root may be violently purgative and cause diarrhea or vomiting. Start with small doses. Avoid if you have bile duct obstruction, gallstones, colitis, or Crohn's, or are pregnant or breastfeeding. Should not be given to children.

DANDELION

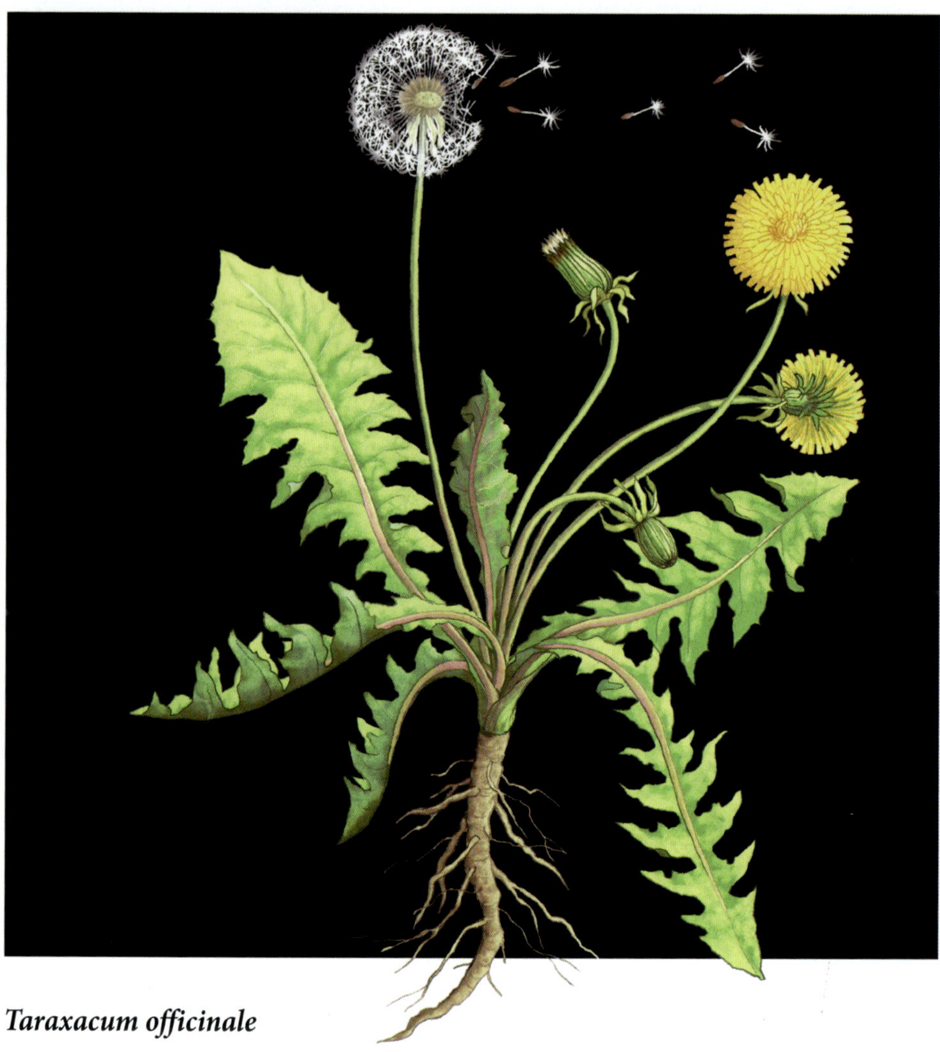

Taraxacum officinale

FAMILY: Asteraceae

OTHER NAMES: Lion's Tooth, *Fr.* Pissenlit, Dent de lion

PARTS USED: Roots, leaves, flowers

CHARACTERISTICS: Leaves: cool, bitter, drying; roots: sweet, bitter, cool

ACTIONS: Diuretic (esp. roots), tonic, alterative, cholagogue, laxative, antioxidant, antiobesity, hepatoprotective, antidiabetic, antiviral, antifungal, anticancer

RANGE: Introduced across Canada

Considered a pesky weed ever since well-groomed lawns became popular, it remains one of the most effective medicinal herbs. Easily identified on every lawn and field in early spring, it is a hardy perennial with a basal rosette of deeply toothed leaves above a central taproot. Several slender hollow stalks emerge from each rosette, containing a milky latex, all leafless with one composite yellow flowerhead, which opens in the morning and closes after sunset. These mature into white fluffy spheres, which are seeds attached to tiny hairy parachutes, easily dispersed in the wind. Harvest leaves in the spring when they are tender; roots can be harvested in fall, split longitudinally and dried for later use.

MEDICINAL USES:

Liver obstructions and stagnation, urinary tract infections, skin eruptions, arthritis, stomach pains

- General cleanser, high in vitamins A, B, C, and D, as well as minerals like potassium, calcium, iron, and zinc. Makes a good spring tonic and encourages elimination of toxins from the body.
- Gentle liver and gallbladder tonic, it helps clear liver and gallbladder obstructions, particularly when there have been bad eating habits and alcohol abuse over the years and digestion is sluggish. Increases bile production, improves digestion, balances digestive enzymes, and encourages elimination of toxins from the body. Used in formulas for cirrhosis, hepatitis, and jaundice. Acts as a mild laxative and increases appetite.
- A powerful diuretic, it can improve elimination of acidic metabolites through the kidneys and urinary tract without depleting the body of potassium like many pharmaceuticals. Helps with joint pain, osteoarthritis, and gout. Reduces edema, high blood pressure, and fluid retention.
- Can clear acne and inflammatory skin conditions like eczema. White latex can be rubbed on the skin to remove warts.
- Powerful antioxidant and anti-inflammatory. May have anticancer and anti-diabetic properties, but more research is needed.
- May be useful in chronic Lyme disease to aid in liver detoxification; however, should be followed closely by a healthcare professional.

OTHER USES:

- The flowers can be made into wine or jelly or added to salads.
- The roasted root makes a nice hot beverage.

DECOCTION: Combine 2–3 tsp. ground root with 1 cup water. Bring to a boil and simmer 10–15 minutes. Cool, drink 3 times a day.

TINCTURE: Fresh root and leaves, 1:2 in 50% alcohol, take up to 1 tsp. 3 times a day.

COMBINATIONS: For congestion in the liver, add Goldenseal, Celandine, or Barberry. Licorice root softens the bitterness. Burdock root helps with acne or rheumatic pain. May be combined with Celery seed for arthritis and gout.

RESEARCH: Both leaf and flower tested on rats were found to modify lipids in the blood, with decreased total of cholesterol and triglycerides attributed to chicoric acid in the herb. Extract was found to have anti-obesity effects in mice and rats, decreasing body weight in animals with a high-fat diet. Roots used in another trial inhibited blood-platelet aggregation or clotting, a risk factor in cardiovascular disease, by 20%. Studies show promise in preventing and treating colitis, combatting viruses, candida, and *Staphylococcus* bacteria, as well as breast and prostate cancers. There is clearly a need for more research on this plant, and much potential for new treatments.

CAUTION: Generally safe, but care should be taken when combined with certain medications. Do not use Dandelions from lawns that have been treated with chemicals.

DEVIL'S CLUB

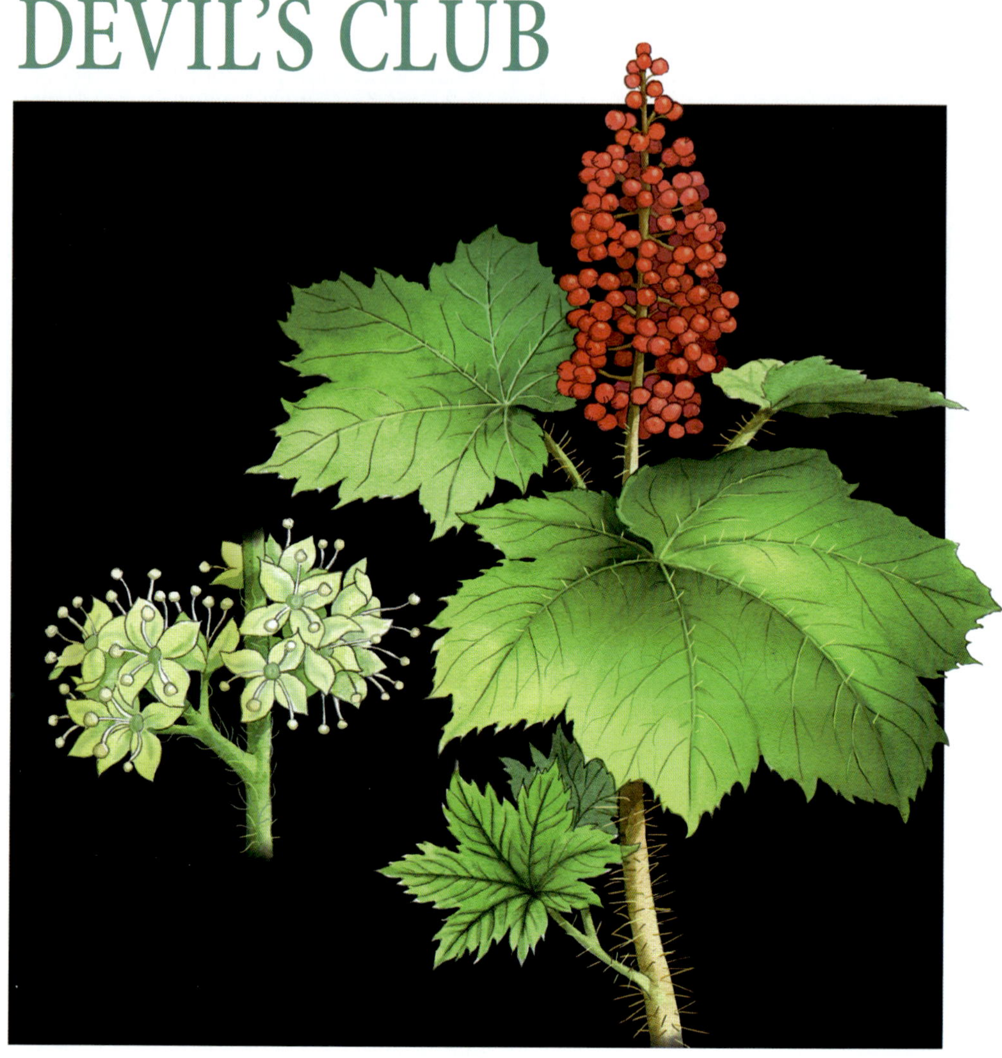

Oplopanax horridus

FAMILY: Araliaceae

OTHER NAMES: Alaskan Ginseng, Devil's Walking Stick, *Fr.* Bois piquant

PARTS USED: Inner bark of roots and stems (preferably green)

CHARACTERISTICS: Cooling, moistening, bitter

ACTIONS: Anti-inflammatory, antirheumatic, diaphoretic, tonic, alterative, antidiabetic, antiviral, antibacterial, expectorant, antipyretic, emetic, purgative, anticancer, antiseptic

RANGE: Native to British Columbia, Alberta, the Yukon, Ontario (sparse)

Many Indigenous Peoples of the Northwest Coast have considered this formidable plant sacred for many years. Its large, maple-shaped leaves, sprawling stalks, and frightening needle-like thorns make it look almost prehistoric, growing to a height of 1–3 m. Its medicine is potent and must be gathered with care and respect. A member of the Ginseng family, it has many of the same properties, affecting general health and vitality. It is usually found in old-growth forests, boggy places, and along streams and low sub-alpine elevations, the long stalks eventually falling over to root and sprout new growth, creating dense colonies. The small, fragrant, whitish-green flowers appear in the spring, growing atop a stalk in pyramid-shaped clusters, then turn to red berries in the summer. Harvest stems and roots in the spring or fall when leaves have died back, being very careful of the sharp spines on the stems and on the veins of the leaves as they can break the skin and become infected. Peel the outer bark, then chip off inner bark and dry before using. Do not harvest more than you need, as it is slow to mature and risks becoming endangered.

MEDICINAL USES:

Arthritis, type 2 diabetes, coughs, colds, arthritis, burnout, tuberculosis

- The inner bark of the root and stem have been used for centuries both for spiritual practices and physical ailments. The presence of a diverse range of phytochemicals, including many anti-inflammatory and antioxidant agents, help to relieve pain, and make it very effective at treating or preventing many inflammatory diseases like arthritis and IBD. It also supports the immune system, inhibiting growth of several types of bacteria, and protects against neurodegenerative diseases such as Alzheimer's and Parkinson's. Studies show it may even have potential as an anticancer treatment.
- Although claims are mostly anecdotal, it shows promise in regulating blood sugar levels and managing type 2 diabetes, particularly among Indigenous Peoples of the Pacific Northwest, where the plant is culturally embedded as a source for healing.
- Decoction helps soothe arthritis and rheumatism. Infused oil can be massaged into joints to relieve pain. Tinctures or infusions may be taken internally to relieve pain.
- Hot tea or tincture in hot water may dispel dampness from the lungs, loosen phlegm, and speed healing. Useful for colds, flu, bronchitis, fevers, and to boost immunity.
- Alkaloids in the extract may relax the blood vessels, lowering blood pressure.
- Antibacterial and antifungal activity, particularly in treatment of tuberculosis.
- Supports adrenals and evens out stress reactions, combating burnout or trauma. Energetically helps strengthen boundaries (symbolized by thorns), particularly against negative external influences.
- Salve, poultices, or infused oil help soothe skin irritations, swellings, and sores, and help prevent infection. Infusion or tincture may help relieve pain.

OTHER USES:

- The inner bark is chewed by shamans or hunters in many west coast Indigenous Peoples during power-seeking rituals to induce a supernatural experience and protect against evil spirits. Devil's Club charcoal is often mixed with red ochre and applied as a face paint.
- Early shoots are edible just after sprouting.

DECOCTION: Standard, ¼–½ cup up to 3 times a day

TINCTURE: Fresh 1:2, dried 1:5, in 60% alcohol. Take 15–30 drops 3 times a day.

COMBINATIONS: With American Ginseng for lethargy, decreased libido, and low immunity, 30 drops 3 times a day.

RESEARCH: Studies show stem extract significantly inhibits growth of breast, lung, and colorectal cancer cells, inducing apoptosis, or cell death, in vitro. Root bark extract found to be effective at slowing growth of several ovarian cancer cell lines. Phenolic compounds and terpenoids may be responsible, interfering with cancer cell growth and division, and may have applications in cancer treatment. Another study found extracts reduced inflammation in human colon, suggesting potential for treating inflammatory bowel disease.

CAUTION: Inner bark can cause vomiting or diarrhea in large doses. Wear gloves when harvesting; sharp spines on the stems and on the veins of the leaves. Berries are toxic. Avoid during pregnancy and breastfeeding. May lower blood sugar and interact with diabetes medications.

DOUGLAS FIR

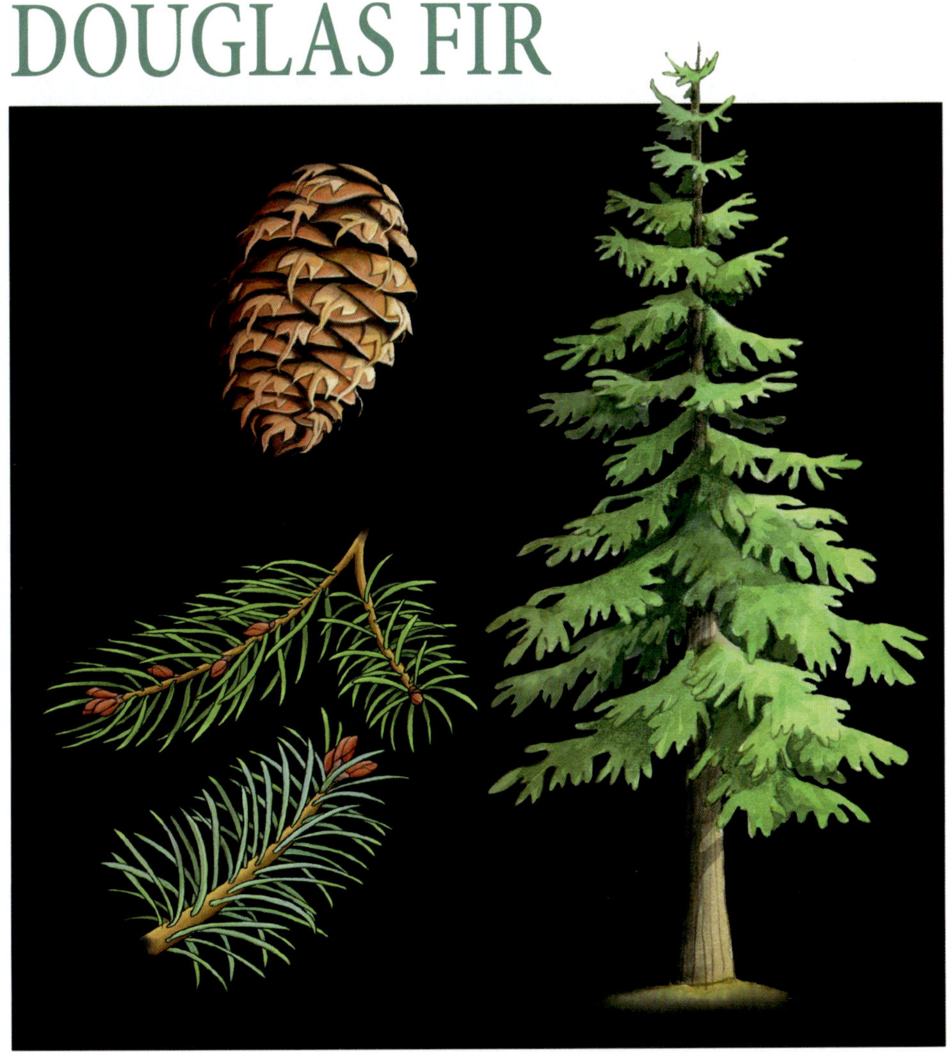

Pseudotsuga menziesii

FAMILY: Pinaceae

OTHER NAMES: Oregon-Pine, *Fr.* Douglas de Menzies, Sapin de Douglas

PARTS USED: Bark, needles, pitch

CHARACTERISTICS: Sweet, fragrant, resinous

ACTIONS: Anti-inflammatory, astringent, antiseptic, antimicrobial, expectorant, sedative, antioxidant

RANGE: Native to British Columbia and Alberta

Douglas Fir, named after the Scottish botanist David Douglas, is a coniferous evergreen of the Pacific Northwest. Often growing up to 80 m. tall, it towers over the other trees in the forest; some have been known to reach over a thousand years old. Not a true fir, its botanical name *Pseudotsuga* means "False Hemlock." Its needles are flat with two white stripes on the underside, and unlike true firs, they spiral around the twig. Bark of the younger trees is smooth with resin blisters, whereas the older trees' bark is ridged and furrowed. The trees are monoecious; both male and female cones grow on the same tree. The seed cones (female) can be 4–10 cm. long with 3-pointed bracts between each scale and they hang down below the branch, turning brown before they fall to the ground. In the spring, the fresh lime-green tips of branches can be picked to make infusions, or to add a woodsy flavour to stews and soups. At certain times in the summer, some trees produce a crystalline sugar from their branch tips, which can be eaten as a confection or added to other foods as a sweetener. The bark is best harvested from thick lower branches, peeled, and dried for later use. Be careful when identifying this tree as it looks similar to the Yew, a poisonous tree which has bright red berries.

MEDICINAL USES:

Colds, coughs, rheumatism, excessive menstruation, kidney and bladder infection, skin inflammation, and wounds

- Astringent, an infusion of the bark will relieve diarrhea or bleeding in the intestine.
- Resin from the bark blisters is antiseptic and will heal cuts, sores, and burns and help prevent infection. It can be added to salves or oil for chest rubs for colds, congestion, or sore muscles.
- Needles and young branch tips are high in vitamin C, and make a nice tea for colds, coughs, and asthma, or simply to quench thirst and give you energy.
- Bark infusion can slow down heavy menstrual bleeding.
- A decoction of the twigs is diuretic and tonic, helping relieve bladder or kidney complaints.
- Rheumatism and arthritis can be treated with a warm infusion compress or infused oil to ease pain and stiffness.

OTHER USES:

- Wood is strong and durable, used for fuel, building and making canoes, tepees, snowshoes, boughs used for bedding and floor coverings.
- Resin used to patch canoes or burned as incense.

DECOCTION: Boil 5 cups of water, reduce heat and add ½–¾ cup needles and young twigs, simmer 10–15 minutes. Strain, add honey if desired.

TINCTURE: Fresh 1:2, dried 1:5, in 50% alcohol. Take 15–30 drops up to 3 times a day.

COMBINATIONS: Often used with Witch Hazel to treat eczema. Add Burdock root or Oregon Grape root to cool down hot skin conditions.

CAUTION: Generally safe but use in moderation.

ECHINACEA

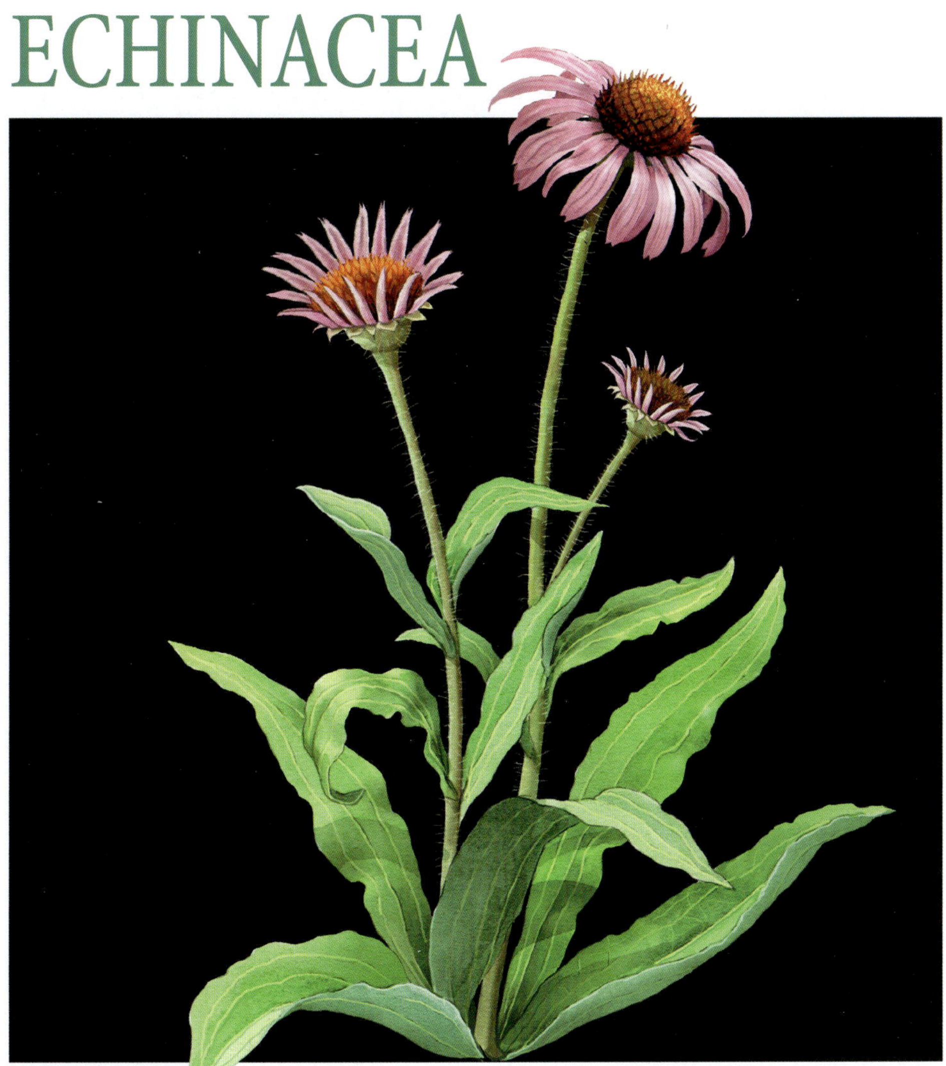

Echinacea angustifolia
Echinacea purpurea

FAMILY: Asteraceae

OTHER NAMES: *E. angustifolia:* Prairie Purple Coneflower, *Fr.* Échinacée à feuilles étroites; *E. purpurea:* Eastern Purple Coneflower, *Fr.* Échinacée pourpre

PARTS USED: Whole plant

CHARACTERISTICS: Sweet, diffusive (tingling), cooling, drying

ACTIONS: Immunostimulant, anti-inflammatory, antiviral, antiseptic, alterative, stimulating, anticatarrhal, lymphatic

RANGE: *E. angustifolia* native to Saskatchewan, Manitoba; *E. purpurea* introduced in Ontario, Quebec

Echinacea's reputation for preventing and lessening the severity of colds and flu is well-known throughout North America. *E. purpurea* has stringy, fibrous roots and its leaves are broader and shorter than *E. angustifolia*'s, which has narrower leaves and petals and a larger taproot. Some consider the latter medicinally superior, as it produces a longer-lasting tingling sensation on the tongue, but both are very effective. Although used for at least the past four hundred years by Indigenous Peoples for infections and snakebites, it only rose in popularity in the seventies as an antiviral. A perennial from the Daisy family, its tall branched stems topped with striking flowers grow up to 1 m. and are popular as a garden flower. *Echinos*, Greek for "hedgehog," refers to its spiny orange-brown seedhead, which is surrounded by pink or purple petals sometimes up to 7.5 cm. long. Aerial parts contain more immune-boosting properties and are harvested in summer when the flowers emerge. Roots, although immune-enhancing as well, contain more volatile oils, and are harvested in the fall. Both may be dried for later use.

MEDICINAL USES:

Respiratory tract infections, fevers, colds, flu, urinary tract infection, ear infection, candida, skin inflammation

- Widely used for immune-boosting properties, it stimulates the white blood cells and inhibits spread of infection, reducing severity and duration of colds and flu. Most effective if taken at first sign of symptoms, and with substantial and frequent doses for no longer than 10 days. Results of studies are inconsistent, which indicates that the freshness of the herb, the species and parts used, dosing, one's overall immune health, diet, and sleep, all impact effectiveness.
- Treats upper respiratory tract infections, flu, colds, sore throat, coughs, fevers, sinusitis, laryngitis, and ear infections.
- Diffusive for strengthening and clearing lymph nodes and to clear infection from the bloodstream. Potent blood tonic, it detoxifies the blood and the liver while reducing inflammation in the body.
- Relieves urinary tract infections and candida or yeast infections.
- Topically helps heal inflammation, eczema, wounds, bites, stings, boils, poison oak, poison ivy, snakebites. May be taken internally as a root tea to increase efficacy. Reduces chance of infection.
- Root chewed to relieve toothache, reduce gum inflammation, and aid digestion.

DECOCTION: ½ tsp. herb in 1 cup water, simmer 10–15 minutes, strain. Take ¼–½ cup every 3–4 hours at onset of symptoms.

TINCTURE: Fresh root, flowerhead, seeds, 1:2, 60% alcohol; dried plant 1:5, 60% alcohol. Take 1 drop for every 2 lbs. body weight (30–100 drops) up to 5 times a day at onset, 3 times a day after.

RESEARCH: New studies on *E. purpurea* confirm it can diminish length and severity of the common cold when taken as recommended, but the mechanism of action is still unknown due to a lack of research, and this effect is only found with certain preparations.

CAUTION: May produce an allergic reaction in some people. Slight risk of gastrointestinal upset, rashes. May reduce the effect of immune-system–suppressing medications. Consult your physician if you have an autoimmune disorder, tuberculosis, diabetes, connective tissue disorders, MS, or HIV/AIDS before using. Avoid long-term use.

ELDER

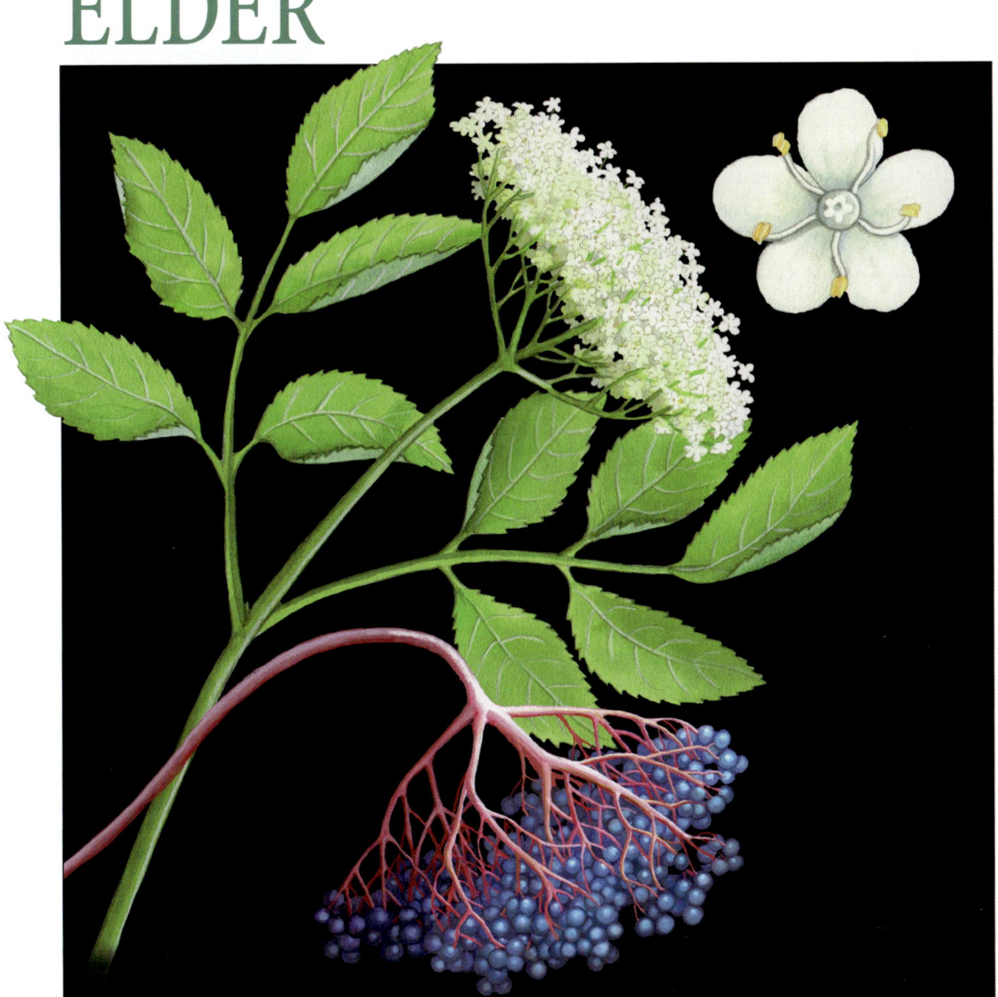

Sambucus canadensis
Sambucus serulea

FAMILY: Viburnaceae (Adoxaceae)

OTHER NAMES: *S. canadensis:* American Black Elder, Canadian Elder; *S. cerulea:* Blue Elder, *Fr.* Sureau

PARTS USED: Flowers, berries, leaves

CHARACTERISTICS: Acrid, bitter, cool; flowers: sweet, cool, drying

ACTIONS: Flowers: diaphoretic, anticatarrhal, mildly sedative; berries: antiviral, anti-inflammatory, diaphoretic, diuretic, laxative, antioxidant; leaves: emollient, vulnerary, purgative, expectorant, diuretic

RANGE: *S. canadensis* native from Manitoba to the Maritimes; *S. cerulean* native to southern British Columbia

Black and Blue Elders closely resemble their European cousin *Sambucus nigra*, both in appearance and medicinal properties. A shrub generally 4–8 m. tall, it has pinnately compound leaves with 5–9 opposite leaflets with one at the tip, each serrated, oval, and pointed. Whitish flowers appear in July, growing in many large umbels and having a somewhat peculiar aroma. They develop blue or black berries at the end of the summer, and should only be used when completely ripe. Do not confuse with the poisonous Red Elderberry. The young branches contain a soft pith, easily removed and once used to make pipes or musical instruments, however the fresh stems are poisonous and should be aged at least a year. Flowers should be harvested gently, removed from their stalks, and dried quickly in a cool oven. The berries may be gathered when ripe in the fall and dried or frozen for later use. They should not be consumed raw. Store in an airtight container.

MEDICINAL USES:

Colds, flu, sinusitis, skin ailments

- Berries are nutritious, rich in vitamin C and other vitamins, anthocyanins and flavonoids, all powerful antioxidants that protect from free radicals. They soothe the mucous membranes of the throat and lungs, relieving irritation. Useful in the first stages of cold or flu, upper respiratory tract infection, sinusitis, or hay fever. Flower infusion promotes expectoration and perspiration when taken hot before bed. It can be mixed with Peppermint leaves if desired. Syrup of the berries has been proven to reduce symptoms and duration of colds and flu if taken at first sign.
- Flowers and leaves are used in ointments and lotions to treat burns, rashes, bruises, sprains, minor skin ailments, and to diminish wrinkles.
- Tea made from the flowers is a mild laxative and diuretic and warm compresses may reduce pain of rheumatism, arthritis, and inflamed swellings. A cold infusion is said to be effective in relief of swollen glands.
- Strained Elder flower tea that has been cooled with ¼ tsp. salt added per cup makes a good eyewash to reduce inflammation.
- Elder berry wine was once used to ease pain associated with arthritis.

FOLKLORE: There are many myths surrounding this bush that date far back and span across many cultures. Medieval beliefs held it to be a symbol of death and bad luck. In Scandinavia it was believed a dryad, Hyldemoer, lived in an Elder tree, and if it was cut or used for furniture she would forever haunt those responsible. In England in the seventeenth century it was thought that the tree would provide protection against witches and people often carried a twig in their pockets to prevent rheumatism.

INFUSION FOR FLU WITH FEVER: Mix equal parts Elder flower, Yarrow, and Peppermint to make 2 tbsp. in 1 cup of boiling water (3 or 4 slices of fresh Ginger root may also be added). Take a warm bath and drink hot before bed.

ELDER BERRY SYRUP: Place 1⅓ cup frozen or 1 cup dried berries in a pot, add enough water to cover. Add 1 tsp. Cinnamon, ½ tsp. cloves, and a few slices of fresh Ginger, and simmer over low heat, stirring and mashing until mixture is mushy and reduced by half. Strain liquid into a measuring cup, and add an equal amount of honey to the juice. Add a squirt of lemon juice and/or brandy if desired (helps to preserve it). Ratio should be 20:80 alcohol to syrup. Store in a jar in the fridge, take 1 tbsp. every hour at the onset of cold or flu, then 3–4 times a day.

RESEARCH: A double-blind, placebo-controlled study from Norway in 2000 where patients showing symptoms of flu who received 15 ml. Elder berry syrup 4 times a day for 5 days were relieved an average of 4 days earlier than the placebo. By blocking the virus from attaching to host cells, the Elder berry inhibits the virus's ability to reproduce. It also activates the immune system by increasing inflammatory and anti-inflammatory cytokines, benefitting both excessive and deficient immunity.

CAUTION: Do not use stems or leaves in preparations, only flowers or berries. Stems are considered mildly poisonous. Raw berries may cause nausea, dizziness, or diarrhea in some people. Do not use berries from Red Elder as they are mildly toxic.

ELECAMPANE

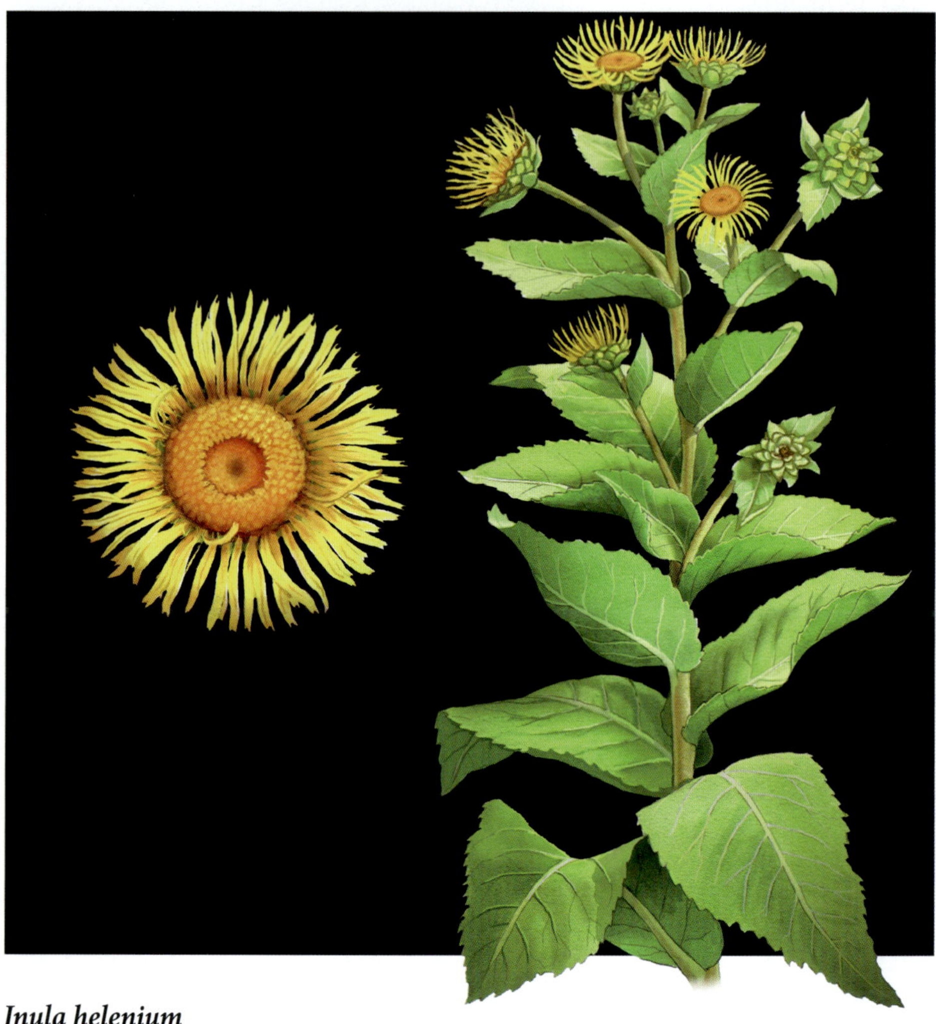

Inula helenium

FAMILY: Asteraceae

OTHER NAMES: Horseheal, Scabwort, Horse Yellowhead, *Fr.* Inule aunée, Grande aunée

PARTS USED: Root, rhizome

CHARACTERISTICS: Slightly bitter, sweet, pungent, warming

ACTIONS: Diuretic, tonic, diaphoretic, expectorant, alterative, antiseptic, astringent, mildly stimulant, carminative, anthelmintic, antimicrobial, antibacterial, anti-inflammatory, antifungal

RANGE: Introduced in British Columbia, Manitoba to Maritimes

This medicinal plant is native to Europe and northwest Asia, coming over to America with the early settlers. Once used by veterinarians for healing lung disorders in horses, hence the name "Horseheal," it has a long history of clearing respiratory problems in animals and humans. It has since been cultivated in herb gardens, mainly for its use as an expectorant in respiratory ailments, and escaped to the wild across central and eastern North America and British Columbia. Growing 1.2–1.5 m. tall, it has soft, hairy stems and large, toothed leaves, 30–45 cm. long, broader at the base and pointed at the tip, with hairy undersides. The large, yellow flowers bloom all summer and resemble a shaggy, yellow daisy, about 7–10 cm. in diameter. Roots are gathered in the fall, typically from 2- or 3-year-old plants. They have a tough, fibrous skin that can easily be peeled off, then sliced and used fresh or dried in various preparations.

MEDICINAL USES:

Respiratory tract infections, indigestion, urinary tract infections, swollen glands, tuberculosis

- Chiefly used for wet coughs, it thins and clears mucus from the lungs, coating and soothing irritation in the mucous membranes and destroying pathogens. Good for asthma, bronchitis, whooping cough, and upper respiratory allergies. Over a longer period of time and in smaller doses, it can strengthen the lungs in cases of chronic bronchitis, asthma, or general weakness.
- High content of inulin, a soluble dietary fibre that works on the intestinal microbiome, helping to maintain regularity, slowing digestion to increase absorption and improving mental health and memory. It helps those who are often cold and tend to have constipation, soothing indigestion and gas, warming and toning the digestive system. Slightly bitter, it increases bile production, acts as a prebiotic, nourishes colon cells, and helps repair leaky gut. May reduce blood glucose spikes, normalizing levels of blood sugar in type 2 diabetes.
- Contains sesquiterpene lactones that are healing, antiseptic and relaxant, and may stop the growth of certain types of cancer.
- Externally may be used as a wash or poultice for skin inflammations or arthritic pain.

DECOCTION: 1–3 tsp. powdered root to 2 cups water. Bring to a boil and simmer 15 minutes, then steep for 1 hour. Take small doses throughout the day.

TINCTURE: Fresh 1:2, dried 1:5, in 60% alcohol, 1–2 ml. 3 times a day.

COUGH SYRUP: Mix ⅓ cup each of Elecampane root, Spikenard, or Sarsaparilla root, and Comfrey root. Mash and combine with 4 cups water, boil and reduce to 1 cup. Strain and add 4 tbsp. brandy and ⅔ cup honey. Take 1 tsp. every 2 hours.

COMBINATIONS: Add Mullein and Licorice root for coughs, Aniseed and Lobelia when there are spasms and constriction in the chest. Works well with White Horehound for bronchitis.

CAUTION: Large amounts may cause vomiting, diarrhea, or cramps. Avoid if pregnant or breastfeeding. May cause contact dermatitis in some people.

EVENING PRIMROSE

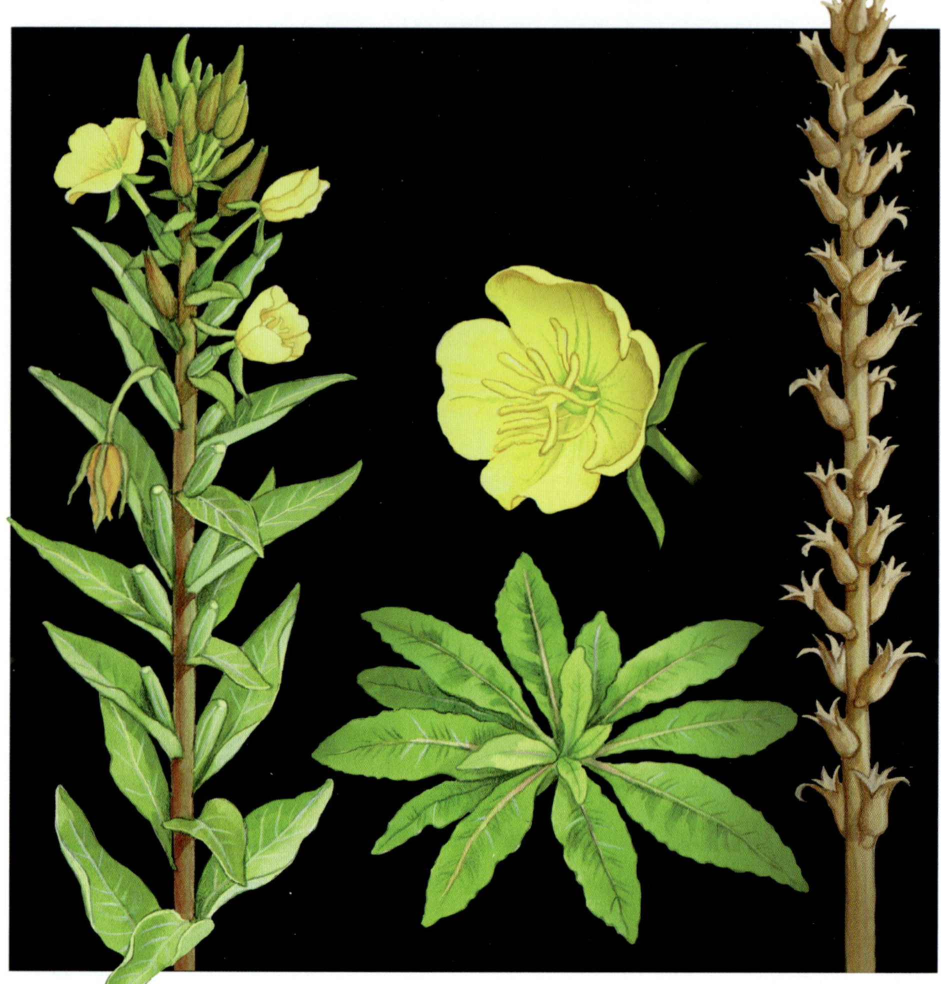

Oenothera biennis

FAMILY: Onagraceae

OTHER NAMES: Sundrop, Evening Star, King's Cure-all, Night Willow, *Fr.* Onagre, Onagre bisannuelle, Herbe aux ânes

PARTS USED: Leaves, oil from seeds, root

CHARACTERISTICS: Sweet, cool and nourishing, slightly bitter, moist, and spicy

ACTIONS: Anti-inflammatory, vulnerary, relaxant, antispasmodic, astringent, sedative

RANGE: Native from Alberta to the Maritimes, introduced in British Columbia, Newfoundland and Labrador

Evening Primrose has a long history in North America, both for its medicinal properties and its use as a vegetable. The entire plant is edible and was a nutritious source of food for pre-contact Indigenous Peoples, particularly the boiled root, which has a peppery taste. An erect biennial, it forms a rosette of basal leaves in the first year. In its second year, the hairy stems arise from the centre to a height of 0.9–1.2 m., bearing yellow, delicately fragrant flowers all along the stalks, with new ones forming until late in the fall. They are replaced by hairy green seed pods that open into four sections to spread their seeds. The common name derives from the flowers, which only open in the evening early in the season to accommodate the flying insects that pollinate them. The root is best when harvested in the plant's first year. The seeds, the most active part medicinally, are gathered when the pods mature late in the summer. The early leaves can be eaten in salads as well as the flowers, or leaves can be cooked and eaten as greens.

MEDICINAL USES:

Hypertension, anxiety, PMS, arthritis, eczema

- The seeds are rich in gamma-linolenic acid (GLA), an unsaturated omega-6 fatty acid which plays an important role in brain function, skin, and hair growth, bone health, and regulates the hormones and reproductive system. It is not made in the body so it needs to be obtained in food.
- Seed oil is used as a muscle relaxant to calm nerves, irritation, headaches, bloating, breast tenderness, and PMS. Sometimes used in midwifery to soften the cervix and ease delivery. Reduces symptoms of menopause, hot flashes, night sweats.
- Some claim it relieves eczema, dermatitis, acne, and inflammation, both topically and orally. May relieve rheumatoid arthritis, but studies are inconclusive.
- Anti-clotting, the seed oil is useful in treating hypertension and preventing heart attacks caused by thrombosis or blood clots; reduces blood pressure. It also helps relieve the pain of diabetic neuropathy. May lessen inflammation and damage caused by multiple sclerosis.
- Mashed root or leaves can be eaten or used as a poultice for healing wounds, bruises, boils, swelling, hemorrhoids, redness, and irritation.

OTHER USES: Roots boiled and eaten like potatoes. Young leaves cooked as greens. Shoots eaten raw.

OIL: 1 tsp. oil daily or as directed.

COUGH SYRUP: Ground dried root may be mixed with warm honey for an effective cough syrup, take as needed.

RESEARCH: Studies have found that Evening Primrose oil was effective at treating PMS symptoms like bloating and cramps, and menopausal symptoms such as night sweats and hot flashes. A combination of vitamin D and Evening Primrose oil was found to reduce symptoms of moderate diabetic neuropathy, and it increased blood flow and reduced inflammation in patients with scleroderma and Raynaud's syndrome. Trials involving conditions like eczema, however, have been inconclusive.

CAUTION: Avoid if you have epilepsy or schizophrenia or are on anticoagulants. May cause headaches or nausea on an empty stomach.

EYEBRIGHT

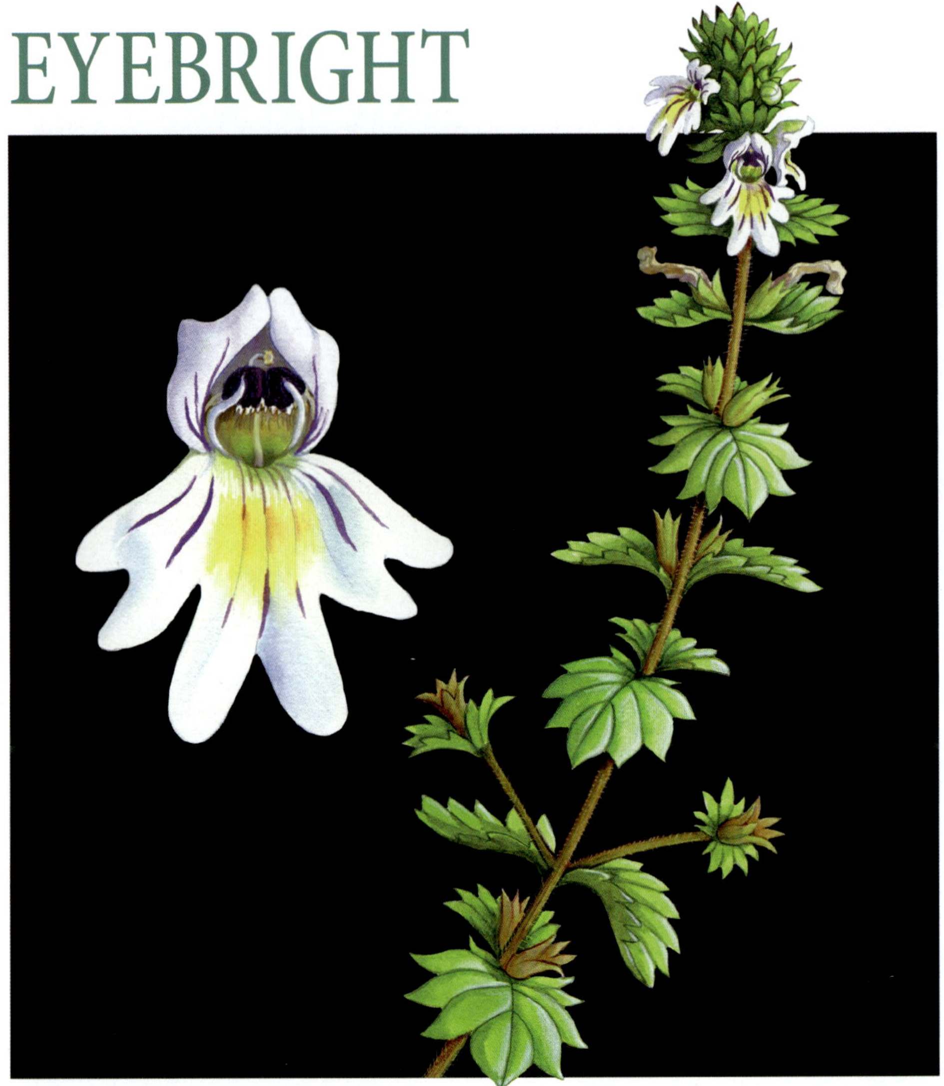

Euphrasia nemorosa

FAMILY: Orobanchaceae

OTHER NAMES: Meadow Eyebright, Canada Eyebright, *Fr.* Euphraise, Casse-lunette

PARTS USED: Aerial, dried

CHARACTERISTICS: Bitter, mildly astringent, cool

ACTIONS: Astringent, anti-inflammatory, expectorant, anticatarrhal, tonic, antioxidant, antihistamine

RANGE: Introduced in Alberta, Ontario to Newfoundland and Labrador

This small, delicate annual, often classified under the more general term *Euphrasia officinalis,* has been used for centuries, particularly in Europe, to treat many eye diseases. Growing up to 20 cm. high, it has square, downy, branching stems with notched leaves that grow in opposite pairs. The tiny white flowers have purplish and yellow markings inside, which herbalists claim resemble a bloodshot eye. There are two lips: the lower has 3 lobes; the upper has 2 that arch over the stamens. Eyebright is semi-parasitic, getting part of its nourishment from surrounding grasses, to which it attaches underground suckers. It is best collected in July and August when the flowers are in bloom; cut just above the root.

MEDICINAL USES:

Eye diseases, sinus congestion, colds, eczema

- Contains aucubin, an iridoid glycoside which is anti-inflammatory, soothing, and reduces swelling. Treats various diseases of the eye, such as pink eye, conjunctivitis, red or irritated eyes, or styes, and can be taken internally and/or externally (should be sterile if applied directly to the eye). Contains vitamins A, B, C, and E, which are known to improve eye health. Increases elasticity in the optic tissues.
- Tea made from leaves, stems, and flowers used to treat symptoms of sinus congestion, allergies, and colds, particularly if the discharge is thin and watery. Relieves inflammation of the mucous membranes.
- Poultice can soothe eczema, acne, and wounds.

INFUSION: Steep 1 tsp. of dried herb in 1 cup of boiling water. Infuse 5 to 10 minutes. Drink 3 times a day.

TINCTURE: Dried herb, 1:5 in 50% alcohol, 6–12 drops, 3 times a day.

EYEWASH: Allow infusion to cool, then strain. Use a sterile eyecup to rinse eyes. Use within 24 hours. Alternatively, pour 2 tbsp. freshly boiled water over 10 drops of tincture. Cool just to lukewarm, fill a sterilized eyecup about a third full and rinse eye in solution. Discard unused liquid.

COMPRESS: Mix 1 tsp. dried herb in 2 cups of water, boil 10 minutes, let cool until lukewarm. Moisten a sterile cloth in liquid, wring slightly, and place over eyes for 15 minutes.

CAUTION: Do not use if you have had eye surgery or wear contact lenses. Test for allergies before using on the eyes. It is preferable to use eye washes under the guidance of a professional to prevent infection.

FALSE SOLOMON'S SEAL

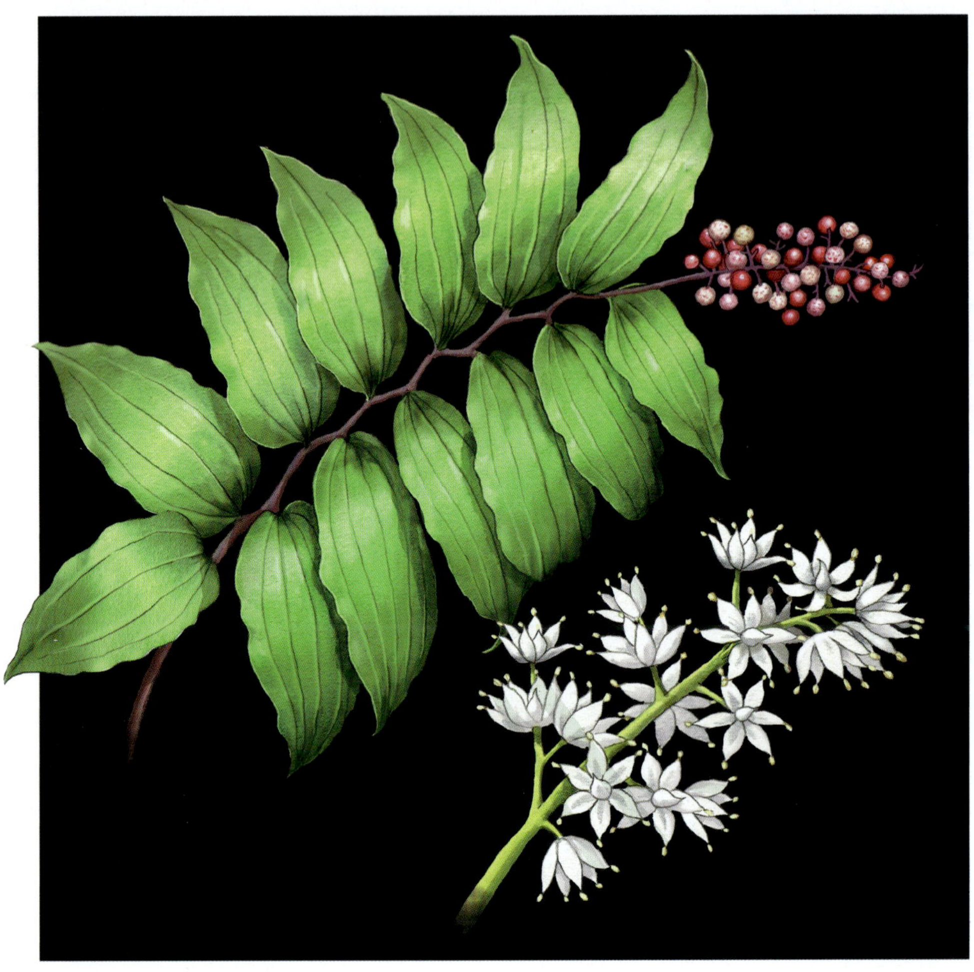

Maianthemum racemosum
***Maianthemum racemosum, ssp.amplexicaule* (Western)**

FAMILY: Asparagaceae

OTHER NAMES: Solomon's Plume, False Spikenard, *Fr.* Smilacine à grappes

PARTS USED: Root, leaves

CHARACTERISTICS: Moistening, bitter, astringent

ACTIONS: Anti-inflammatory, analgesic, astringent, demulcent, blood purifier, tonic, cathartic

RANGE: Native across all provinces and the Northwest Territories

This native perennial has been used by Indigenous Peoples for centuries, but it is rarely used in modern herbal medicine. It typically grows in partial shade and in moist, soft soil such as woodlands, shaded ravines, and streamsides. Named for its resemblance to Solomon's Seal, it usually has 7 to 12 alternate leaves growing in a similar zigzag formation; however, the flowers are very different, growing in a plume at the end of the stalk rather than the characteristic bell-shaped flowers that hang from the underside of the stem of Solomon's Seal. False Solomon's Seal also produces a cluster of berries that are mottled beige or green at first, turning to deep red in the fall, and although bitter raw, may be cooked and eaten in jams or jellies. They should not be confused with Solomon's Seal berries, which usually are found in pairs, and are dark blue or black and poisonous. The western subspecies *amplexicaule* is very similar to the eastern variety except for a more erect stem and leaves that clasp the stem. Harvest the root in the fall when foliage has died back, leaving a 7.5 cm piece with sprout in the soil for future germination.

MEDICINAL USES:

Arthritis, sore joints and ligaments, coughs, sore throat

- Decoction of root used by Indigenous Peoples to ease pain of arthritis, inflamed joints, torn ligaments, injuries, kidney issues, and back pain. It restores flexibility, lubricates and moistens connective tissue.
- Fresh root may be chewed for coughs, colds, and sore throats.
- Poultice of fresh crushed leaves or dried powdered root can be applied to wounds, bruises, and hemorrhoids to stop bleeding and ease pain.
- Tea or tincture from roots used to help some menstrual disorders and regulate the cycle.
- Eases headache pain.

OTHER USES:
- Berries can be eaten in small amounts or made into jams.
- Young shoots can be picked in spring and cooked like asparagus.

DECOCTION: Standard, take 2-6 tbsp. 3 times a day.

TINCTURE: Fresh root 1:2, in 50% alcohol. Take 10–30 drops 4 times a day.

CAUTION: Berries are laxative and emetic if eaten in large amounts. Avoid if pregnant. May cause contact dermatitis in some people.

FALSE UNICORN

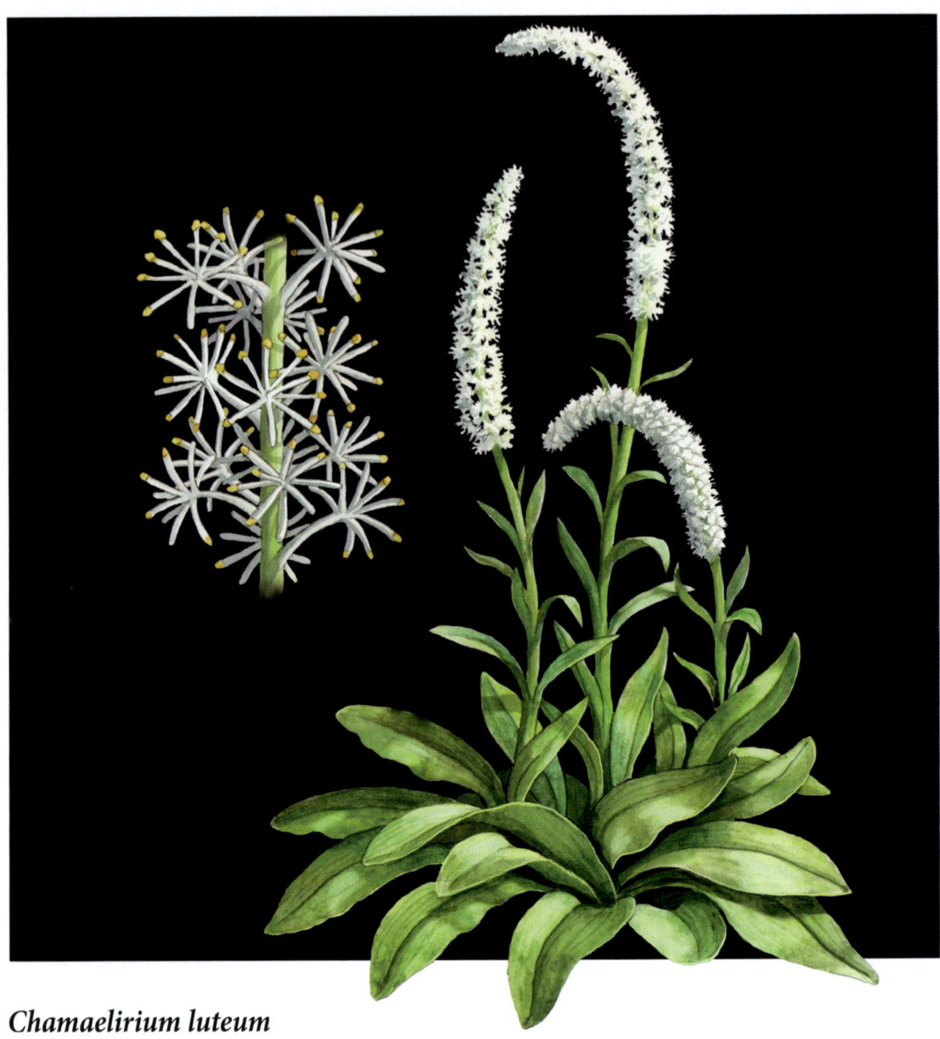

Chamaelirium luteum

FAMILY: Melanthiaceae

OTHER NAMES: Blazing Star, Fairy Wand, Starwort, Devil's Bit, *Fr.* Chamaelire doré

PARTS USED: Root and rhizomes

CHARACTERISTICS: Astringent, bitter, cooling

ACTIONS: Adaptogen, diuretic, digestive, emetic, uterine tonic

RANGE: Native to Ontario

False Unicorn root is a medicine that has been used traditionally for centuries by Indigenous Peoples in North America as a tonic for reproductive problems. It was adopted by Europeans, and eventually led to exporting and overharvesting. Now considered an endangered species, there are very few left in the wild and harvesting is strongly discouraged. It is a slow-growing perennial with a bulbous root that takes 4–6 years growth before it can be used as medicine. Its stems grow to a height of up to 1 m., with leaves that are lance-shaped and small, with those growing from the root longer and wider. Flowers are tiny and greenish-white on long plume-like racemes, often drooping. Male and female grow as separate plants, the male inflorescences usually shorter and withering after flowering. Both are needed to produce seeds. Do not use unless it has been cultivated or grown in your own garden, as the plant is endangered. Alternative herbs with similar medicinal properties include Motherwort (*Leonurus cardiac*), Raspberry leaf (*Rubus idaeus*), Chaste Berry (*Vitex agnus-castus*), Dang Gui (*Angelica sinensis*), and Lady's Mantle (*Alchemical vulgaris*).

MEDICINAL USES:

Prolapsed uterus, infertility, leukorrhea, dysmenorrhea, menorrhagia

- Nourishes and strengthens the endothelium and uterine lining, increases circulation to the pelvic area, supports the mucous membranes, reducing dryness in the cervix. One of the best tonics for the ovaries and uterus, it helps in prolapse, increases fertility, and is often used to prevent miscarriage.
- Strengthens and tones reproductive tissues in both males and females, particularly where there is stagnation, pelvic congestion or pain before periods, leukorrhea, dysmenorrhea, amenorrhea, hemorrhoids, varicose veins in the legs, or urinary or digestive weakness.
- May prevent miscarriage and ease nausea during pregnancy. However, it should only be used during pregnancy under supervision of an experienced herbal practitioner.

DECOCTION: ½ tsp. dried root simmered in 1 cup water for 15 minutes. Strain and take twice a day.

TINCTURE: 1:5 in 45% alcohol, 2–5 ml. 3 times a day diluted in water.

CAUTION: Use only under supervision of a healthcare professional if using while pregnant. Avoid if breastfeeding. May cause nausea in large doses. Do not use if taking lithium.

FERNLEAF BISCUITROOT

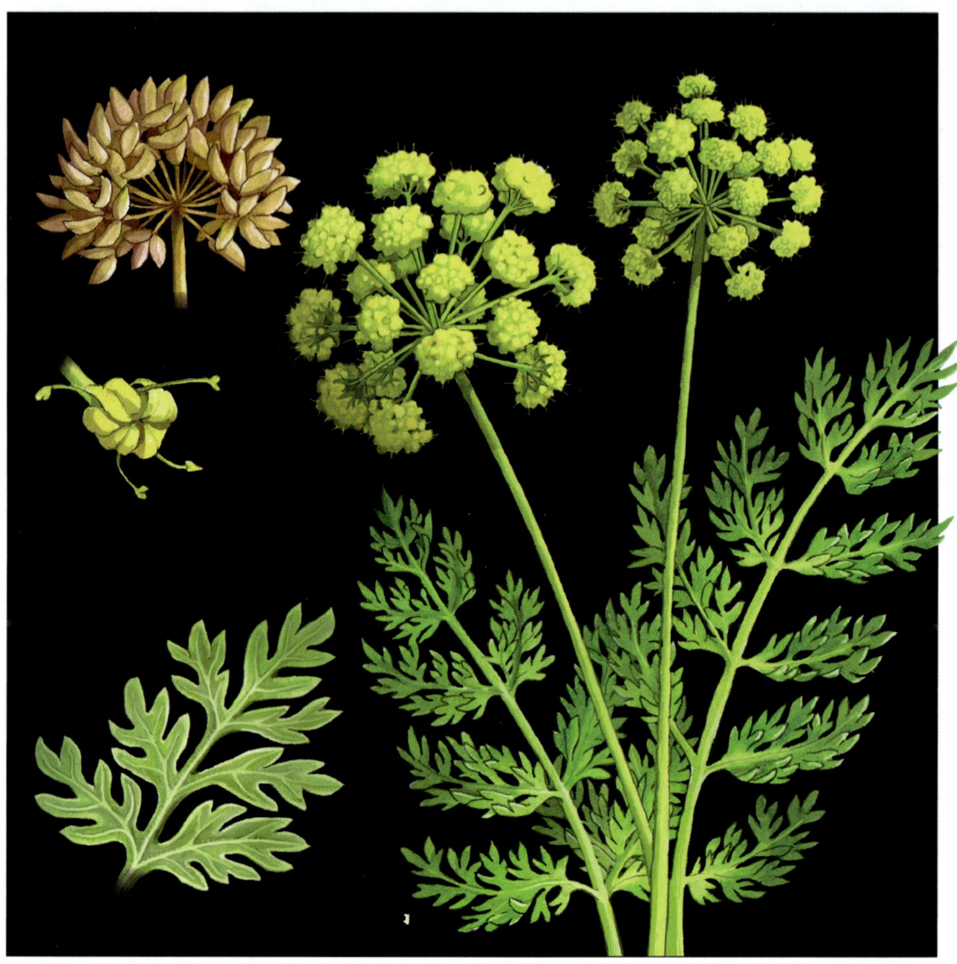

Lomatium dissectum

FAMILY: Apiaceae

OTHER NAMES: Desert Parsley, Lomatium, Indian Parsley, Toza, *Fr.* Lomatium à feuilles découpées

PARTS USED: Root, seed

CHARACTERISTICS: Pungent, bitter, warm, drying, resinous

ACTIONS: Antibacterial, antiviral, antifungal, stimulating expectorant, immune stimulant

RANGE: Native to British Columbia, southern Alberta, Saskatchewan (rare)

Lomatium has been highly regarded by Indigenous Peoples of the Pacific Northwest for centuries, both as food and as a potent medicine. During the pandemic of 1918–1920, an American doctor working with the Washoe people of Nevada noticed a dramatically decreased rate of infection among those who were using this herb. A native perennial of the carrot family with a long woody taproot, it is still found along the dry, rocky slopes and meadows of western Canada, although its numbers have dwindled. Its fragrant yellow or purple flowers bloom from April to May and grow in umbels of 10–30 rays atop a hollow stalk that can reach up to 1.8 m. tall. The leaves are mostly basal and divided, with fine hairs along the veins of the underside. For a time it was little used in modern herbalism; however, with the recent resurgence of new deadly viruses, interest in *Lomatium* has increased, some herbalists claiming it is probably our strongest and most effective antiviral herb, particularly with respiratory tract infections. The root should be at least 3 years old to be medicinally effective. Dig up in late spring or fall, slice longitudinally and hang to dry. Only take what you need, as it is becoming endangered.

MEDICINAL USES:

Respiratory tract infections, colds, flu, stomach disorders, fungal infections, sores, arthritis

- Tincture or decoction used as a powerful remedy for flus or colds, high fevers, coughs, bronchitis, pneumonia, and asthma, where the respiratory tract is involved. Dramatically reduces viral count, proven effective against many types of bacteria, mold, and fungi.
- Anecdotal evidence among herbalists has shown success in eliminating some cases of rotavirus, shingles, Epstein–Barr, cytomegalovirus, chronic fatigue, HIV, hepatitis C, candidiasis, urinary tract infection, and H1N1, although few clinical trials have been done to date.
- Decoctions of the root have been used internally to treat stomach disorders, and as a dietary tonic to help gain weight or build immunity.
- Decoctions used externally as a poultice for arthritis, sores, boils, bruises, wounds, or as a rinse for mouth or gum infections. Effective against periodontal disease. A few drops of tincture placed on a Band-Aid and kept on for 4 or 5 days may get rid of warts.

OTHER USES: Young shoots can be cooked as greens, and the root can be boiled and eaten, or dried and ground to a powder and added to flours or soups.

FOLKLORE: Some American Indigenous men used to carry the seed as a love charm.

TINCTURE: Use 3 parts Everclear alcohol to 1 part distilled water. Chop dried root finely and fill a mason jar about ¼ full (fresh root ½ full), cover with alcohol mixture to the top and cap. Shake vigorously and store in a dark place for at least 2 weeks. Strain and bottle. Start with 5–10 drops diluted in water, once a day for a week, and increase if well tolerated, up to 30 drops 4 times a day.

CAUTION: May cause itchy rashes in a small percentage of patients taking it for the first time. To reduce likelihood of rash, take Dandelion root, and discontinue use if rash becomes severe. Safety during pregnancy unknown so not recommended.

FEVERFEW

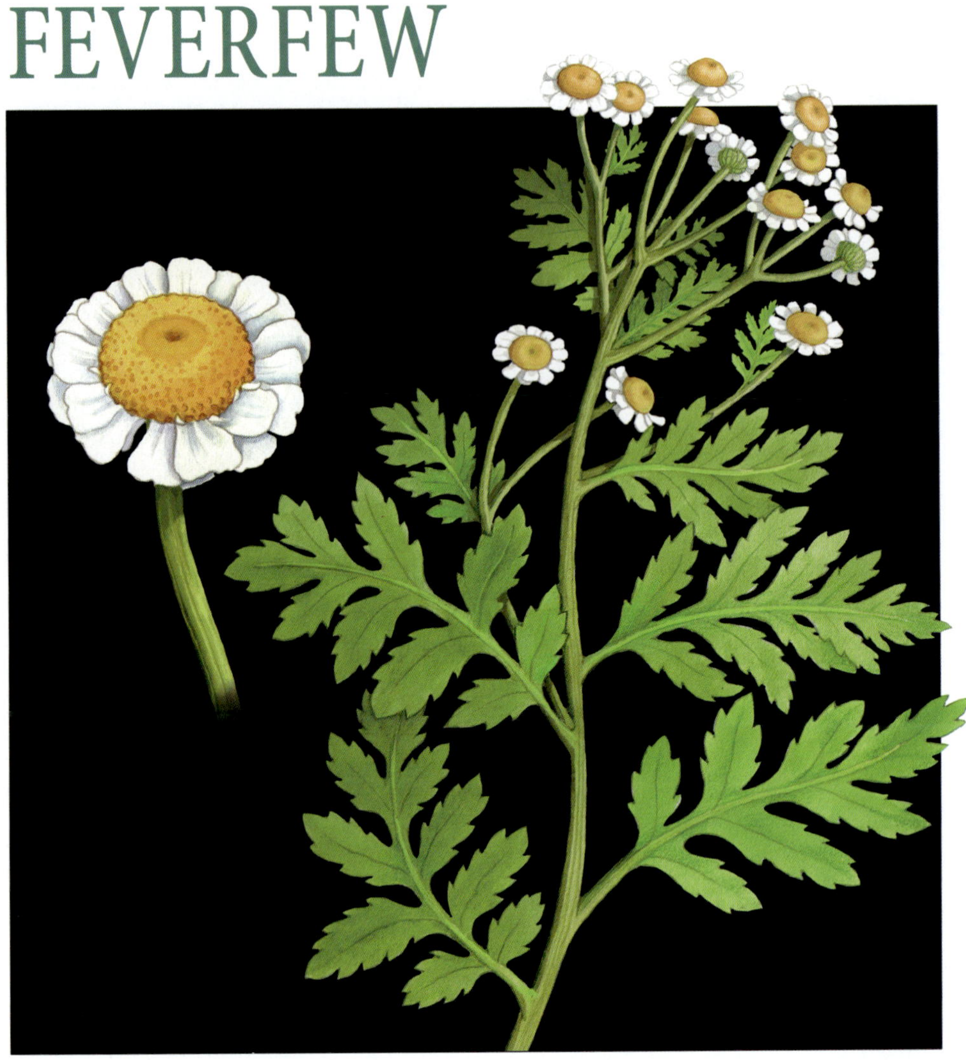

Tanacetum (Chrysanthemum) parthenium

FAMILY: Asteraceae

OTHER NAMES: Featherfew, Featherfoil, Flintwort, Bachelor's Buttons, *Fr.* Grande camomile, Pyrèthre doré

PARTS USED: Aerial

CHARACTERISTICS: Aromatic, bitter, astringent, cooling

ACTIONS: Febrifuge, anti-inflammatory, emmenagogue, tonic, analgesic, aperient, carminative, vermifuge, antimicrobial, antipyretic, antirheumatic, diaphoretic, diuretic, nervine, stomachic, vasodilator

RANGE: Introduced across all provinces except Alberta and Saskatchewan

This erect perennial or biennial European native, now common throughout North America, grows mostly in gardens, occasionally escaping into the wild or remaining around old homesteads. Its branched, leafy stem is furrowed, about 60 cm. high, with alternate pinnate leaves, its leaflets gashed and toothed. The compound flower resembles a small Daisy, its centre convex and bright yellow, petals often doubled. It flowers throughout the summer and is aromatic, but bees dislike it and will keep their distance. Gather in early summer and dry for later use.

MEDICINAL USES:

Migraines, fevers, irregular menstruation, stomach upset, arthritis

- Once known for its fever-reducing properties and usefulness for the common cold, but there are more effective herbs. Its main use now is in preventing and treating migraines and has been proven effective in several scientific studies. Its analgesic and anti-inflammatory properties make it a useful pain reliever for headaches, arthritis, and rheumatism.
- Bitter compounds stimulate digestion, increase appetite and help relieve colic, nausea, indigestion, and colitis.
- May help reduce skin inflammation and relieve dermatitis and psoriasis.
- Uterine stimulant, promotes menstruation, eases irregularities and cramps. Tones the womb after childbirth.
- There is some promising research into using Feverfew and St. John's Wort for diabetic peripheral neuropathy.
- Anti-inflammatory action may relieve the pain of arthritis and rheumatism.
- Some claim it will relieve tinnitus and Meniere's disease.

FOLKLORE: Planted around one's dwelling was said to purify the air and prevent disease. Often used to ward off insects.

TINCTURE: Fresh herb 1:2, dried herb 1:5, in 60% alcohol, take 1–4 ml. in water, twice a day.

INFUSION: Fresh herb 1 tsp. per day; dried herb: ½ tsp. per day. (Works on a deeper level when used in small amounts over a longer period of time, so be patient if you don't see immediate results.)

COMBINATIONS: With Ginko Biloba and Black Cohosh for tinnitis or dizziness. With Ginger, Garlic, Prickly Ash, or Cayenne to improve circulation. With Peppermint and Elder flower for fevers. Add Lemon Balm or Skullcap for headaches, stress, and tension.

RESEARCH: Studies on rats investigated the use of Feverfew and St. John's Wort for the management of pain associated with diabetic peripheral neuropathy, a common problem in diabetics. An extract of the aerial parts of St. John's Wort, which contains hyperforin and hypericin, combined with an extract from the Feverfew flower, which contains parthenolide, relieved neuropathic pain, whereas separately they were ineffective. There were no apparent side effects. In another study, patients who took capsules of Feverfew every day had fewer migraines after 12 weeks and they were less intense, with less nausea and vomiting. Acts as a vasodilator, which opens the blood vessels and improves circulation.

CAUTION: Not recommended if pregnant or nursing. Fresh herb may cause mouth ulcerations in some people, avoid if allergic to plants in the Daisy family. If taking for more than a week and wish to stop, reduce gradually, as stopping all at once may cause headaches, anxiety, muscle stiffness, and joint pain. May increase the risk of bleeding. Avoid if you are on blood thinners. Ask your doctor before taking if you are on any medications. Do not give to children under two years of age.

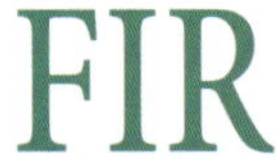

FIR

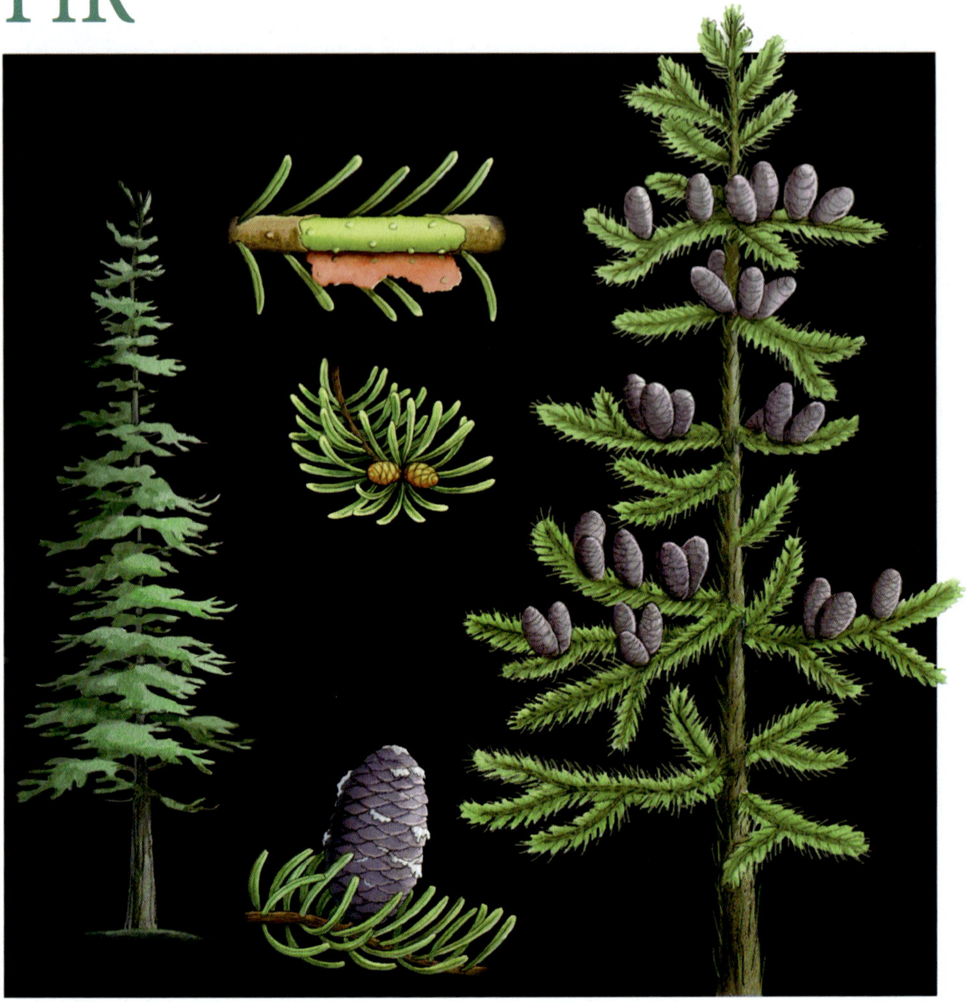

Abies lasiocarpa (Subalpine Fir)
Abies balsamea (Balsam Fir)

FAMILY: Pinaceae

OTHER NAMES: *A. lasiocarpa:* Mountain Balsam Fir, Alpine Fir, White Fir, Rocky Mountain Fir, *Fr.* Sapin de montagne, Sapin concolore; *A. balsamea*: *Fr.* Sapin Baumier

PARTS USED: Resin, needles, bark

ACTIONS: Antioxidant, antiseptic, antifungal, diuretic, expectorant, diaphoretic, laxative, tonic, analgesic, stimulant, anti-inflammatory

RANGE: *A. lasiocarpa* native to British Columbia, southern Yukon, Alberta; *A. balsamea* native from Alberta to Newfoundland and Labrador

Known as the "Medicine Tree" by some Indigenous Peoples, the Subalpine Fir has been a traditional medicine for lung ailments for centuries. This native evergreen is the smallest of the true firs, growing up to 50 m. in height, but usually smaller, and shrub-like close to the timberline. Mostly found above 600 m., it prefers the higher elevations but can occasionally be found along the coastline, its short, rigid branches making it look more slender and spire-like than other conifers. The needles are about 2.5 cm. long, soft, flat, and blunt or sometimes notched at the tip, usually curving upwards. The dark purple cones stand upward on the branch and often have globs of pitch stuck to them, which tend to drip when the weather gets warm. The grey, smooth bark on young trees has resin blisters, but as the trees get older the bark becomes cracked and fissured, with reddish scales. Balsam Fir needles tend to lie flatter than the Subalpine Fir, but is otherwise very similar. Bark and needles can be harvested at any time, but the vitamin C content is higher in the winter.

MEDICINAL USES:

Colds and flu, fever, lung ailments, insomnia, wounds, burns, muscle pain

- Antiseptic and analgesic, the resin from blisters on the bark may be applied to wounds, sores, and burns. Speeds healing.
- Decoction of bark and needles is high in vitamin C, works as a tonic for colds and flu, lung ailments, fevers, and trouble sleeping. Poultice of needles can be applied to the chest for coughs and chest colds and to induce sweating.
- Pitch can be chewed to clean the teeth, or made into an infusion for gargling for a sore throat or bad breath. May be emetic if taken internally.
- Essential oil can be diluted in a carrier oil and used as a massage oil to relieve muscle tension and pain, or a few drops added to the bath to reduce tension.

OTHER USES:

- Cones may be ground to a powder, mixed with fat, and eaten as a snack. Aids digestion.
- Inner bark can be dried, ground, and mixed with flour for bread-making.
- An infusion made from the needles can be used as a deodorant.
- Boughs often strewn onto floors of teepees or sweat lodges or burned as incense in ceremonies.
- Powdered needles mixed with bear grease to make a pleasant-smelling hair tonic, and to help dandruff.
- An aromatic massage oil can be made by infusing needles in olive oil for 4–6 weeks and then straining.

DECOCTION: Break up branches and put into a pot, cover with water, and bring to a boil, simmer for 20 minutes until the aroma fills the room. Breathe in steam. Once liquid has cooled slightly, strain into a container. Drink 2–3 cups a day. Add honey if desired.

CAUTION: Pitch can induce vomiting in strong doses. May cause skin reactions in some people. Use in moderation.

FIREWEED

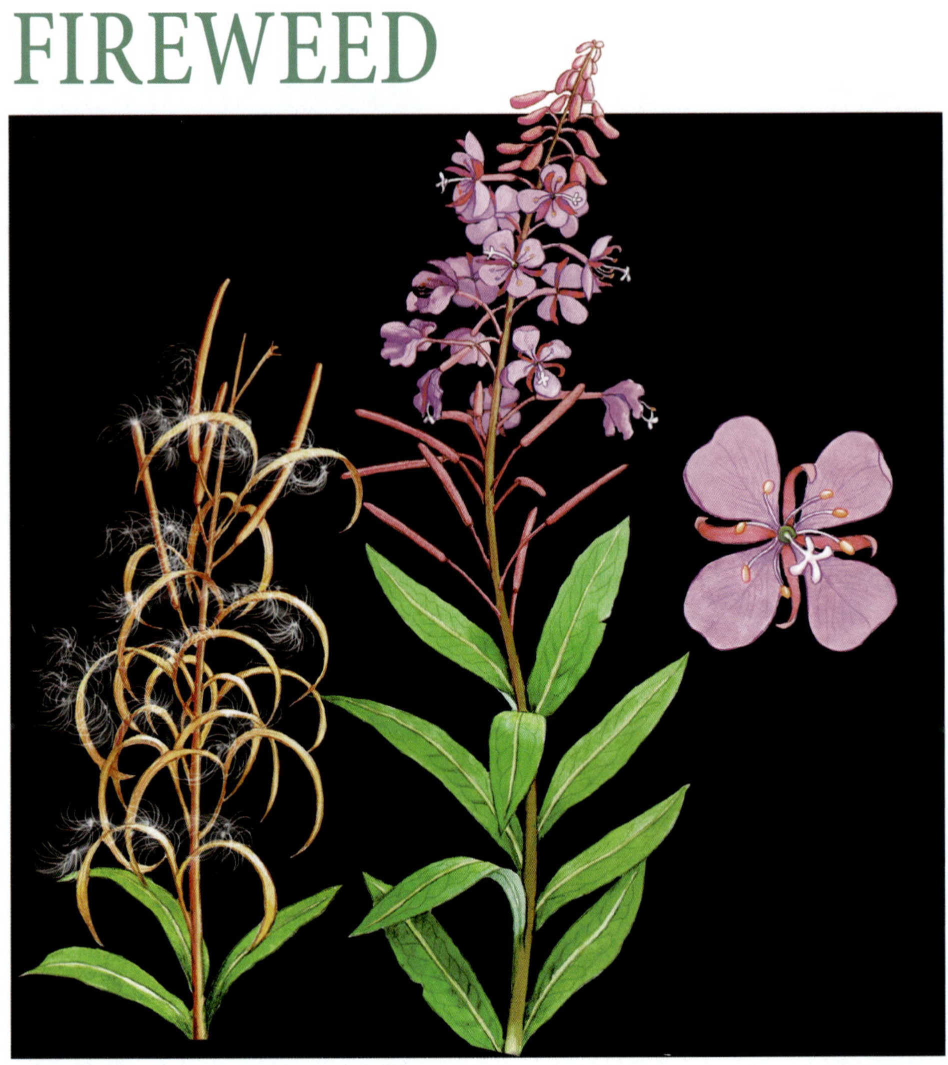

Chamaenerion (Epilobium) angustifolium

FAMILY: Onagraceae

OTHER NAMES: Willow Herb, Purple Firetop, Blooming Sally, *Fr.* Épilobe, Herbe-à-feu

PARTS USED: Roots, leaves, flowers

CHARACTERISTICS: Sweet, cool, drying

ACTIONS: Anti-spasmodic, antifungal, antioxidant, antibacterial, anthelmintic, antiseptic, astringent, anti-inflammatory, demulcent, emollient, laxative

RANGE: Native across Canada

This colourful flower is noted for being one of the first plants to appear after a fire; it thrives on burnt or disturbed land and can become invasive very quickly as it spreads both by self-seeding and rhizomes. Native to North America, it is a perennial herb growing up to 1.8 m. tall with magenta flowers that bloom from July through to September. They bloom low on the stem at first, then throughout the summer they work their way up to the top. In the fall the seedpods split open and the plant tops become white and feathery, the tufts of white hair distributing the seeds on the wind. The willow-like alternate leaves are dark green above and silvery underneath with a lighter central vein. The lateral veins are unique, as they don't extend to the outer edge but loop together near the margin. Young shoots may be picked in the spring and eaten fresh in salads. Leaves can be picked early in the summer and dried in a paper bag, then stored in a glass jar for later use. The root should be dug in the fall and may be used fresh, mashed as a poultice for inflammations.

MEDICINAL USES:

Asthma, coughs, irritable bowel, diarrhea, skin problems

- Whole plant is edible and is a gentle but effective anti-inflammatory. Rich in vitamins A and C, calcium, and iron. Tannins tighten tissues and dry out "dampness" or mucous production.
- Antispasmodic, demulcent, high in mucilage, soothes mucous membranes. A cool decoction of the whole plant used to treat sore throats, hiccups, lung congestion, whooping cough, asthma. Flowers can be infused and gargled to ease a sore throat or laryngitis.
- Leaf decoctions are anti-inflammatory and antispasmodic, good for the stomach and digestive tract; soothe ulcers, gastritis, colitis, diarrhea, irritable bowel, intestinal spasms. As a gargle they help with mouth sores and swollen or bleeding gums. Normalizes gut flora and mucilage calms an irritated digestive tract.
- Antifungal properties help with candida overgrowth.
- The root can be macerated and applied to boils, abscesses, or skin infections. Leaves and flowers are cooling and drying and can be used in poultices for psoriasis, eczema, hemorrhoids, acne, burns, and wounds.

OTHER USES:

- Young shoots and flowers are good in salads or as a potherb.
- Dried leaves make a nice tea.
- Yields a delicious honey.
- Cordage made from fibrous stems.
- Cottony seed hairs can be used as stuffing or tinder.

TINCTURE: Fresh herb, 1:2 in 50% alcohol, 10–60 drops, 1–3 times a day

INFUSION: 1–2 tsp. dried herb in 1 cup of boiling water. Drink as needed.

IVAN CHAI (FERMENTED) TEA: Collect stalks before or during flowering. Remove leaves and allow to wilt for about 12–18 hours on a sheet of cloth. Take 4 or 5 leaves at a time and roll together between the palms to bruise, then place loosely into a bowl and cover with a lid or plate, stirring often to aerate. When they become fragrant and dark in colour, stop the fermentation process (usually 3–5 days). Place in oven at lowest temperature setting until completely dry. Store in airtight container.

RESEARCH: Leaves and flowering tops show strong activity against *Staphylococcus aureus* and *Candida albicans*, and moderate activity against *E. coli* and *Pseudomonas aeruginosa*. Rhizomes contain fewer tannins and no mucilage, but do contain anti-inflammatory flavonoids, and have proven useful for urinary problems associated with prostatitis and benign prostatic hyperplasia. The tannin oenothein B, which has antiviral and anti-tumour properties, may also be useful in treating many hormone-sensitive cancers and conditions like polycystic ovaries, menorrhagia, chronic cystitis, and acute prostatitis. A biotech company in Saskatoon has produced a Fireweed extract that outperformed cortisone cream on irritated skin, reducing redness and soreness in much less time. The flavonol glucuronide is believed to be responsible.

CAUTION: Avoid if pregnant or breastfeeding. Do not exceed recommended dose. Avoid use 2 weeks before or after surgery.

FULLER'S TEASEL

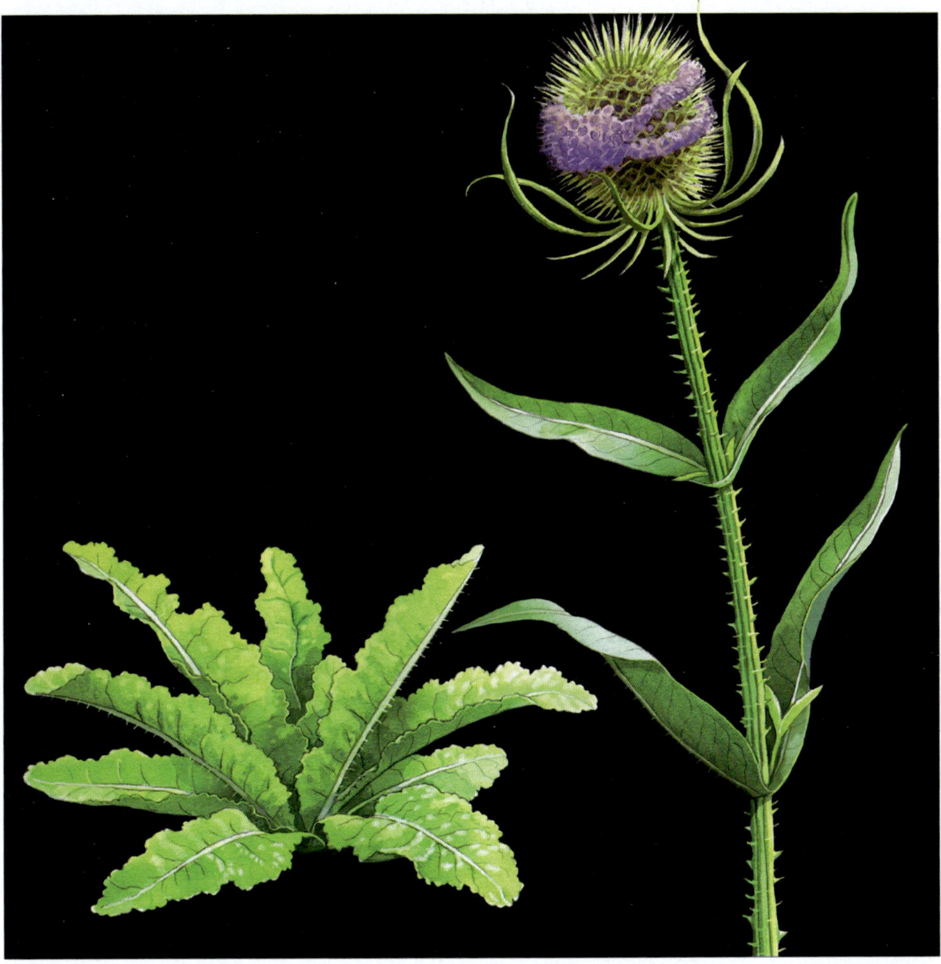

Dipsacus fullonum
Dipsacus sylvestris

FAMILY: Dipsacaceae

OTHER NAMES: Draper's Teasel, Venus Cup Teasel, Common or Wild Teasel, Barber's Brush, Card Thistle, Church Broom, *Fr.* Cardère des bois, Cardère sylvestre

PARTS USED: Root, leaves

CHARACTERISTICS: Warming

ACTIONS: Antimicrobial, anti-inflammatory, antibacterial, diaphoretic, diuretic, stomachic, kidney tonic, antioxidant, antipyretic, analgesic, antiviral

RANGE: Introduced in British Columbia, Alberta, Ontario, Quebec, Nova Scotia

Fuller's Teasel does not have a long history of use in Western herbal medicine, but it has recently gained popularity for its potential effectiveness in treating Lyme disease. A native of Europe/Eurasia introduced to North America, it usually grows in wet ditches, fields, and waste places throughout British Columbia and Central and Eastern Canada. Sometimes reaching up to 1.8 m. tall, it is easily recognized by its spiky oval flowerhead with rings of mauve-coloured blooms and long spiny bracts. A biennial plant, its first year of growth consists of a rosette of prickly basal leaves and a taproot that can extend 60 cm. or more into the ground. In the second year, a prickly stem emerges, with erect branches terminated by the flowerhead. Lance-shaped opposite leaves may measure up to 30 cm. long and have toothed or wavy edges and spines along the central vein. Flowerhead turns brown in the fall but stem remains stiff throughout the winter and is often used in dried flower arrangements. Roots are best harvested before the flower stem emerges in the second year, between fall and spring, and tinctured fresh.

MEDICINAL USES:

Lyme disease, nerve pain, stiff joints and muscles, brittle bones, fever

- Shown to be effective in treating Lyme disease. After treatments with antibiotics, sometimes symptoms remain, as the bacteria will often hide in the body's tissues and continue reinfecting the patient for months or years after treatment. Teasel coaxes them out into the bloodstream, where the immune system can tackle them more effectively.
- Diuretic and diaphoretic action helps rid the body of toxins and reduces intermittent fevers.
- Tonifies the liver and kidneys, improves circulation, and treats jaundice.
- Soothes nerve pain and helps chronic inflammation. Strengthens connective tissue, eases pain in the joints and back, reduces arthritic pain and stiffness. May ease some of the symptoms of multiple sclerosis and chronic fatigue. Helps build bone mass and restores porous bones.
- Infusion strengthens the stomach, improves the appetite.
- Infusion of the leaves applied externally can help acne.
- Ointment made from the roots has been used to remove warts.

OTHER USES:

- Blue dye obtained from the dried plant.
- Early wool manufacturers attached the dried seed heads to a spindle to comb, or tease, the wool to raise the nap.

TINCTURE: Fresh leaves and roots, 1:2 in 50% alcohol. Start with 1–3 drops 3 times a day, add one more drop daily until symptoms decrease.

DECOCTION: ½ tsp. dried leaves and roots in 1 cup water, drink up to twice daily.

RESEARCH: Trials conducted in 2022 concluded that ethanolic extract from leaves of *D. fullonum* showed great potential against *Borrelia burgdorferi*, or Lyme disease, a tick-borne bacterial disease that can develop very serious symptoms if not met with immediate and aggressive treatments. Although in its acute stage it is treated with antibiotics, it can develop into relapsing chronic form that is resistant to antibiotics. An iridoid-glycoside fraction of *D. fullonum* leaf extract showed remarkable anti-Borrelia effect and reduced cytotoxicity. Studies have also established the antioxidant and antimicrobial activity and in vivo effectiveness of Teasel leaf extracts against several cancer strains.

CAUTION: Rash may develop with use; reduce dosage if this occurs. May react with anti-inflammatory drugs and antidepressants. Avoid if pregnant or breastfeeding due to lack of research.

GENTIAN

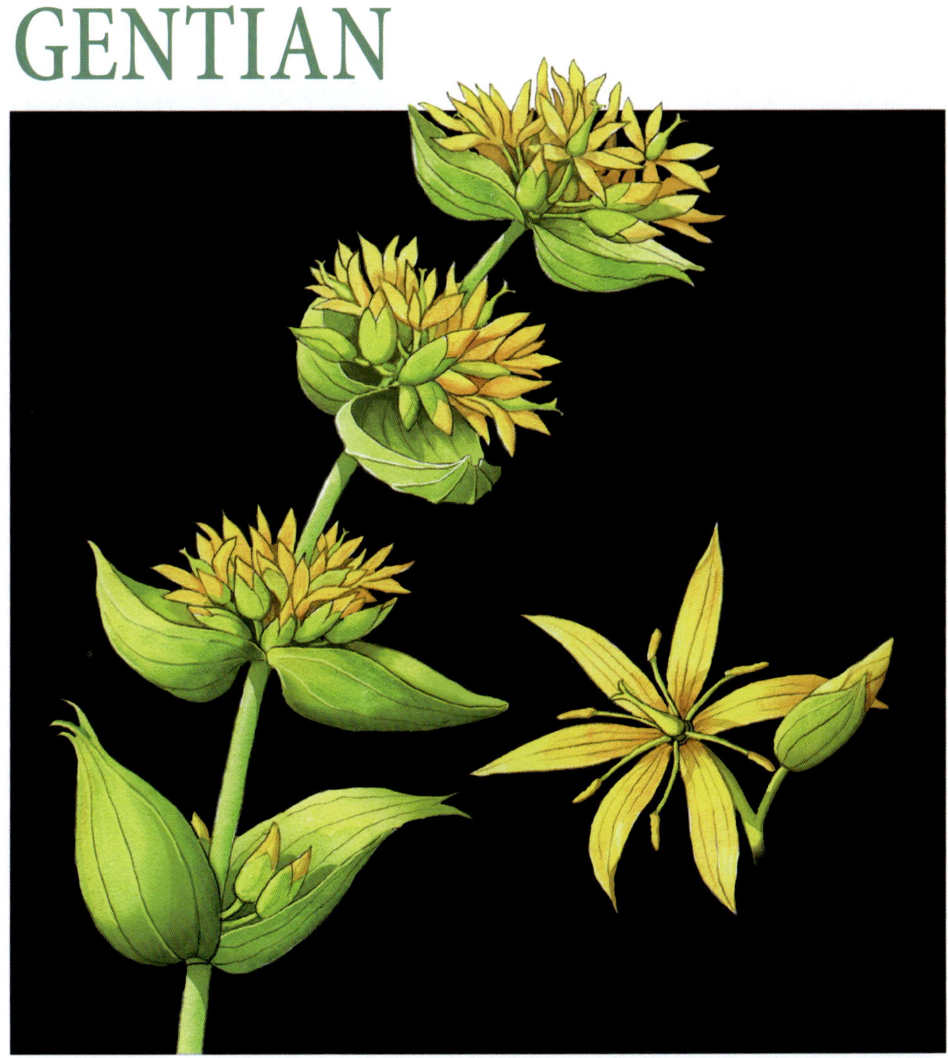

Gentiana lutea

FAMILY: Gentianaceae

OTHER NAMES: Bitterroot, Gall Weed, Yellow Gentian, *Fr.* Gentiane jaune

PARTS USED: Root, rhizomes

CHARACTERISTICS: Bitter, cool, sweet, aromatic

ACTIONS: Anthelmintic, anti-inflammatory, antiseptic, cholagogue, tonic, gastric stimulant, stomachic, digestive tonic, antioxidant, antimicrobial

RANGE: *G. lutea* introduced in Alberta

Gentian, one of the strongest bitter herb tonics available, is well-known in herbal medicine for treating digestive problems. A native of Europe, Africa, and Asia, many of its species were used by the ancient Egyptians, Romans, and Greeks for centuries. Across Canada, Yellow Gentian is often cultivated but has only been found growing wild in a few locations in Alberta. It is most often in alpine meadows, moist grasslands, and pastures, and can reach a height of about a metre. Its large oval or lance-shaped basal leaves have deep ribbed veins, and the flower stalk emerges in summer with whorled clusters of star-shaped blooms growing from the axils of the upper leaves. The large taproot can be at least 30 cm. long and is often 5 cm. thick. Harvest in the fall after several years of growth but preferably before flowering, which takes about three years. Dry for later use.

MEDICINAL USES:

Digestive problems, constipation, worms, liver congestion and jaundice, upper respiratory tract infections, food allergies and cravings, loss of appetite, exhaustion

- The root of Yellow Gentian is so bitter it can be detected even in a dilution of 1:12,000, however, this allows it to tone the digestive system better than any other herb, stimulating saliva in the mouth, gastric acid in the stomach, and bile in the digestive tract, making for a more efficient digestive process. Normally used in small doses where there is debilitation, recovery from long-term illness, and loss of appetite. By improving the digestive process, this may also improve mental clarity, mood, and focus.
- Treats stomachaches, heartburn, flatulence, anemia, anorexia, food intolerances, slow and sluggish digestion, nausea, and constipation. It works particularly well for children who are not thriving, and for people with a weakened or stressed digestive system.
- Anti-inflammatory action makes it useful in healing wounds and other inflamed tissues and reducing pain, and its antibacterial properties speed healing. May be applied topically as a poultice or cream for eczema, sores, and swellings.
- A study using a German supplement containing Gentian was found to improve sinusitis after 8 days, reducing inflammation and bacterial count, however more research is needed.
- Several species of Gentian were once used by Indigenous Peoples as a vermifuge, to treat snakebites, and as an antidote for witchcraft.

TINCTURE: Dried root 1:5 in 50% alcohol. Take 3–12 drops 3–5 minutes before meals; start with 3 drops and add more if well tolerated. It is recommended to take 2 parts Gentian with 1 part Ginger tincture to add warmth and prevent nausea.

DECOCTION: ⅛–½ tsp. dried root in 1 cup water, simmer for 10 minutes. Strain and sip before meals. Add Ginger, Cinnamon, Orange peel, Cardamon seed, or honey to improve taste.

COMBINATIONS: May be used with Dandelion root, Barberry, Burdock root, Celandine, or Yellow Dock root.

CAUTION: Avoid during pregnancy and breastfeeding. Do not exceed recommended doses or use over long periods of time, particularly if you have ulcers or heartburn as it may exacerbate the problem. May cause nausea in large doses. Use only dried root.

GHOST PIPE

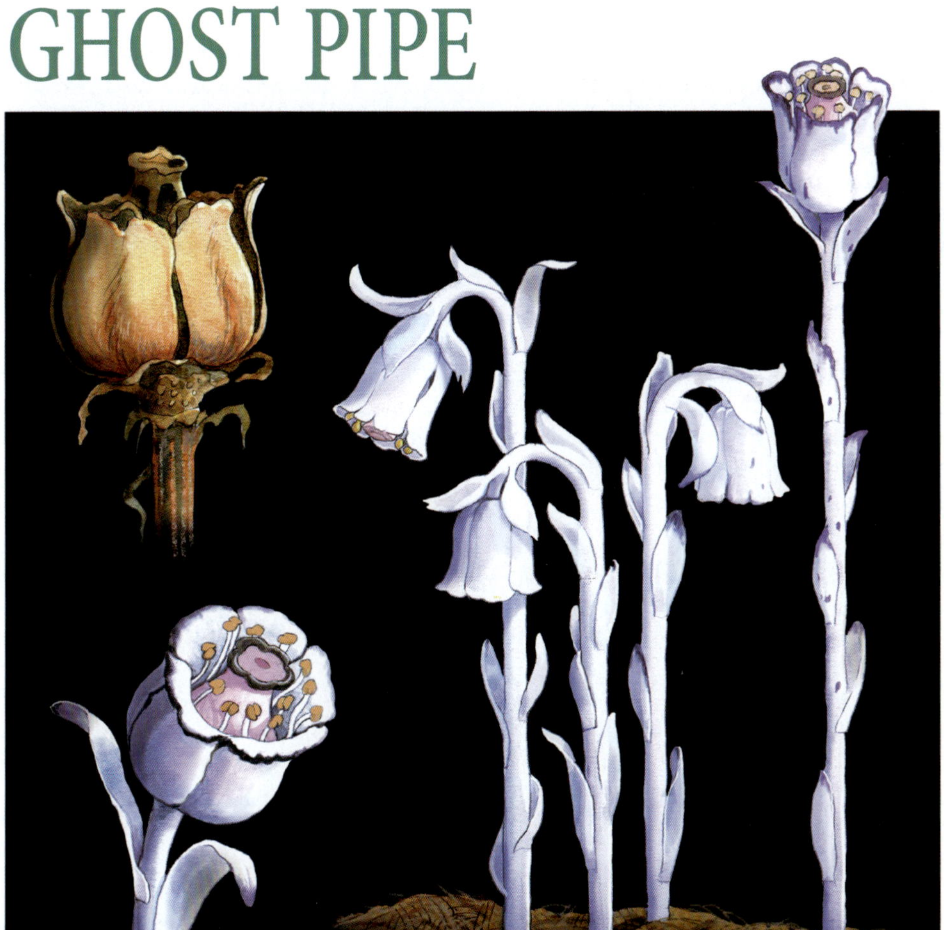

Monotropa uniflora

FAMILY: Ericaceae

OTHER NAMES: Indian Pipe, Corpse Plant, Ghostflower, Fairy Smoke, *Fr.* Monotrope uniflore, Pipe Indienne, Plante fantôme

PARTS USED: Aerial

CHARACTERISTICS: Relaxing, cooling, acrid, slightly sweet

ACTIONS: Antispasmodic, antibacterial, hypnotic, nervine, sedative, tonic, diaphoretic, anodyne

RANGE: Native across all provinces and Northwest Territories

This strange, ghostly perennial is typically found growing in clumps under trees in moist, shaded forests across North America. Reaching a height of 10–30 cm., its unique white colour is due to its lack of chlorophyll. It depends instead on a parasitic relationship with the mycelial networks or fungi below the surface for its nutrients. These fungi, which grow amongst the fine roots and rhizomes of the neighbouring trees, pull water and minerals from the soil, which are then taken in by the tree, pulling them up the trunk to nourish the leaves so photosynthesis can occur. The sugars created then flow back down the trunk to the roots, where they are absorbed by the mycelium, creating a symbiotic network where each communicates and feeds off the other. Ghost Pipes tap into the nodes connecting the tree roots to the fungus, drawing nutrients from both. The mass of roots sends up several white, waxy stalks with scale-like leaves that turn black when touched, and terminates in a solitary flower, which curves downward. As they mature, the flower turns up, the plant turns black or brown, and its seedpod dries out, releasing tiny seeds over the forest floor. Pick only the aerial parts, as the roots will produce more plants if not disturbed, and only take a small percentage, as these plants are becoming rare.

MEDICINAL USES:

Seizures, anxiety, panic attacks, spasms, toothache, eye inflammation, chronic pain

- Long history of use by Indigenous Peoples; an infusion can be used as a remedy for convulsions, panic attacks, anxiety, fainting, or any condition where there is emotional or sensory overload. Relieves spasms and calms the nervous system.
- The tincture has a mild analgesic action on pain, but it's more useful at helping deal with chronic or acute pain by reducing sensitivity to it without being completely overwhelming. It eases emotional pain by helping people detach from it so they can deal with it more effectively. Can bring people down from a bad drug-induced experience, helping them feel more grounded.
- Infusion can be used for colds and to bring down a fever.
- Crushed plant can be rubbed on bunions or warts, poultice used on sores that are taking a long time to heal.
- Flowers chewed for toothaches.
- Juice of the plant mixed with rosewater can be ingested to soothe bladder inflammation and ulcers. It can also be applied to the eyes with a sterile cloth to ease conjunctivitis, pinkeye, or inflammation.

TINCTURE: Fresh herb 1:2 in 50% alcohol. Tincture turns purple. Start with 3 drops, increase to 1 ml. in cases of severe panic or anxiety.

CAUTION: Contains glycosides, and may be poisonous if eaten in large doses. May cause vivid dreams. May lower blood pressure and heart rate. Do not use if pregnant or breastfeeding.

GOLDENROD

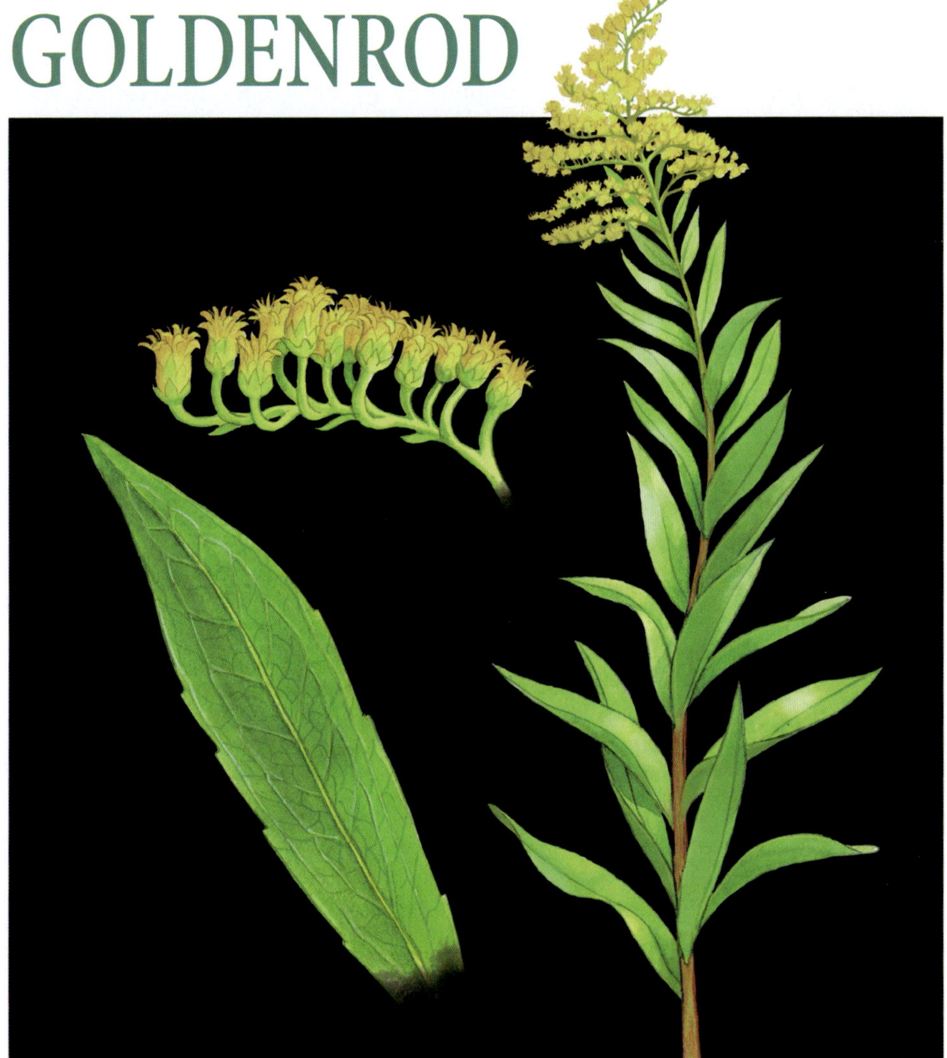

Solidago canadensis

FAMILY: Asteraceae

OTHER NAMES: Canada Goldenrod, *Fr.* Verge d'or, Solidage

PARTS USED: Aerial

CHARACTERISTICS: Slightly bitter, astringent, sweet, slightly aromatic, dry

ACTIONS: Anticatarrhal, anti-inflammatory, antifungal, antiseptic, diaphoretic, carminative, diuretic, astringent, vulnerary, expectorant, antispasmodic, antilithic, antimicrobial, antioxidant

RANGE: Native from Saskatchewan to the Maritimes

Goldenrod's botanical name *Solidago*, meaning "to make whole," refers to its ability to restore the body to health and wholeness. There are over a hundred different species across North America, *S. canadensis* being one of the native ones, used for centuries by Indigenous Peoples as a wound herb. Goldenrod grows in many different habitats, depending on the species; some prefer dry fields, others wetlands or marshes. It is a perennial with erect, often downy stems, branching at the top. The leaves are alternate, elliptical, toothed and stalked, the upper ones smaller. There are clusters of small, yellow flowers; the European variety, *S. virgaurea*, has blooms all around the stem, the Canadian variety on only one side. Harvest top third of the plant when there are buds and open flowers, but avoid plants that have wilted flowers. Pick only the top third of the plant, then hang to dry in the shade.

MEDICINAL USES:

Urinary tract infections and stones, upper respiratory problems, sore throat, skin inflammations, stomach upset, candida

- Contains tannins, flavonoids, and volatile oils, which work together to tighten, dry, and reduce permeability and inflammation in tissues, disperse stuck mucus, and promote healing. Particularly useful when there is heat and dampness and lack of tone in the respiratory or urinary tracts.
- Useful in the treatment of urinary tract infections, where there is burning pain, urgent and frequent urination, mucus, and incontinence. Diuretic action, when taken with lots of fluids, helps reduce inflammation, and may help expel stones.
- Effective for flu, colds, and upper respiratory infections in hot infusion, it reduces fevers, expels mucus where it is thin and copious, decongests, and soothes coughs. Also useful in treating chronic bronchitis and asthma.
- Anti-inflammatory action useful for arthritic pain, aching joints, and rheumatism. Take with plenty of water.
- A good source of rutin, a powerful flavonoid that increases the strength of capillaries and improves the tone of the cardiovascular system.
- Infusion may be used as a gargle for sore throats or laryngitis.
- Used for centuries as a wound herb, it is effective in poultices, ointments, and baths for treating slow-healing wounds, burns, eczema, and varicose veins.
- Soothes upset stomach, flatulence, colic.
- Tincture may be used to desensitize from seasonal allergies like Ragweed.
- Prevents and treats urogenital disorders like yeast infections, infusion may be drunk as a tea or used as a douche.

OTHER USES: Flowers produce a strong yellow dye.

INFUSION: 1 tbsp. fresh or 2 tsp. dried herb, infused in 1 cup boiling water for 10 to 15 minutes. Mint or honey may also be added. Drink 3 times a day. May increase urination or coughing/sneezing when you first start using it. If using long-term for allergies or urinary irritation, watch for dryness in people who have a tendency toward a dry constitution.

COMBINATIONS: With Bearberry, Elder flower, Yarrow, Usnea, or Marshmallow for urinary tract infections. With Elder flower, Echinacea, Thyme or Mullein for cold or upper respiratory tract infections. With Ash or Poplar bark for arthritis and rheumatism.

CAUTION: Avoid if you have kidney disease or are taking heart medications, due to its diuretic effect.

GOLDENSEAL

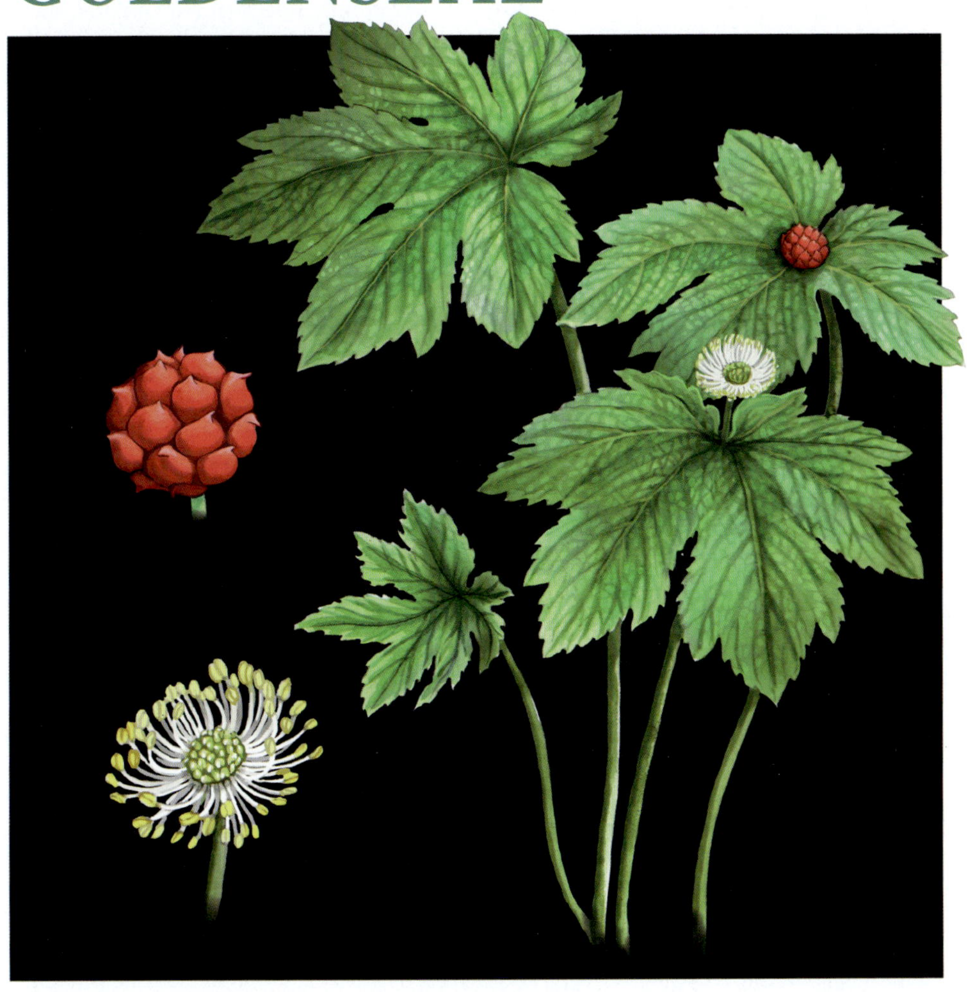

Hydrastis canadensis

FAMILY: Ranunculaceae

OTHER NAMES: Ground Raspberry, Orange Root, Yellow Root, *Fr.* Sceau d'or

PARTS USED: Roots, leaves

CHARACTERISTICS: Bitter, cool

ACTIONS: Antimicrobial, antifungal, anti-inflammatory, digestive, tonic, alterative, anticatarrhal, hypertensive, emmenagogue, diuretic, cholagogue, stimulant

RANGE: Native to southwestern Ontario and Quebec (rare and endangered)

Goldenseal has had a long history of use by Indigenous Peoples and was more recently adopted by the European settlers. Overharvesting and habitat loss have resulted in it becoming endangered, so it is now mostly grown commercially in North America. A low-growing perennial that prefers shady places, it has a single hairy stem that grows up to a height of 10–50 cm. There are 3 leaves, one at the base and two on the upper stem, terminated by a single greenish-white flower. The leaves have 5 or more lobes and are doubly-toothed, and the flower becomes a small, inedible fruit resembling a raspberry. The yellow root bears scars from previous stems and should be 3–5 years old before harvesting. Lift out in the fall after the foliage has died down.

MEDICINAL USES:

Colds, upper respiratory problems, indigestion, diarrhea, urinary tract infections

- Antiviral and antibacterial, used to fight infections, and is a popular treatment for colds, upper respiratory tract infections and hay fever, diarrhea, stomach flu, urinary tract infections, and vaginitis, particularly when there is overproduction of mucus.
- Its bitter properties protect and heal the digestive tract, stimulate digestive enzymes, and enhance growth of beneficial bacteria.
- Used topically for eye and skin infections, sore gums, cankers.
- The Iroquois used a decoction of the root for whooping cough, diarrhea, fever, and indigestion. It was mixed with bear grease as an insect repellent. The Cherokee used it to improve appetite and in a poultice, wash, or salve for skin diseases.
- Potentially beneficial in treating diabetes and cancer, toning the circulatory system, and improving heart health, but there is very little research supporting these claims.
- Reduces heavy menstrual bleeding and can be used as a douche for vaginal infections.

TINCTURE: Fresh 1:2, 15–30 drops 4 times per day. Dry 1:5 in 60% alcohol, 20–50 drops 4 times per day.

INFUSION: Dried leaf 2–6 tbsp., up to 4 times a day

COMBINATIONS: Often combined with Echinacea for colds or flu. For urinary tract infections, may be combined or substituted with Stinging Nettles, Marshmallow root, Burdock, Slippery Elm, or Dandelion.

RESEARCH: Up until recently, very few studies have proven the efficacy of Goldenseal. Since only a small amount of its active ingredient, berberine, is absorbed when taken orally, results from studies on berberine may not apply to Goldenseal. However, it is now known to contain compounds that are relatively ineffective when used in isolation but when combined they work in synergy to enhance their antimicrobial activity. The alkaloid berberine, which is in higher concentration in the roots, and 3 flavonoids which are more prevalent in the leaves, work together, so to obtain the full power of the medicine or potentiation, the whole plant should be used. One study on commercial supplements found that many didn't contain enough of the plant to be effective and often had unlisted ingredients. Very little research has been done on the other alkaloids, hydrastine, canadine, and palmatine, which may also increase the effectiveness of the other components.

CAUTION: Avoid if pregnant or breastfeeding. Should not be given to infants as it may cause neonatal jaundice. May interfere with some medications, check with your healthcare provider. Avoid long-term use, large doses may cause vomiting, diarrhea, nervousness, and depression.

GOLDTHREAD

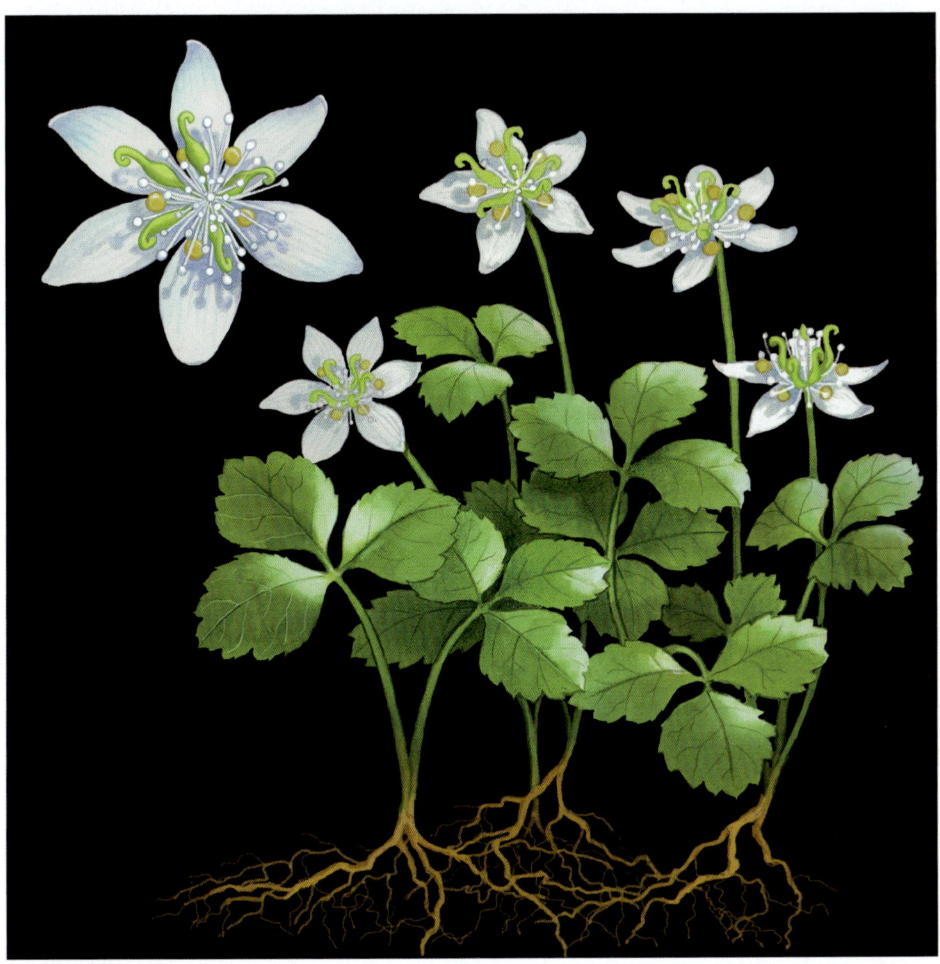

Coptis trifolia
Coptis groenlandica

FAMILY: Ranunculaceae

OTHER NAMES: Golden Root, Canker Root, Fr. Savoyane, Sabouillane, Coptide du Groenland

PARTS USED: Dried rhizome, roots, stems, leaves

CHARACTERISTICS: Bitter

ACTIONS: Bitter tonic, antibacterial, stomachic, anti-inflammatory, astringent, antiphlogistic, sedative, antifungal

RANGE: Native across all provinces and Nunavut

Goldthread is a tiny native perennial herb that has been over-picked to the point where it is now difficult to find. The roots look like a tangled mass of gold thread, and the leaves are evergreen and shiny, somewhat resembling wild strawberry leaves with 3 leaflets and slightly scalloped edges. The flowers bloom from May to August; a single flower atop a long stem of 7.5–15 cm., with 5–7 delicate white petals. It is found in damp, shaded woods, but keep in mind that it is endangered, and unless it is found in abundance, it should be left where it is.

MEDICINAL USES:

Mouth sores, digestive disorders, wounds

- Indigenous Peoples have been chewing fresh Goldthread root for centuries to cure mouth sores and thrush; works also for trench mouth and topically for herpes.
- In a sitz bath for rectal fissures or vaginitis, and topically for skin ulcers in general.
- Contains a strong, bitter alkaloid called berberine, which acts as an antibacterial and blood purifier. Good for indigestion and other digestive disorders, jaundice, and general recovery from illness.
- When used with Goldenseal, is said to be effective in helping to destroy one's appetite for alcohol.
- Some studies claim it may be promising in treating HIV, infectious hepatitis, some strains of flu, and even cancer.
- Some Mi'kmaw people use Goldthread to treat external sores and wounds by boiling it with sheep fat to make a salve.

DECOCTION: 1 tbsp. fresh finely chopped root (or 1 tsp. dried), add 1 cup of water and boil for 20 minutes. Cool and use as a gargle for mouth sores, or drink 1 tbsp. 3–6 times a day for chronic stomach and digestive inflammation.

TINCTURE: Finely chop entire plant and place in a jar. Cover with 100-proof vodka. Put on lid and leave for 6 weeks, shaking daily. Strain. Drink 1 ml. in a bit of water 3 times a day.

CAUTION: Mildly toxic, not recommended during pregnancy or breastfeeding.

GROUND IVY

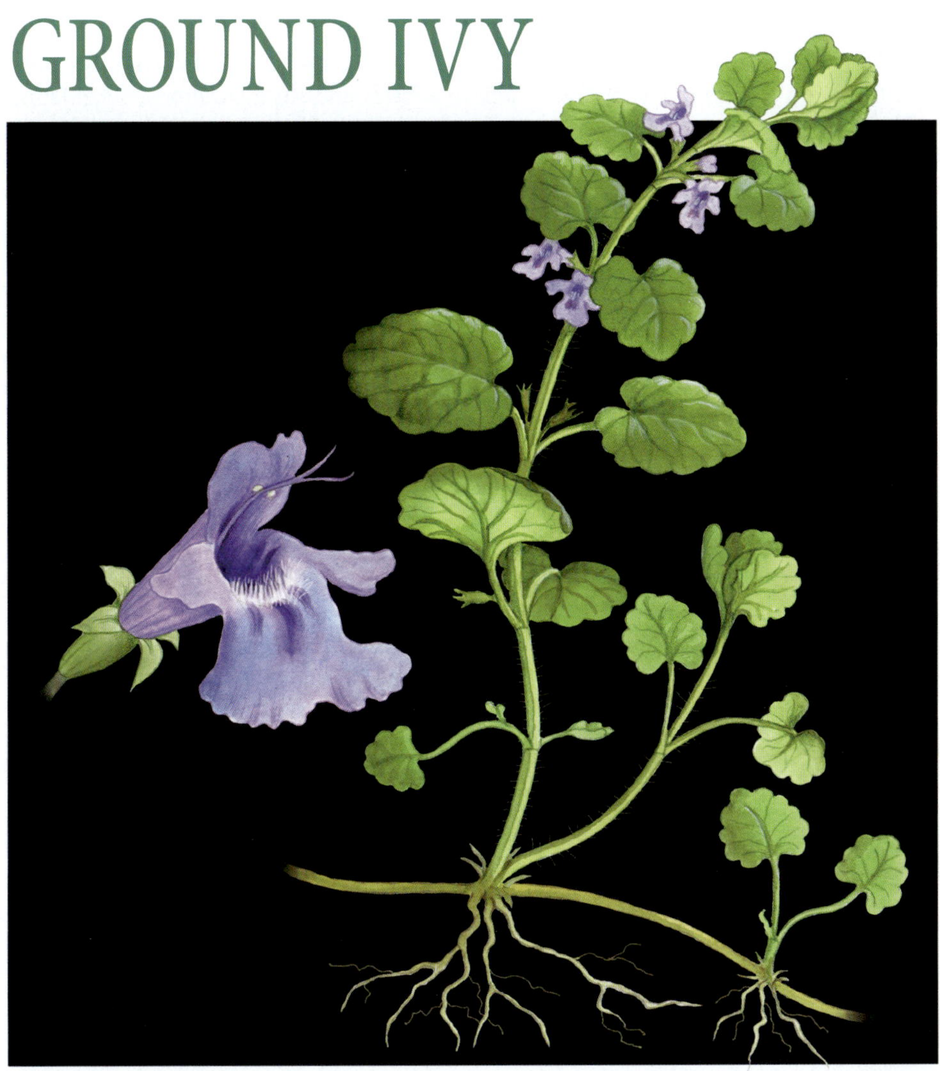

Glechoma hederacea

FAMILY: Lamiaceae

OTHER NAMES: Creeping Charlie, Alehoof, Field Balm, Hedgemaids, *Fr.* Lierre terrestre

PARTS USED: Aerial

CHARACTERISTICS: Salty, sweet, warm, dry, aromatic, astringent

ACTIONS: Anticatarrhal, antibacterial, antihistamine, antioxidant, antispasmodic, astringent, carminative, cholagogue, expectorant, diuretic, vulnerary, decongestant, diaphoretic, anti-inflammatory, tonic

RANGE: Introduced across all Canadian provinces

Ground Ivy is a tenacious little weed that has been cursed at relentlessly by gardeners over the years, but if you search into its history you will discover herbalists once held it in high esteem for its ability to relieve sciatica and skin irritations. Originating in Europe, it is a perennial ground creeper that forms a thick mat and literally takes over lawns and fields. Its leaves are kidney-shaped, stalked, and somewhat downy, with rounded indentations. The tiny flowers are purplish, two-lipped, and grow in clusters. Stems are square, downy, and trailing. It continues to bloom throughout the summer and fall, and the leaves remain green even through the winter. The plant has a balsamic smell due to oil glands on the underside of the leaves. The early Saxons used it to clarify beer before the advent of hops, giving it the name Alehoof. It is best gathered in late May to mid-June when the flowers are fresh. Harvest only the top 50% of the plant, and only from clean areas.

MEDICINAL USES:

Upper respiratory infections, digestive problems, mouth infections, kidney stones, tinnitus

- A fragrant, pleasant tasting aromatic herb used primarily for upper respiratory tract and nasal congestion. High in vitamin C, its expectorant properties help to treat damp coughs with fever and aids in clearing up mucus and congestion in sinuses, ear infections, and tinnitus. Useful when there is a chronic, persistent cough, treated over a longer period of time. Usually combined with other herbs in formulas.
- Fresh juice or tea soothes digestive tract in cases of gastritis, enteritis, diarrhea, intestinal gas, colic, and hemorrhoids. May be beneficial to the liver and for removing kidney stones.
- Infusion used as a gargle for mouth infections, gingivitis, sore throat. Especially effective for receding gums and after dental surgery.
- Eases the pain of sciatica, gout, and arthritis, can be added to bathwater to soften skin and ease backaches.
- Used as a poultice, its anti-inflammatory action makes it soothing for Stinging Nettle stings, wounds, sunburn, and irritation from other skin conditions.

FOLKLORE: Tea was believed to be effective for overcoming shyness. Strewing the leaves over the floor is said to create good dreams and peaceful sleep. A garland of Ground Ivy was often worn during the pagan festival of Beltane held on May 1 to celebrate the return of the spring flowers.

TINCTURE: Fresh leaves, 1:2 in 40% alcohol. Take 5–10 drops in water up to 4 times a day.

INFUSION: Steep 2 tsp. fresh (or 1 tsp. dried) herb in 1 cup of boiling water covered for 10 minutes. Flavour with honey or Peppermint leaves, as it is quite bitter. Makes a nice spring tonic.

COMBINATIONS: With Echinacea, Thyme, Goldenrod, or Calendula for ear, nose, or throat infections or sinusitis. With Elder flower, Stinging Nettle, or Plantain for hay fever. With Eyebright, Elder flower, Goldenrod, or Ginger for catarrhal tinnitus. With Dandelion or Gentian roots for indigestion. In poultices with Yarrow and Chamomile for sores and abscesses.

CAUTION: Contains pulegone, which can irritate the digestive tract, liver, and kidneys. Avoid if you have renal or hepatic disease. Not recommended during pregnancy or breastfeeding. Avoid if taking anticonvulsants, sedatives, or mood-altering drugs. May cause throat irritation.

HAWTHORN

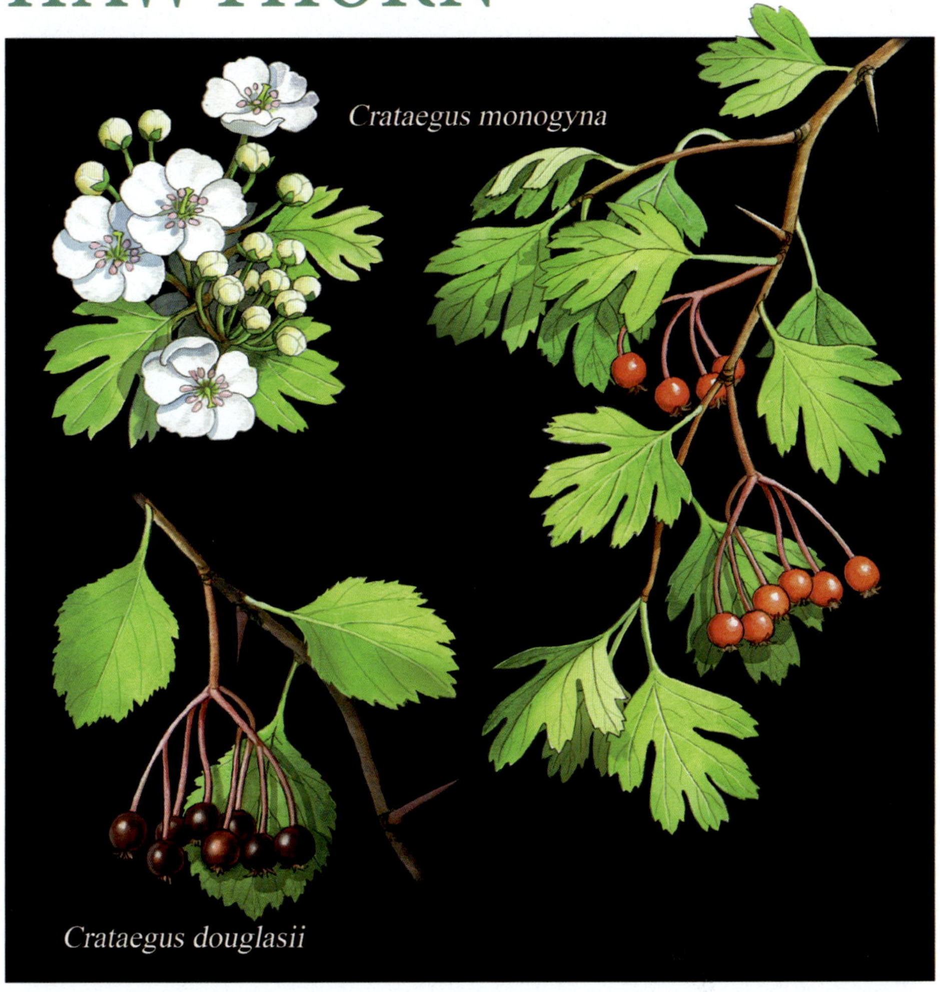

Crataegus monogyna; Crataegus douglasii

FAMILY: Rosaceae

OTHER NAMES: *C. monogyna*: One-seeded Hawthorn, English Hawthorn, May Thorn, White Thorn, *Fr.* Aubépine; *C. douglasii*: Black Hawthorn, River Hawthorn, Columbia Hawthorn, *Fr.* Aubépine noire

PARTS USED: Leaves, flowering tips of branches, berries, bark

CHARACTERISTICS: Sour, slightly warm, sweet (berries); cool, astringent (flowering tips)

ACTIONS: Anti-inflammatory, antioxidant, antihypertensive, adaptogen, cardiotonic, diuretic, astringent

RANGE: *C. monogyna* introduced in British Columbia, Ontario, Quebec, Maritimes; *C. douglasii* native to British Columbia, Alberta, Saskatchewan, Ontario

Hawthorn is a deciduous shrub or small tree from the Rose family that has been a favoured heart remedy in Europe for centuries. There are over 100 species in North America, however *C. monogyna*, and occasionally our native *C. douglasii* are the ones most often used for medicines. Their thorny branches and pretty white flowers make them ideal for hedgerows if you wish to keep out unwanted visitors. English Hawthorn grows up to 10 m. tall, it has alternate toothed leaves with 3–7 lobes and thorns about 1.3 cm. long. The white or pink flowers usually emerge in May, giving off a slight fishy odour that attracts pollinators then fades when the flowers are dried. Black Hawthorn is slightly smaller, its leaves are not lobed and are finely toothed, and the "haws," or berries, are black when fully ripe. The branch tips and flowers can be hung upside down or placed in a paper bag until crisp. The haws are gathered in late August or September and can be dried for later use. Both can be tinctured fresh if desired.

MEDICINAL USES:

High blood pressure, angina, atherosclerosis, high cholesterol, digestive problems, poor circulation, anxiety

- Used historically for hundreds of years for relatively mild heart conditions, Hawthorn provides a safe remedy and cardiotonic, particularly when stress and anxiety are key factors. Contains flavonoids, which reduce inflammation and cause dilation of the coronary arteries, subsequently increasing blood flow to the heart. This makes heart contractions more efficient, bringing more oxygen and nutrients into the heart cells. Antioxidants help to strengthen arterial walls, making them more pliable. Flowers and berries have similar actions, however, the berries are slightly better for lowering blood pressure, whereas the flowers are thought to be better for improving circulation to the peripheries. Slow-acting and nourishing, it should be taken for at least 3 months to see the full effect. There is no known risk with long-term use.
- Improves conditions like mild arrhythmia, angina, palpitations, hypertension, tachycardia, and atherosclerosis.
- Reduces anxiety and insomnia associated with stress and palpitations. Helps when dealing with grief and loss, bringing a sense of calm to stressful situations.
- Fruit extract soothes digestive problems, helping to break down fats and providing fibre and probiotic action to improve transit time. Helps relieve stomach ulcers. Astringency helps settle diarrhea and irritation in the gut.
- Improves circulation to the extremities.

OTHER USES:

- Berries rich in vitamin C and can be eaten (remove seeds) or used to make jams, jellies, candy, wine, or cordials.
- Europeans used it for spiritual protection and to decorate the maypole, a pagan symbol of renewal and fertility.

TINCTURE: Fresh leaves, flowers 1:2, dried plant and/or berries 1:5, in 60% alcohol. Take 10–30 drops up to 3 times a day. Should be continued for at least 4 months to get maximum benefit.

INFUSION: Steep 1–2 tsp. leaves and flowers 15–30 min. in boiling water. Drink up to 3 cups a day. Cold infusion of berries, 2–4 tbsp. up to twice a day.

RESEARCH:

- In human clinical trials with people who have had chronic heart failure, it was shown to improve exercise tolerance and reduce fatigue and shortness of breath when taken for 3–6 weeks, with only minor adverse effects.
- In a 2006 study, 79 people with type 2 diabetes and high blood pressure were given 1200 mg. of Hawthorn extract for 16 weeks. They experienced significantly more improvement than the placebo group. Polyphenols and flavonoids have been shown to have hypoglycemic effects, reducing blood glucose and increasing plasma insulin release from the pancreas in trial on mice.
- A 6-month study of 64 people with atherosclerosis found that taking Hawthorn extract reduced the thickness of plaque buildup in the arteries.
- Triterpenoids in Hawthorn may have an anticancer function, showing promising research in breast, liver, colon, and gastric cancers.

CAUTION: May interfere with digoxin or other heart medications. Consult doctor before use. May cause vertigo, dizziness, mild nausea, agitation.

HEAL-ALL

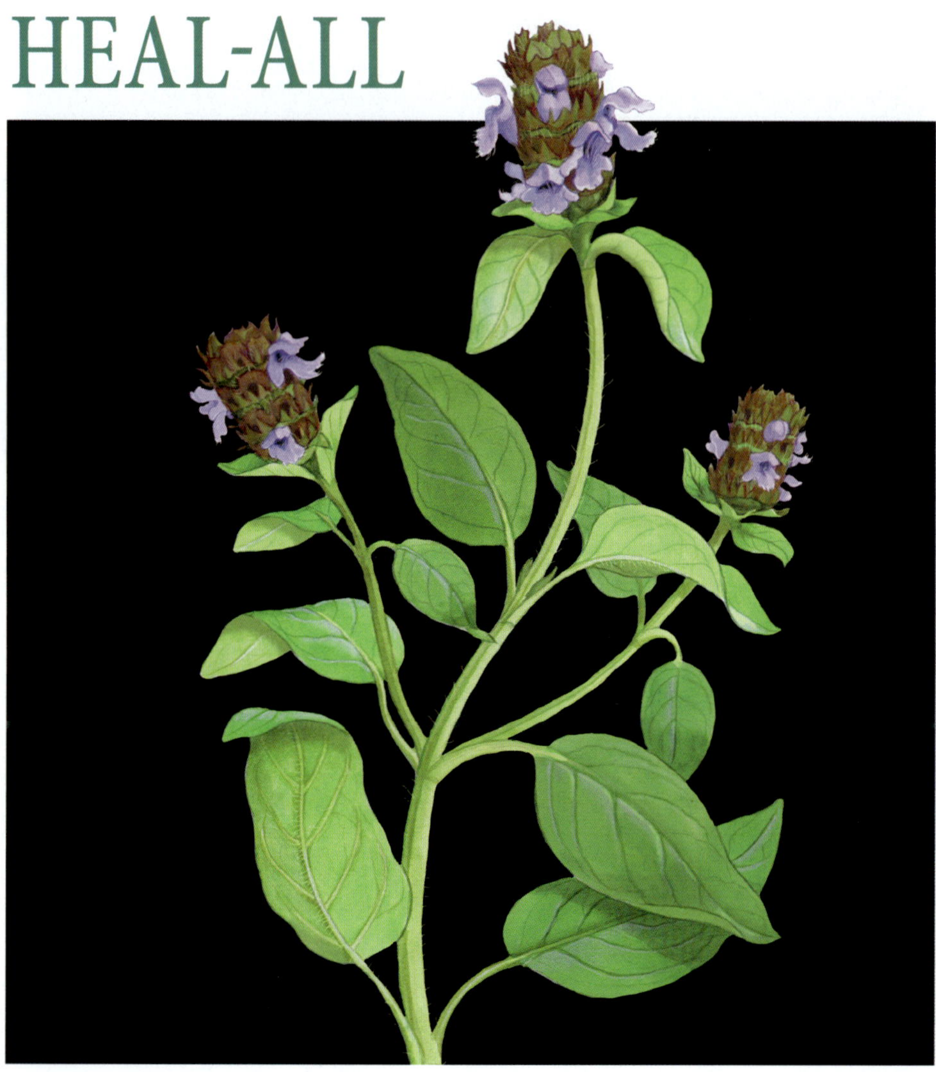

Prunella vulgaris

FAMILY: Lamiaceae

OTHER NAMES: Self-heal, All-heal, Prunella, Woundwort, Carpenter Weed, *Fr.* Brunelle, Herbe au charpentier, Prunelle commune

PARTS USED: Aerial

CHARACTERISTICS: Slightly bitter, pungent, cold, moistening, acrid

ACTIONS: Astringent, vulnerary, tonic, anti-inflammatory, diuretic, haemostatic, antiseptic, antibacterial, antioxidant, antiviral, demulcent, sedative, anti-tumour, hypotensive, hypoglycemic, hepatoprotective, antipyretic

RANGE: Native across all provinces, introduced in the Yukon

Although this native perennial herb of the Mint family was once used, as its name suggests, to heal just about anything, it has somewhat lost its popularity with Western herbalists over the years, but new research suggests it could prove to be quite useful. It grows up to 30 cm. high, and is easily identified by its dense cluster of purple flowers at the top of a square stem. They grow in rings around the fat cylindrical spike, looking somewhat ragged since they are never all in bloom at once, and each tubular flower is composed of a two-lipped calyx with dark red tips and a two-lipped purple corolla resembling a throat. Below the flower spike is a set of two stalkless leaves and then more paired opposite leaves on stems branching off of a creeping stem, which sends roots into the soil at intervals. It grows in fields and waste places, and can be picked in the summer or fall and dried for later use.

MEDICINAL USES:

Wounds, sore throat, swollen lymph nodes, hemorrhoids

- Loaded with antioxidants and anti-inflammatory compounds, Heal-all makes a delicious, nourishing and immune-boosting tea that can be used regularly as a healthy drink for the liver, skin, and the whole body. The young plants can be eaten raw or cooked, are high in vitamins A, B, C, and K and make a great spring tonic. Helpful during allergy season to relieve irritation and congestion.
- Before the Second World War it was used extensively to clean wounds and stop hemorrhaging; the fresh leaf can be used as a poultice or in a compress. Soothes inflamed wounds or sores.
- Used internally for diarrhea, colitis, hemorrhoids, or internal bleeding.
- May be infused in oil and made into lotions or ointments for hemorrhoids, burns, skin ulcers, boils, eczema, and other skin irritations.
- Popular in Asia since the fourteenth century, it has been used as a wound herb, for swollen glands and goiter, eye inflammations, liver problems, and high blood pressure. Included in many formulas for fever, infections, and digestive problems.
- Its immune-boosting properties make it effective at the onset of colds and flu, upper respiratory infections, fevers, and sore throats.
- Lymphatic stimulant and diuretic, it clears swollen lymph nodes and relieves mastitis.
- Has anti-viral properties, inhibits the binding ability of a virus so it can't replicate. Effective against Herpes Simplex virus (cold sores), HPV, and HIV.

FOLKLORE: Once believed to be a holy herb and that it could drive away the devil.

INFUSION: Infuse 1–2 tsp. dried herb in 1 cup boiling water. Steep 1 hour. Drink 3 times a day or use as a gargle or lotion.

COMBINATIONS: With Lemon Balm and St. John's Wort for cold sores. With Stinging Nettle, Goldenrod, or Marshmallow leaf for allergies.

RESEARCH: Triterpenoids were found to be the main active ingredients, responsible for its anti-inflammatory, anti-tumour, and antiviral properties. Flavonoids have activity against osteoporosis and osteoarthritis. Has been studied extensively for its anticancer properties. An aqueous extract was shown to inhibit invasion and migration of human liver carcinoma and oleanic acid induces cell apoptosis of lung adenocarcinoma cells. It had significant inhibitory effects on several infectious viruses, as well as a variety of antibacterial activities. It also improves liver injury from alcohol abuse, autoimmune hepatitis, and thyroid disease. However, since it is such a complex herb, further research and development are needed to fully understand its potential as a medicinal herb.

CAUTION: Generally considered safe, although excessive use may cause diarrhea or abdominal pain.

HEMLOCK

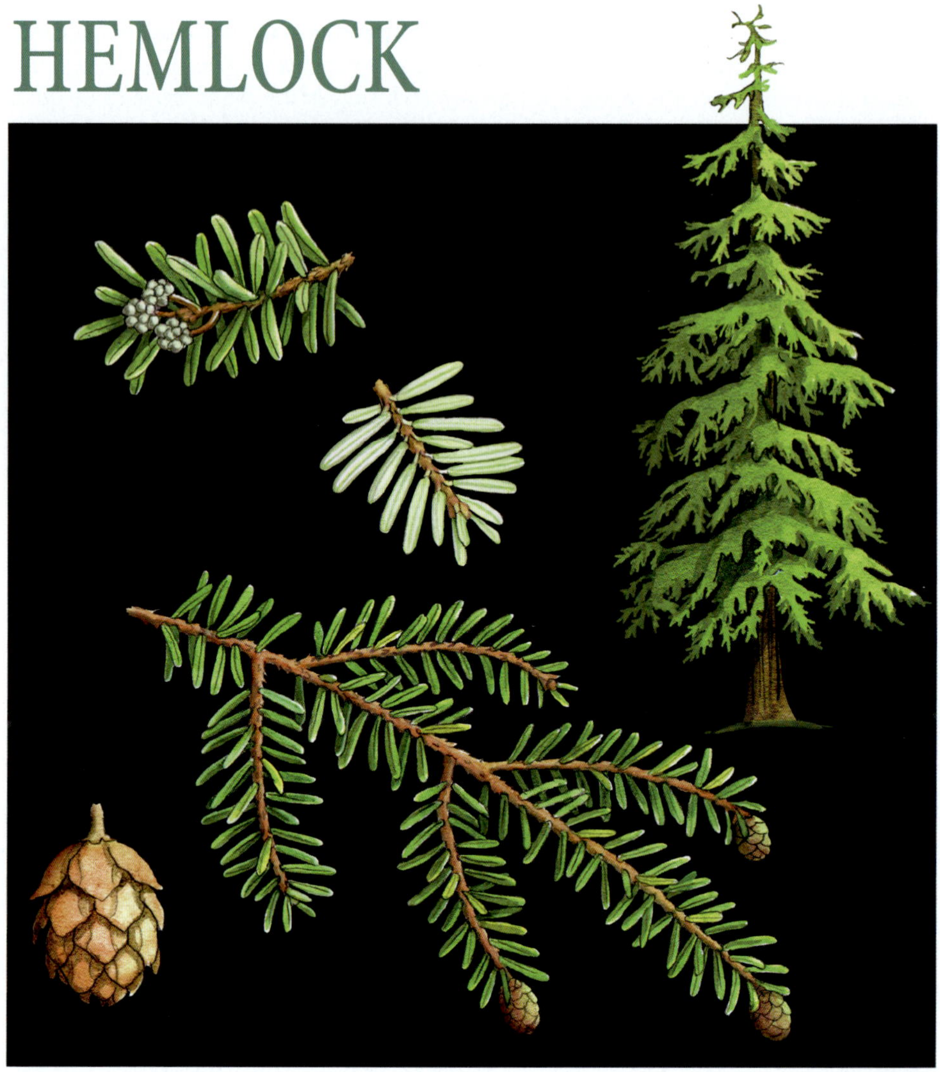

Tsuga canadensis
Tsuga heterophylla

FAMILY: Pinaceae

OTHER NAMES: *T. canadensis:* Eastern Hemlock; *T. heterophylla:* Western Hemlock; *Fr.* Pruche, Tsuga.

PARTS USED: Light green tips, inner bark, resin

CHARACTERISTICS: Sweet, pungent, warming, astringent

ACTIONS: Antioxidant, antimicrobial, astringent, diuretic, diaphoretic

RANGE: *T. canadensis* native from Ontario to Maritimes; *T. heterophylla* native to British Columbia and Alberta

These tall, graceful conifers might bring to mind the poisonous herb *Conium maculatum* that killed Socrates, but it is in no way poisonous, and was simply given the name because of its odour, which resembles that of the herb. The western variety can be one of the tallest and most common in British Columbia, reaching up to 70 m., whereas the eastern species is less common and usually only reaches 20–30 m. Both tolerate cool, moist conditions, acidic soil, and high elevations. It is usually recognizable by its drooping, feathery crown, as well as the blunt soft needles of varying lengths with two white stripes on their underside. The male cones are tiny and yellow, the female cones are 2–5 cm. in length and can be purple-green when young or brown as they get older. The bark also changes with age, being reddish brown and smooth when young and becoming grey and more furrowed as it ages. It is tolerant of a wide variety of growing conditions, and the Western variety has been known to reach 1,200 years of age. Collect bark only from branches close to the ground and within reach so as not to harm the tree. Light green branch tips can be harvested in the spring and used fresh.

MEDICINAL USES:

Hemorrhages, tuberculosis, kidney and bladder problems, diarrhea, colds, fever, sores, sunburn, rheumatism

- Bark can be peeled easily from young branches; starchy, sweet inner bark is scraped off, pounded and dried to be used as medicine or food.
- Infusion or decoction of the inner bark or twigs is diuretic and astringent, used internally for kidney and bladder complaints, diarrhea, hemorrhaging, tuberculosis, and fevers.
- Used externally in a decoction of the bark for sores, ulcers, or rashes, or in a poultice for bleeding wounds. Some Indigenous Peoples also chew the needles and use them as a poultice for burns.
- Sap or resin can be heated with fat to make a salve or with oil as a chest rub for colds and sore muscles. Sometimes the warm sap is applied to wounds or use it in a poultice to ease the pain of rheumatism.
- Needles are rich in vitamin C and can be drunk as an infusion. Sour leaf buds can be eaten fresh in the spring or brewed as a tea. Relieves colds, coughs, and fevers.
- Liniments from bark decoction rubbed on the chest for colds, or mixed with deer tallow to prevent sunburn.

OTHER USES:

- Inner bark dried to a powder and used as thickener for soups or mixed with flours for bread.
- Pounded and steamed into a paste, it is used to make cakes, often mixed with berries and roasted in a pit oven or eaten in winter as survival food.
- Powdered bark is put into shoes for sweaty feet and to reduce foot odour.
- Wood is often carved for utensils. The bark is rich in tannin and used for tanning hides, and it also yields a red or brown dye.

BARK DECOCTION: Drink ½–¾ cups to 3 times a day.

TIP INFUSION: Standard infusion, drink ½–¾ cups up to 3 times a day.

OIL: Place 2 tbsp. ground pitch into a mason jar with 1 cup of olive oil, a few twigs may be added if desired. Place in a crockpot with a couple of inches of water and heat for 3 or 4 days at lowest temperature, strain, and bottle.

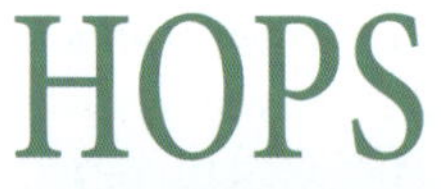

female flowers

male flowers

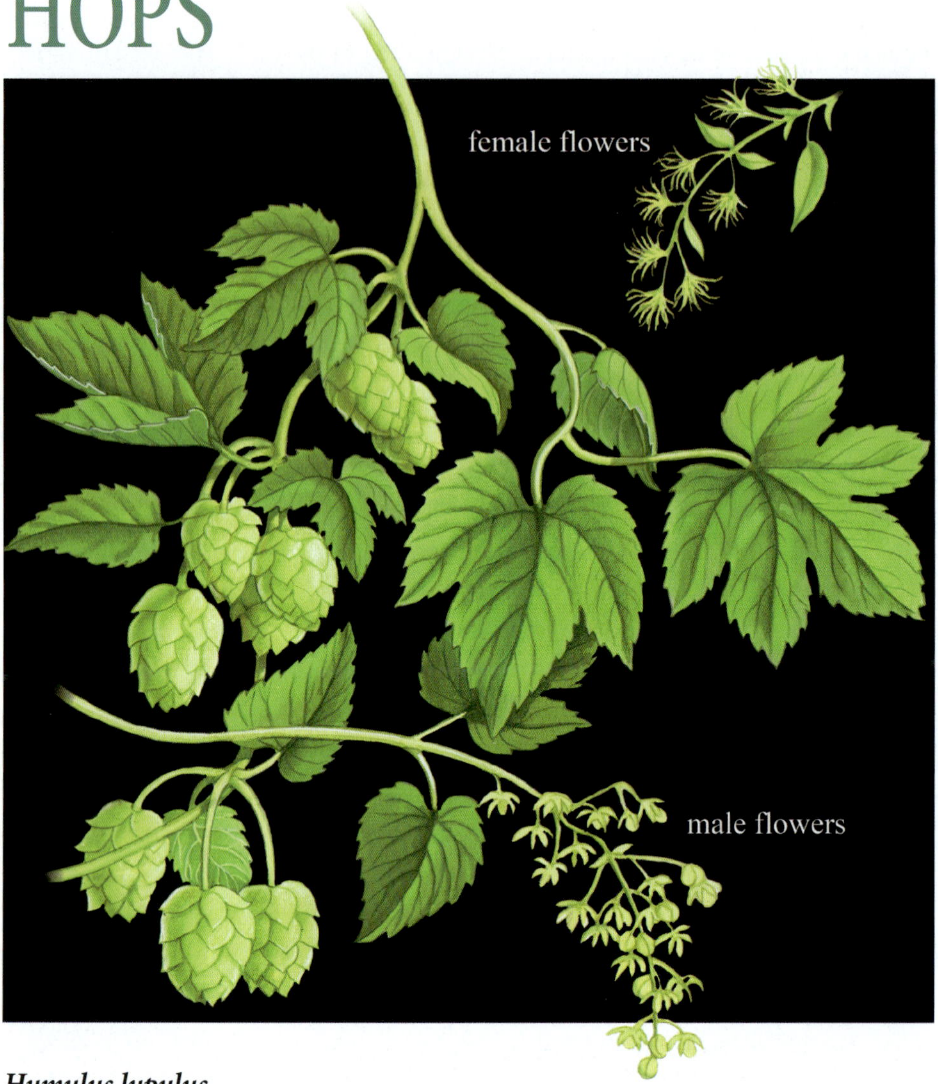

Humulus lupulus

FAMILY: Cannabaceae (Hemp)

OTHER NAMES: Common Hops, *Fr.* Houblon

PARTS USED: Fruit (cones)

CHARACTERISTICS: Bitter, cold, dry, slightly pungent, astringent, sweet

ACTIONS: Sedative, diuretic, tonic, antiseptic, nervine, antispasmodic, cholagogue, antirheumatic, antioxidant, anodyne, anti-inflammatory

RANGE: Introduced in British Columbia, native from Alberta to Newfoundland and Labrador

Hops may be well-known as a stabilizer, preservative, and bitter flavouring for beer, but it is also a potent medicinal herb. This climbing perennial vine, often growing up to 6 m. long, is native to North America but is also cultivated all over the world. Typically it is found growing wild along old railway sites and farmlands. The leaves are opposite, dark green, and heart-shaped with finely toothed edges, the larger ones having 3–5 sharply toothed lobes. The flowers, like hemp, grow male and female on separate plants. The male flowers grow in bunches 7.5–12 cm. long; the females grow in cone-like strobiles about 3 cm. long. Only the females are used for brewing beer and as a medicine, as the medicine is in the flowers. The strobiles are gathered when they turn an amber-brown colour, in August or September, and should be dried gently in an oven to preserve their volatile oils. Should be used within 6 months as they quickly lose their potency.

MEDICINAL USES:

Anxiety, nervous indigestion, rheumatism, menopausal symptoms

- Hops have a long history of use as a medicine both in Europe and amongst Indigenous healers. They were predominantly used for their effects on the nervous system, as their antispasmodic action relieves tension and constriction, on both a physical and emotional level. Often after sickness or a traumatic experience, the body will go into a state of imbalance that can persist, manifesting as chills, indigestion, ulcers, diarrhea, IBS, spasms and difficulty sleeping. Hops are sedative and relaxant, easing nervous tension and anxiety on a visceral level and bringing a calmer state of mind.
- Dried strobiles used in infusions or put into pillows to promote sleep.
- Slightly heated, they may be used to relieve toothaches or earaches.
- Eases restlessness, headache, anxiety, nerve pain. May be added to cough syrups to calm irritable coughs.
- Has a relaxing influence over the digestive tract, relieves nervous indigestion, increases bile production, stimulates appetite, eases cramps, IBS or mucous colitis, sluggish liver, jaundice.
- Contains estrogen-like chemicals that promote menstruation and flow of breast milk, and relieves vaginal dryness or discomforts of menopause. Eases hot flashes.
- When combined with Chamomile flowers and applied as a poultice or ointment, Hops are an effective anti-inflammatory, and can relieve pain from swelling, bruises, and boils. For rheumatic pains and neuralgia, apply as a hot poultice, or take internally as an infusion.
- Believed by some to encourage hair growth.

TINCTURE: Dried strobiles 1:5, 65% alcohol, take 1–4 ml. per day.

INFUSION: Add 2 tsp. dried hops to 1 cup boiling water. Steep covered for 15 minutes.

COMBINATIONS: Add Passionflower, Lemon Balm, or Valerian for insomnia or anxiety.

RESEARCH: Rich in bioactive substances, Hops prove to be promising in the treatment of some chronic diseases, particularly due to anti-inflammatory and antioxidant effects on the cardiovascular system and a reduction in blood glucose levels in patients with type 2 diabetes. The presence of xanthohumol has been found to act synergestically with chemo treatments in some cancers, reducing the doses needed, increasing apoptosis of cancer cells and inhibiting metastasis. However, more studies are needed to increase absorption and bioavailability.

CAUTION: May aggravate feelings of depression in people with low energy and anxiety. Frequent contact may cause dermatitis in some people.

HORSETAIL

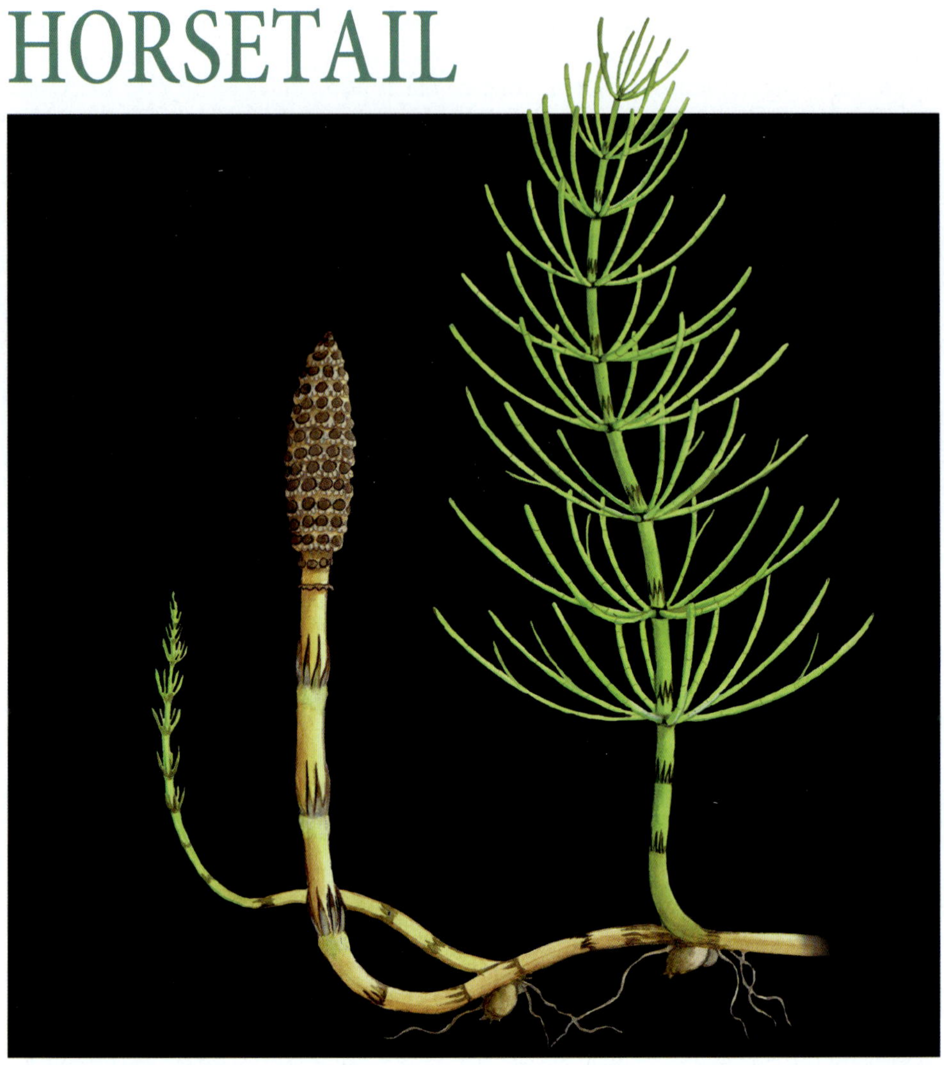

Equisetum arvense

FAMILY: Equisetaceae

OTHER NAMES: Field horsetail, Bottlebrush, Pewter Wort, Scouring Rush, *Fr.* Prêle des champs, Queue de renard

PARTS USED: Green sterile stalk

CHARACTERISTICS: Cool, dry, slightly bitter, astringent, salty

ACTIONS: Antibiotic, diuretic, astringent, vulnerary

RANGE: Native across Canada

Horsetail is a rather odd-looking, prehistoric-like, non-flowering native plant that reproduces by spores located under the scales of the edible, asparagus-like shoots, a spike of around 20 cm. tall which appears in the spring. In summer the spike disappears and is replaced by a green sterile stalk that grows to about 30 cm. and is used as medicine, with whorls of thin branches, resembling a smaller version of the large tree-like plants that covered the earth 400 million years ago. These stems and branches contain silicon crystals which help strengthen bones, and also make it useful for cleaning and polishing metal objects and kitchen utensils. It is usually found in swamps, damp woods, and fields. Gather the young green stalks after fruiting stems have died down in spring or early summer before branches begin to droop. To make sure you have *E. arvense,* and not *E. palustre*, or Marsh Horsetail, cut the central stem crosswise. The central hollow should be at least twice the size of the peripheral hollows. Bundle together, and hang to dry where there is good airflow.

MEDICINAL USES:

Urinary tract infections, osteoporosis, joint problems, wounds, kidney and bladder disorders

- The use of this herb in Europe dates back to Greek and Roman times, but was also used extensively by Indigenous Peoples throughout North America. Not only high in silica, Horsetail contains many minerals like manganese and potassium that are important for bone health and maintaining and repairing connective tissues. It can increase the body's ability to absorb calcium, repair bone loss and fractures, build cartilage in the joints, and help prevent osteoarthritis, however it is not recommended for long-term use.
- Traditionally used as a diuretic to increase urine output and relieve chronic urinary tract infections and kidney complaints. Has a tonic and anti-inflammatory effect on mucous membranes and strengthens against recurrence of infections. May flush out kidney stones. Helps incontinence, bedwetting, and benign prostate inflammation. Tightens and tones tissues in cases of diarrhea, hemorrhoids, and dysentery.
- Crushed sterile stems are astringent, and when used as a poultice or ointment it will stop bleeding and heal cuts, sores, and other minor wounds, assist tissue regeneration, and reduce inflammation.
- Because of the presence of silica, a mineral essential to bone health, it strengthens and heals joints and bones. It has been suggested that it may be used as a treatment for osteoporosis, however, there is no scientific evidence yet.
- Dissolved in the bath, it can be soothing for rheumatic pain, rashes, or other wounds. In a foot bath it can ease infections.
- Liquid obtained from boiling stems often used as a mouthwash or gargle for oral infections, cankers, or sore throats. Add salt if desired.
- High mineral content provides nutrients for hair loss and brittle nails, encourages growth and regeneration. A few drops of tincture mixed with liquid coconut oil (MCT) used topically keeps hair shiny, strengthens nails, and moisturizes the skin.

OTHER USES: As an abrasive for scouring pots and pans or polishing metal.

BATH SOAK: Steep 1 cup of Horsetail in hot water for 1 hour. Add liquid to bath water.

COMPRESS: Crush dried herb and soak in enough warm water to make a paste. Mix with crushed Plantain if desired. Apply to boils or other sores twice a day.

INFUSION: 2 tsp. dried plant infused in 1 cup boiling water for 15 minutes. Strain. Drink 3 times a day. This can be mixed with lemon juice and salt to be used as a gargle.

TINCTURE: Dried herb, 1:5 in 25% alcohol. Take 1–3 ml. in a little water up to 3 times a day.

COMBINATIONS: With Rosemary or Stinging Nettle in infused oil for hair and scalp. (Leave on overnight, 2–3 times a week.) With Bearberry or Juniper berry for urinary tract infections. With Stinging Nettle as a blood tonic.

CAUTION: Generally safe used for short periods of time. May cause diarrhea, abdominal discomfort, or nausea in some people. Prolonged use or large doses may cause kidney toxicity due to its diuretic action, and lead to electrolyte imbalances or thiamine deficiencies. Avoid if you have kidney or liver disease or edema or are taking diuretics. Due to lack of data, avoid during pregnancy or breastfeeding. May be toxic to horses.

HYSSOP

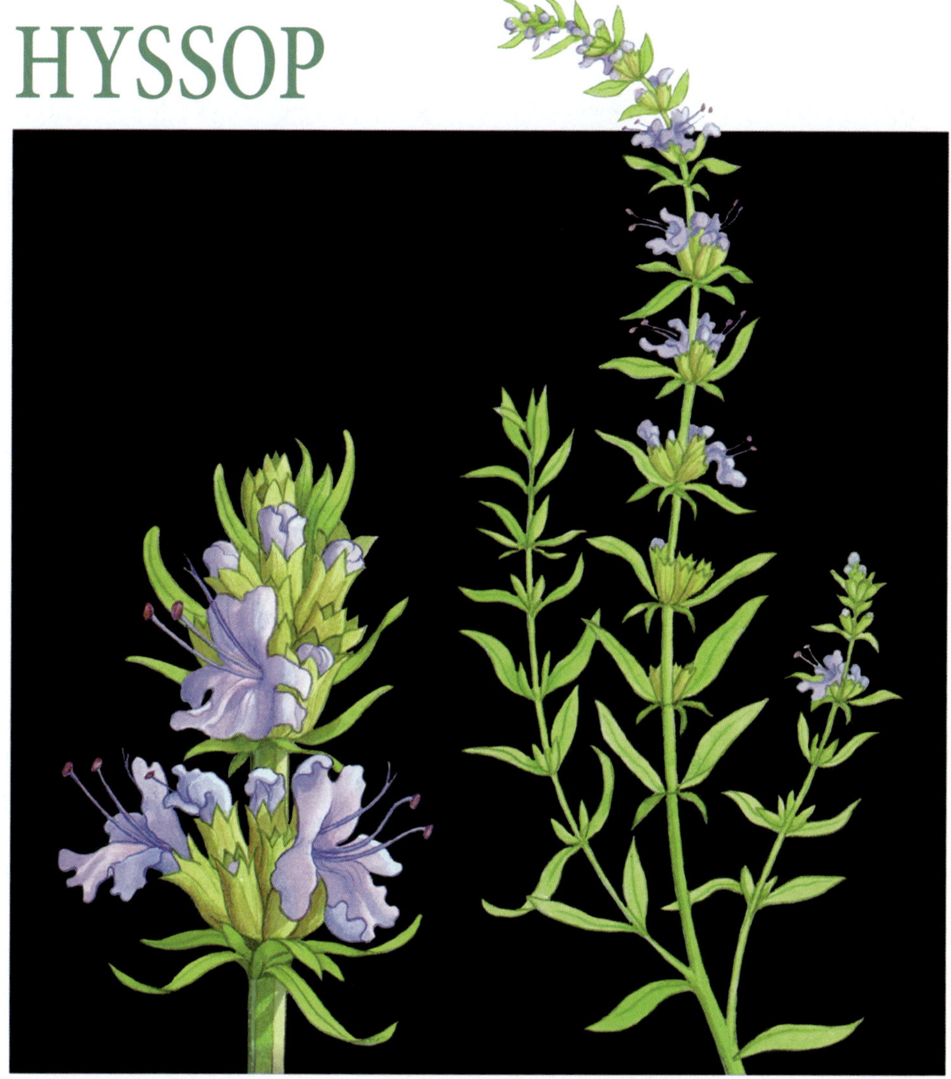

Hyssopus officinalis

FAMILY: Lamiaceae

OTHER NAMES: *Fr.* Hysope

PARTS USED: Aerial, dried

CHARACTERISTICS: Bitter, pungent, dry, slightly warming

ACTIONS: Demulcent, anti-spasmodic, antiseptic, expectorant, diaphoretic, sedative, carminative, aromatic, tonic, vulnerary, relaxant, nervine, anti-inflammatory, antifungal, antimicrobial

RANGE: Introduced in Quebec, Ontario, and Nova Scotia

Hyssop is an aromatic shrubby perennial from the Mint family that grows in clumps along fields and roadsides throughout the summer. It has stalks growing up to 60 cm. tall with shiny dark-green opposite toothed leaves along a square stem and many tiny 2-lipped purple flowers that run up one side of the top part of the erect stalk. It has been used since ancient times for ritual cleaning of sacred places because of its unusual odour, and when planted in a garden, it attracts bees and butterflies. Harvest the flowering tops in August when in flower.

MEDICINAL USES:

Respiratory and sinus infections, indigestion, fevers

- Contains the terpenoid marubiin, which helps unproductive coughs deep within the chest by loosening mucus so it can be coughed up more easily. Generally taken after the infection has peaked as an infusion or decoction, and often combined with other herbs. Patient should drink lots of water as well to help with expectoration.
- Mainly used for respiratory infections like colds, bronchitis, tickling cough, sinusitis, and hoarseness, but also effective for asthma. Diaphoretic, it promotes perspiration and relieves fevers.
- For childhood illnesses like chickenpox and measles it can be used with Calendula, both externally as a compress to relieve skin inflammation and internally for fever.
- Its carminative action helps relieve sluggish digestion, gas, and colic. A gentle laxative, it soothes the mucous membrane of the digestive tract.
- Antiviral action may help with herpes infections.
- Relieves dryness of the skin, may remove discolouration from bruises.
- Improves circulation, poultice may be applied to the skin to heal wounds or ease pain from rheumatism.

FOLKLORE: Once believed to be a holy plant, Hyssop was said to purify sacred places and forgive one's sins. It was also used to disinfect against the plague.

OTHER USES:

- Fresh flowers and young shoots may be eaten in salads.
- Crushed dried leaves and flowers may be used in potpourris or as a strewing herb to mask odours.

COMPRESS: 2 tbsp. dried herb mixed with 2 cups of boiling water, steep for 15 minutes. Soak a clean cloth in liquid and apply to skin.

INFUSION: Mix 2 tsp. dried herb per cup of boiling water; steep 10 minutes covered. Drink up to 3 times a day. Add sugar or honey if desired.

COMBINATIONS: With Thyme, Mullein, Licorice, or Elecampane for coughs, with Elder flower, Calendula, or Chamomile for children's colds, and with Boneset, Yarrow, or Peppermint for asthma.

CAUTION: Should not be used by pregnant women as it can cause a miscarriage. Essential oil should always be diluted and should not be used by people with a history of epilepsy. Do not exceed recommended doses.

JAPANESE KNOTWEED

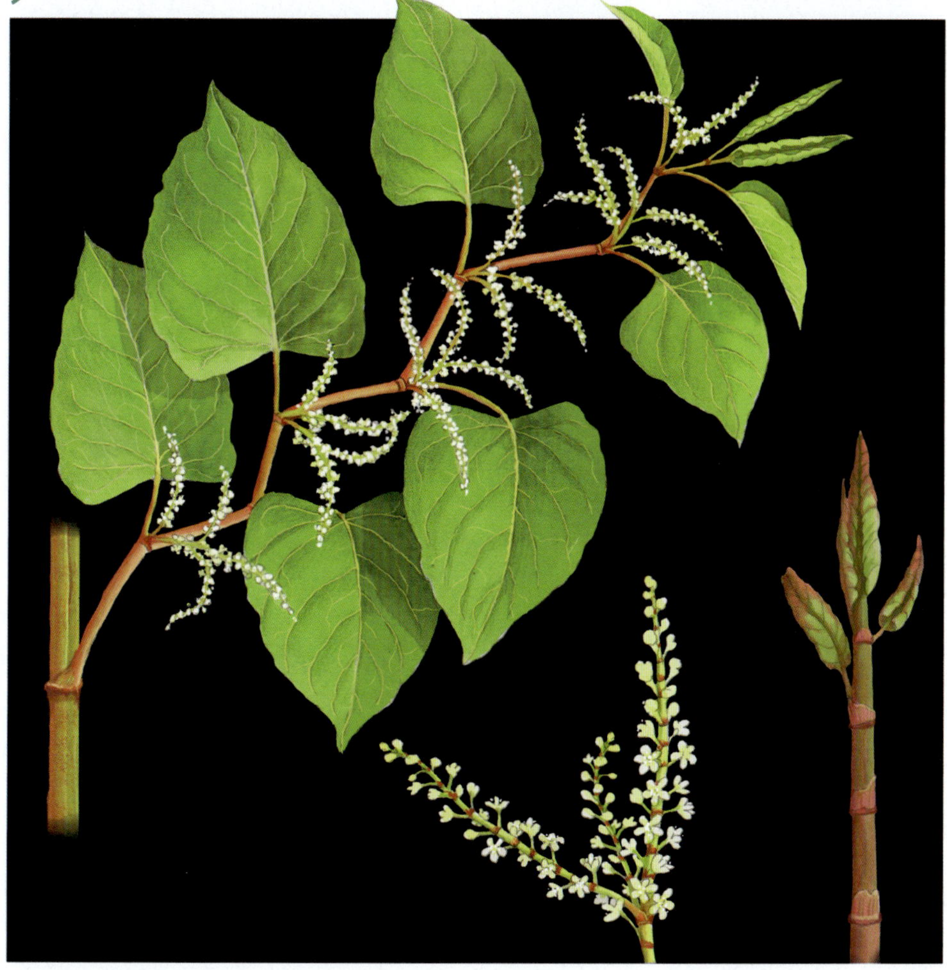

Fallopia japonica

FAMILY: Polygonaceae

OTHER NAMES: Hu Zhang, American Bamboo, Mexican Bamboo, Fleeceflower, *Fr.* Renouée de japon

PARTS USED: Roots, rhizome, young stalks

CHARACTERISTICS: Bitter, cold, dry, sweet

ACTIONS: Analgesic, antiarthritic, antioxidant, antibacterial, anticancer, antiviral, laxative, tonic, anti-inflammatory, antimicrobial, astringent, neuroprotective, hemostatic, vasodilator

RANGE: Introduced across Canadian provinces except Saskatchewan

Japanese Knotweed, a native to Eastern Asia first introduced in North America in the nineteenth century, has become a highly invasive plant across the continent as well as in Europe and Australia and is now regarded as being in the top one hundred invasive plants in the world. Growing to a height of up to 3 m. with a root system that can extend 2–3 m. deep and 14–18 m. in length, it can spread quickly and even break through concrete, making it almost impossible to eradicate.

However, it does have some redeeming qualities. Firstly, its young shoots and leaves taste good and are highly nutritious. It is also a valuable medicinal herb, its root being high in resveratrol, which is important in brain function and heart health, and the whole plant is recently being considered in the protocol for treatment of Lyme and other bacterial infections.

It grows in large clumps along roadsides and streams, its purple or green stems hollow and smooth, about 2.5 cm. in diameter. Its reddish nodes are surrounded by papery sheaths. New stems emerge in April, the shoots reddish to purple and fading to green as they mature. They grow quickly, and the bamboo-like stems can reach 1 m. in 3 weeks or up to 3 m. tall in a season. The alternate leaves are oval to triangular with a flat base and pointed tip. Rhizomes are brown with an orange interior and can be harvested in the fall; chop up finely before drying or tincturing as they become rock-hard after a few days. Shoots should be picked when they are about 15 cm. tall and green with red tips. Make sure the area where you harvest has not been sprayed with herbicides and do not discard root pieces into compost as even the smallest piece can regenerate into new plants.

MEDICINAL USES:

Alzheimer's, heart disease, Lyme disease, gingivitis

- High in resveratrol, a polyphenolic compound with antioxidant properties, it is useful in slowing the aging process and preventing neurodegeneration. But it seems to work best when the whole plant is used due to the synergistic action of all its constituents. It stimulates circulation and disperses blood stasis, promoting vasodilation of the arteries, reducing blood pressure, lowering chance of stroke, and improving cardiovascular health. It also enhances blood flow to the eyes, heart, skin and joints, and crosses the blood-brain barrier, protecting from inflammatory damage.
- Considered as a preventative for neurodegenerative diseases like Alzheimer's, improves memory and brain health.
- Resveratrol acts as a blood sugar regulator, preventing insulin resistance.
- Antibacterial, a decoction may be used for sore throat, gingivitis, or plaque build-up on the teeth.
- Regulates bowel motility. A gentle laxative, it can relieve constipation and ease diarrhea. Often combined with other herbs.
- A popular herb in Chinese medicine, its ability to clear heat, blood stasis, and dampness make it useful in several conditions, including coughs with yellow phlegm and heat symptoms, menstrual pain, jaundice, leukorrhea, and muscle or joint pain. Bolsters the immune system and reduces congestion.
- May be effective in treating Lyme disease and other bacterial infections. Recent research has supported anecdotal findings of its effectiveness.
- Can be used externally for burns, abscesses, and chronic inflammations like rheumatoid arthritis. Reduces pain and risk of infection.

OTHER USES: Young shoots can be cooked in salted water and eaten like asparagus. Young leaves can also be steamed and eaten. Not very palatable raw.

TINCTURE: Fresh root, 1:3 in 40% alcohol, 1–2 ml up to 3 times a day.

DECOCTION: Mix 1 tsp. of dried root in 1 cup of water; simmer 10 minutes. Let stand to steep for half an hour. Take ½ cup 2 times a day.

COMBINATIONS: With Hawthorn for cardiovascular health, with Yellow Dock for constipation, with Reishi and Chaga, ground and decocted overnight, to increase mental clarity.

CAUTION: Avoid taking in large amounts as it could cause nausea and vomiting. Don't use with blood-thinning medications. Do not use during pregnancy.

JUNIPER

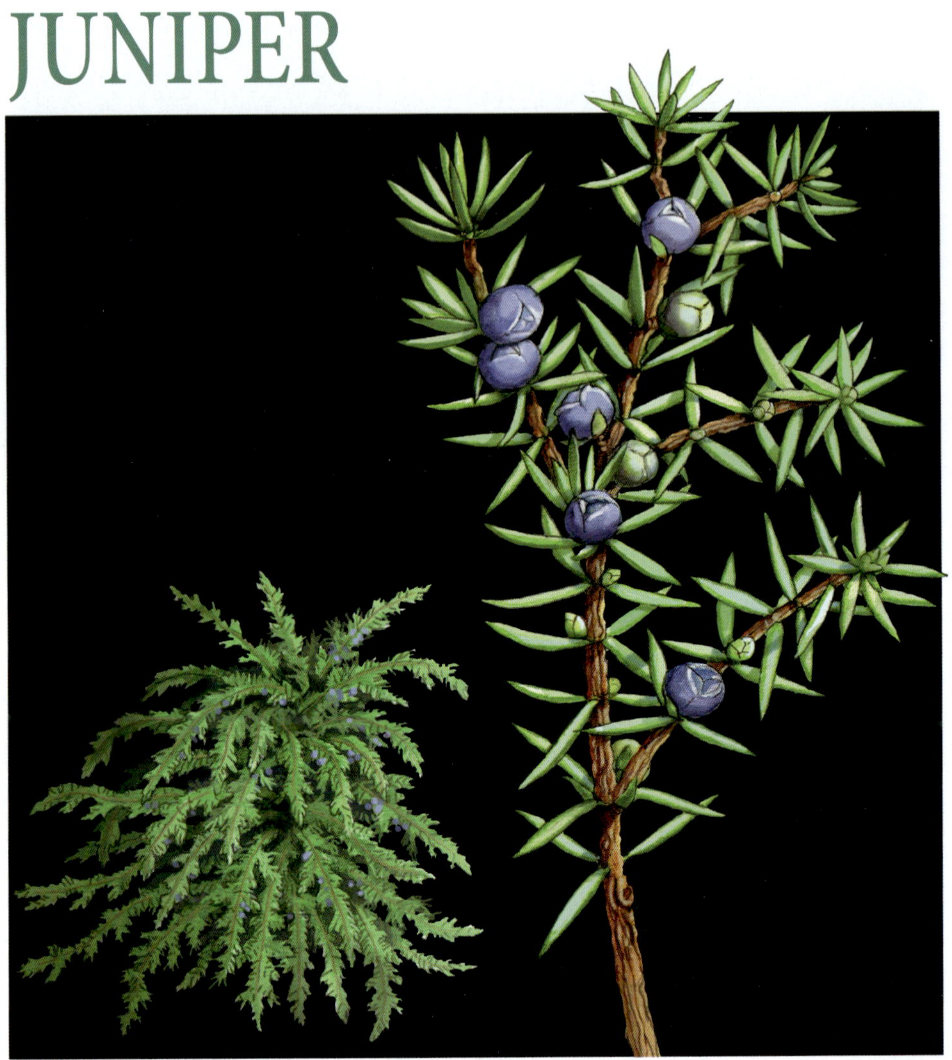

***Juniperus communis* (Common)**
***Juniperus horizontalis* (Creeping)**

FAMILY: Cupressaceae

OTHER NAMES: *Fr.* Genévrier

PARTS USED: Berries (cones), needles

CHARACTERISTICS: Warming, spicy, pungent, drying

ACTIONS: Antibacterial, alterative, aromatic, carminative, diaphoretic, diuretic, stomachic, tonic, anti-inflammatory, antimicrobial, emmenagogue, antioxidant, antifungal, antiviral, analgesic

RANGE: Native across Canada

This coniferous evergreen is one of the most widely distributed across the world, including sixty species just in the Northern Hemisphere. In Canada, they grow mostly as shrubs from 0.9 to 1.2 m. in height, although they have been known to reach 9 m. Its use as a purifying herb began with the ancient Greeks and continued in Europe where it was highly regarded as a kidney tonic. The Egyptians also used it in their mummification process. The Common variety usually used medicinally has needle-like leaves that grow in whorls of three around the branch, and unlike other varieties such as Creeping Juniper, they do not become scale-like as they mature. The bark is reddish-brown and peels off in thin, vertical strips. Its resinous, fragrant berries, the part primarily used as medicine, are actually female cones that take three years to mature, turning a dark blue with a powdery coating when ready to harvest, usually in the fall. They can be eaten raw, tasting a bit like gin, or they can be dried and ground as flavouring or medicine.

MEDICINAL USES:

Urinary tract infections, liver stagnation, digestive problems, diabetes, gout, menstrual cramps, colds and flu, coughs, burns

- Berries are a powerful diuretic; clear bladder and kidneys of excess uric acid, cleanse and strengthen the kidneys and remove kidney stones. Useful in the treatment of urinary tract infections due to antimicrobial action. Relieves gout, arthritis, and joint pain.
- Useful when there is "dampness" and congestion, with a coating on the tongue. Warms and dries up mucous as in colds, flu, and sinus infection and bronchitis. Helps relieve coughs and clears phlegm, strengthens immunity.
- Aids sluggish digestion, expels gas, relieves heartburn, stimulates appetite. Where there is stagnation, it will stimulate the liver and gallbladder.
- Increases menstrual bleeding, avoid using if you have heavy periods.
- Externally, a poultice of leaves pounded to a paste may be applied to burns or boils, or to ease toothaches or sore gums.
- Dried berries are astringent, decoction may be used to clear acne, eczema, dandruff. Diluted essential oil rubbed on the skin warms and soothes arthritic joints.
- Testing with Chinese Juniper berries has shown it may have antidiabetic properties, lowering blood sugar levels in rats, but more research is needed on humans.

OTHER USES:
- Added to cooking meats, stews, sauerkraut, soups.
- Burned as smudge in Indigenous ceremonies to cleanse a space of negative energies.
- The Dutch use the berries to flavour their gin.
- A bush planted near the front door was once believed to repel witches.
- Can be used as a substitute for synthetic antioxidants to preserve meats.

INFUSION: Steep ½–1 tsp. powdered berries in 1 cup boiled water, covered, for 30 minutes. Strain and drink ½ cup 2–3 times a day

TINCTURE: Dried powdered berries 1:5 in 75% alcohol, take 2–3 ml., 2–3 times a day.

COMBINATIONS: For coughs and colds, may be combined with demulcents like Coltsfoot, Slippery Elm, or Marshmallow to reduce irritation of the kidneys. With Celandine to increase cleansing effect, Dandelion root for a gentle blood purification, Burdock root for more chronic conditions, and Cleavers for cooling inflammation and congestion.

RESEARCH: May reduce LDL (bad) cholesterol and increase HDL (good) cholesterol, reducing risk of heart disease. Has also shown a protective effect on nerve tissue, making it a potential alternative treatment in diseases like Alzheimer's, Parkinson's and other neurological disorders, but more human trials are needed. The flavonoids present in Juniper berries have been found to relieve inflammation by down-regulating the inflammatory stages of autoimmune diseases and arthritis.

CAUTION: Can be irritating to the kidneys. Consult a professional if you have kidney problems or are on medication for diabetes. Avoid if pregnant or breastfeeding. Not for use by children. Use only ripe berries. Essential oil can cause blistering if undiluted. May interact with some medications, particularly diuretics and lithium. Avoid taking larger doses than recommended or using for more than 4–6 weeks in succession.

LABRADOR TEA

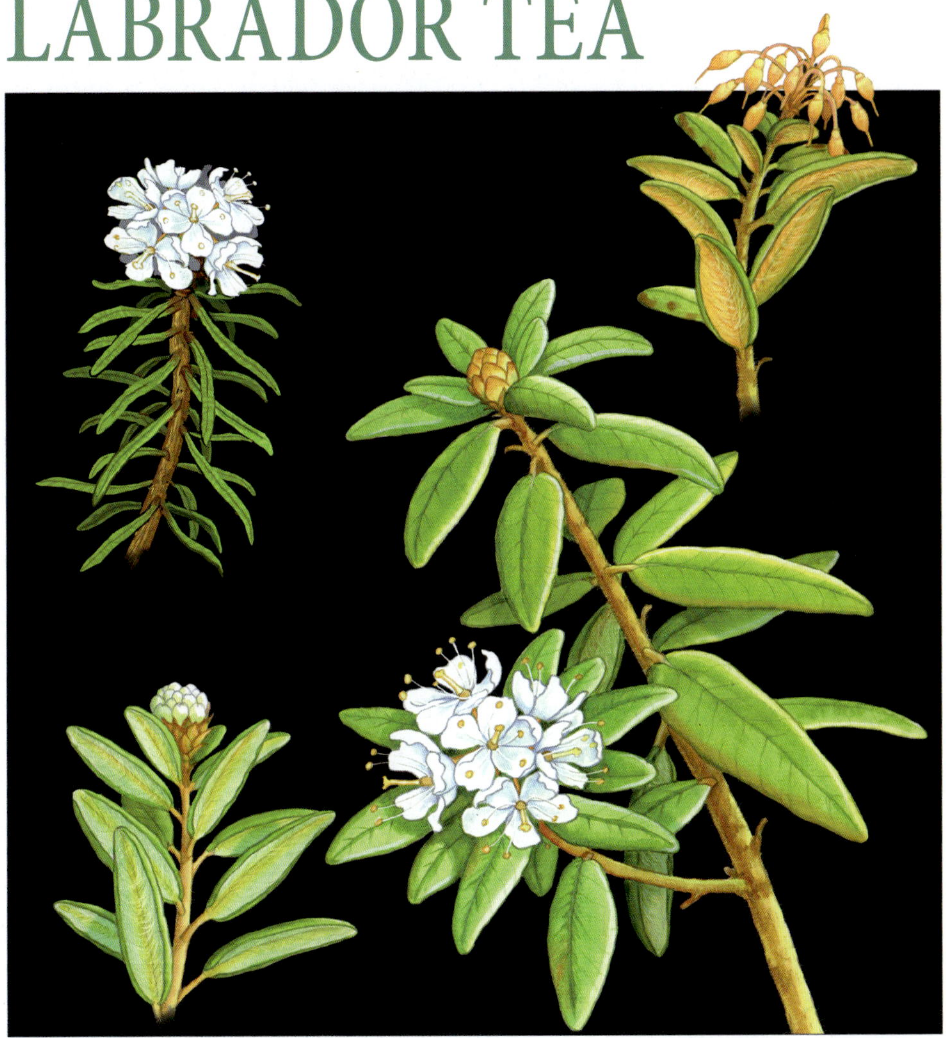

Rhododendron groenlandicum

FAMILY: Ericaceae

OTHER NAMES: Bog Labrador Tea, Muskeg Tea, Marsh Tea, Swamp Tea, Muskeg Herb, *Fr.* Thé du Labrador, Lédon de Groenland

PARTS USED: Leaves, flowers

CHARACTERISTICS: Spicy, fragrant

PROPERTIES: Tonic, diaphoretic, astringent, analgesic, diuretic, narcotic, insecticide, anti-inflammatory, antioxidant, antimicrobial, antifungal, antiviral

RANGE: Native across Canada

Labrador Tea is a native evergreen shrub that has long been used, both by Indigenous Peoples as a soothing tea and medicine, and by European settlers as a tea replacement during shortages throughout North America. It grows in bogs, moist forests, and along roadsides to a height of up to 1.5–2 m., with alternate elliptical leaves that are green and leathery on top and rusty coloured and woolly underneath. They droop slightly on the branch and their edges are rolled under. In June and July there are tiny clusters of white flowers that form on the end of each hairy stalk. The leaves can be collected at any time, but most herbalists usually wait until early fall, taking only a handful of leaves from the top of several different plants. They can be dried whole in a paper bag and chopped just before brewing.

MEDICINAL USES:

Respiratory infections, skin irritations, diabetes, headaches, kidney ailments

- Rich in essential oil, this fragrant tea has been used for centuries by many northern Indigenous Peoples. Its vitamin C content was also important for its role in preventing scurvy. It is most commonly used to treat colds, flu, diarrhea, respiratory infections, or stomach upsets, as well as for its diuretic action, its effectiveness at removing kidney stones and as a blood tonic. However, it should be used with caution due to its ledol and grayanotoxin content, which make it toxic in high doses, although less toxic than other similar species. Use internally only in infusions, and reserve decoctions only for external use.
- A poultice or a strong decoction may be used externally for burns, scalds, or wounds. Its astringent action also helps in cases of eczema or psoriasis, and may help get rid of scabies, ringworm, or lice.

OTHER USES:

- Leaves strewn in closets keep moths away.
- Tincture used to kill lice, mosquitoes, and fleas, repels mice.
- Brown dye obtained from plant.
- Used as flavouring in stews and marinades

INFUSION: Put a small handful of leaves in a pint of boiling water, turn heat down, and simmer 5–10 minutes. Drink no more than 2 cups a day.

RESEARCH: Was found to improve insulin sensitivity and diminish the effects of obesity and hyperglycemia on the health of some Cree diabetics when used as a complementary treatment. Studies show *R. tomentosum* may also be effective in treating acute myeloid leukemia using a variety of solvents to maximize extraction of ursolic acid and quercetin, believed to be responsible for its anti-AML activity. However, more studies are needed.

CAUTION: Do not boil tea if using internally. Brew for only a short period of time in an open container. Contains ledol, a toxic terpene which may cause headaches, cramping, or paralysis in high doses. Not recommended for pregnant or lactating women. Do not consume in excess as it is slightly narcotic.

LADY'S MANTLE

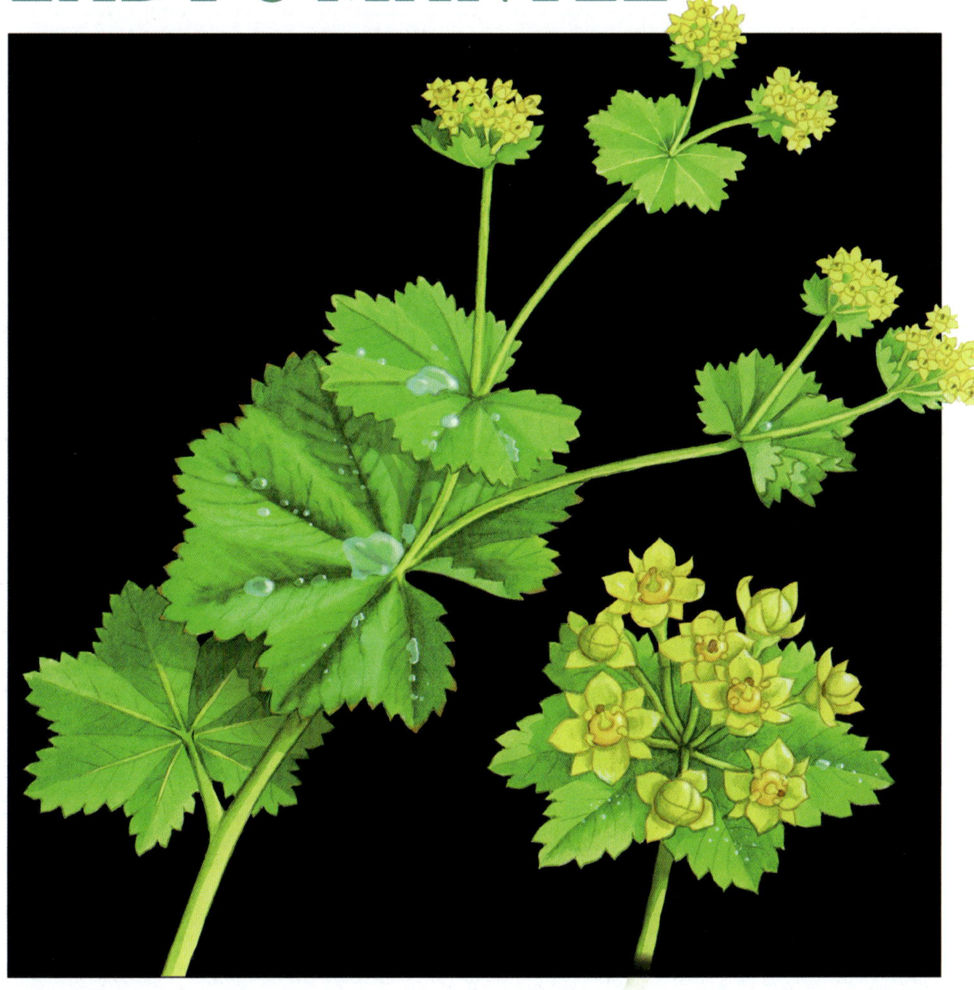

Alchemilla vulgaris

FAMILY: Rosaceae

OTHER NAMES: Dew-cup, Lion's Foot, Bear's Foot, *Fr.* Alchémille, Pied-de-lion

PARTS USED: Leaves and flowers

CHARACTERISTICS: Bitter, astringent, neutral, dry

ACTIONS: Astringent, depurative, emmenagogue, tonic, vulnerary, antibacterial, antifungal, antiviral, anticancer, antioxidant, neuroprotective, diuretic, uterine tonic

RANGE: Introduced in British Columbia, native and introduced (depending on variant) Ontario, Quebec, New Brunswick, Nova Scotia, Prince Edward Island, and Newfoundland and Labrador

Lady's Mantle is a low-growing meadow plant found in cool and wet climates around the world, but in Canada most are found in gardens or have escaped into the wild. It gets its name from the Arab word "alkemelych," meaning alchemy, which refers to the belief that the dewdrops that bead up on its leaves held magical powers of transformation. It is a perennial with an erect stem standing about 30 cm. high. The lower kidney-shaped leaves have 7 or 9 lobes, and are finely toothed at the edges; upper leaves are notched and toothed and folded somewhat like a fan. The small green/yellow flowers grow in clusters from June to August. The whole plant is covered with soft tiny hairs. The leaves and flowers should be gathered early in the summer and dried for later use.

MEDICINAL USES:

Heavy menstruation, wounds, prolapsed uterus, childbirth, arthritis, vaginitis

- This herb has been used for centuries, primarily as a woman's herb, but it is also a potent astringent, its compounds having a tonic effect on skin and weak tissues in the reproductive and digestive systems. Tannins modify and control outflow of fluids while salicylates relieve spasms and pain. Dries out damp tissues, toning, strengthening, and reducing inflammation.
- Restores tone in the female reproductive system, stimulates production of progesterone, which balances hormones to reduce heavy menstruation, cramps, and PMS, helps recovery from trauma to the uterus, miscarriage, IUD removal, endometriosis, prolapse, or childbirth. May reverse infertility, and strengthens the womb. A poultice of the leaves are soothing for engorged breasts after childbirth. Treats candida, leukorrhea, and vaginitis.
- Heals wounds, bruises, rectal tears, hemorrhoids, episiotomies. Reduces infections, dries, tones, and stimulates regeneration of skin cells and connective tissues.
- Tonic to the digestive tract, strengthens mucous membranes, assists digestion of fats, eases cramping, mild diarrhea, nausea, and indigestion.
- Mild diuretic, good for wet coughs, edema, fluid retention.
- A mild infusion can be used as an eye wash to reduce inflammation of conjunctivitis. A stronger infusion has been proven to be effective as a gargle or mouthwash for mouth sores or laryngitis.

FOLKLORE: This plant's name was once associated with the Virgin Mary, and dewdrops that gathered on its leaves were used in potions. The herb placed under a pillow at night was said to promote a good night's sleep. Connected to female creativity, it may be burned to overcome artistic blockages.

TINCTURE: Dried herb 1:5 in 25% alcohol, take 2–3 ml. in a little water, repeat every 2–3 hours if taking for excess bleeding, less often if using as a tonic.

INFUSION: 1–2 tsp. dried herb in 1 cup boiling water, infuse 10–15 minutes. Take 3 times a day.

COMBINATIONS: Used with Yarrow or Calendula for irregular periods, endometriosis, or postpartum problems. With Shepherd's Purse or Raspberry leaf as a uterine tonic. With Agrimony or Tormentil for digestive tract infection.

RESEARCH: Salicylates present in the aerial parts have been found to thin blood and increase circulation, having significant hypotensive effects. Also, forty-five active compounds have been found in Lady's Mantle that have free radical scavenging properties and the ability to suppress tumour cell growth. An ethanolic extract decreased the malignant potential of hormone-independant and estrogen-dependent tumours of the female reproductive organs.

CAUTION: Not recommended for use during pregnancy or lactation. Avoid use 2 weeks before surgery or if taking blood-thinning medication.

LARCH

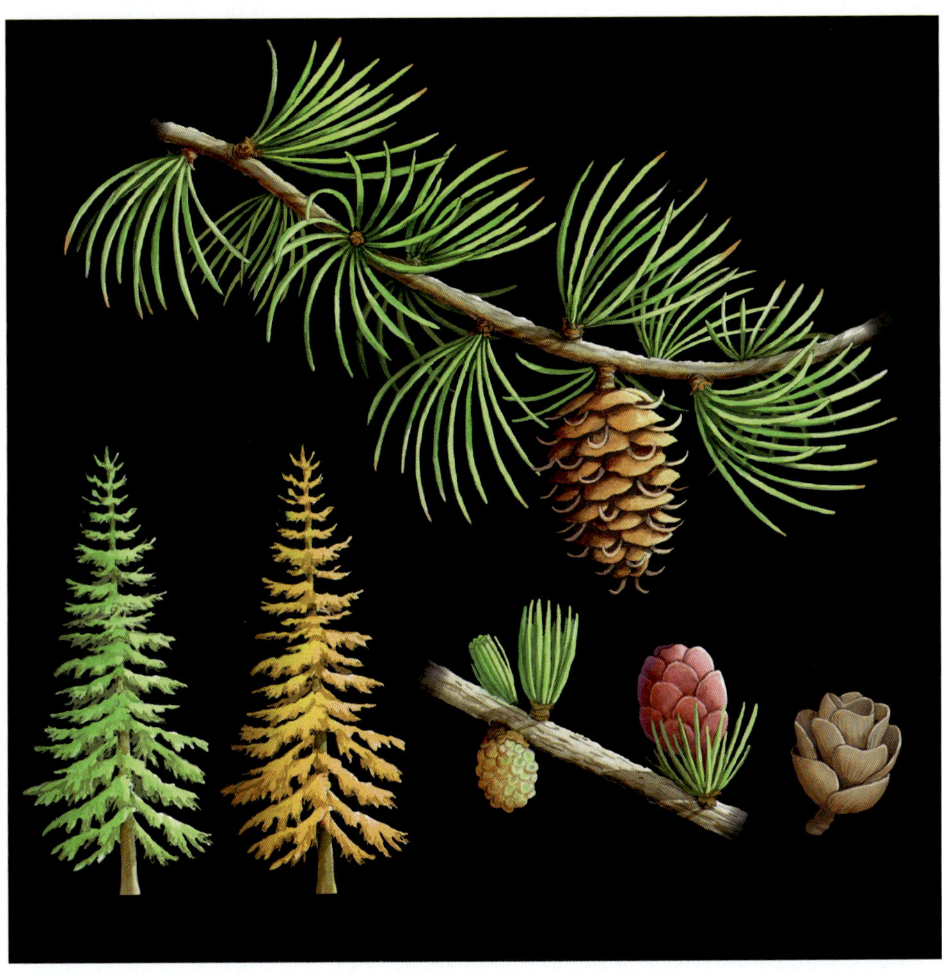

Larix occidentalis
Larix laricina

FAMILY: Pinaceae

OTHER NAMES: *L. occidentalis*: Western Larch, *Fr.* Mélèze de l'Ouest; *L. laricina*: Tamarack, Eastern Larch, Black Larch, Hackmatack, *Fr.* Mélèze laricin

PARTS USED: Resin, needles, bark, wood

ACTIONS: Alterative, antiseptic, anti-inflammatory, diuretic, expectorant, immune stimulant, laxative, vulnerary, probiotic, anticancer, anti-rheumatic

RANGE: *L. occidentalis* native to British Columbia, Alberta; *L. laricina* native across Canada

Larch or Hackmatack, derived from the Algonquin word *akemantak*, meaning "wood used for snowshoes," is a deciduous conifer that grows throughout most of Canada. Where other conifers remain green and keep their needles all year round, Larches turn bright yellow in the fall and lose their needles over the winter. They grow to a height of 20–60 m. depending on the species, and prefer sun and moist soil, tolerating cold temperatures. Western Larch, the largest of the Larches and most used medicinally, grows in the mountainous regions of western Canada. It is very fire-tolerant, its bark resistant to sparks. It often sheds its lower branches as it matures, and it can live for hundreds of years. Its needles are flat on top and ridged beneath, growing in clusters along the branch. Female cones grow above the male cones and vary between red and purple when young, appearing from May to July and maturing in the fall. Fresh green tips are best gathered in early spring.

MEDICINAL USES:

Wounds, coughs, colds, irritable bowel, cancer, chronic viral infections, ear infections, chronic fatigue

- An infusion of the gum of these unusual conifers was used traditionally for many years by Indigenous Peoples in the treatment of colds and tuberculosis. A decoction or poultice of the branch tips was used to wash and disinfect wounds, burns, and bruises, and the gum was chewed or made into teas for coughs or sore throats.
- Contains an excellent source of dietary fibre, Larch arabinogalactan (LA), which increases appetite, helps cancer patients gain weight, and boosts immunity. It improves stress-induced gastrointestinal problems and may hold promise in treating many diseases such as Alzheimer's, irritable bowel syndrome, and chronic fatigue.
- Decoction taken internally is effective against colds, flu, sore throats, and sinus and ear infections.
- Decoction of stem tips used as a soak reduces pain and stiffness of arthritis.

OTHER USES:

- Gum is a thickening agent, sap can be boiled down to make a syrup.
- Bark contains tannins, wood is used for building material, as it doesn't rot as fast as other wood.

SUPPLEMENTS (LARCH ARABINOGALACTAN): Typically 1,000–2,000 mg. per day; take as directed on the product.

DECOCTION: Leaves, stem tips, and gum, put a handful in a pan and cover with water, simmer covered for 20 minutes.

INFUSION: Gather fresh spring tips, cover with boiling water, and steep, covered, for 20 minutes. Drink as desired.

RESEARCH: Recent research has validated traditional uses, confirming not only that Larch reduces symptoms of colds by 23%, but also that it's anti-inflammatory, effective in stimulating the immune system and increasing the body's ability to defend itself against viral infections. The wood contains Larch arabinogalactan (LA), a polysaccharide and rich source of dietary fibre in the form of a white powder extracted from the wood, particularly the Western Larch. An effective prebiotic, it resists digestion by enzymes in the saliva and small intestine and enters the large intestine intact, where the microflora slowly ferment it, promoting the growth of beneficial microflora such as *Bifidobacterium* and *Lactobacillus acidophilus*. It stimulates natural killer cell cytotoxicity against tumour cells, and increases macrophages, T-cells, and the release of interferon, which inhibits the metastasis of tumour cells in the liver and enhances immune function. This could make it a potent support in the treatment of cancer, in preventative medicine, and to treat chronic viral infections and other diseases.

CAUTION: Immune stimulant. Avoid if you have an autoimmune disease such as Lupus, Crohn's, or rheumatoid arthritis. Might decrease the effectiveness of medications that suppress the immune system. Avoid if pregnant or breastfeeding as there is currently no information on safety.

LEMON BALM

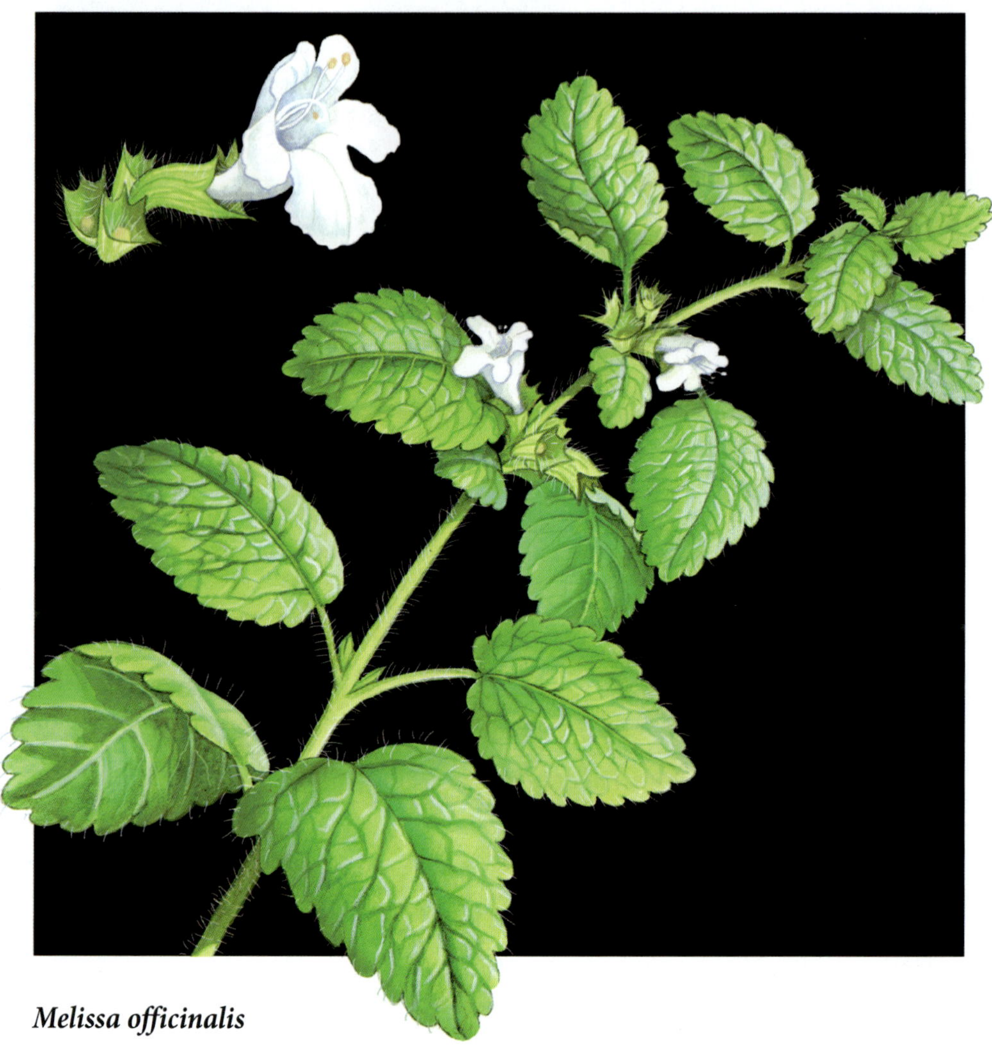

Melissa officinalis

FAMILY: Lamiaceae

OTHER NAMES: Sweet Balm, *Fr.* Mélisse

PARTS USED: Leaves

CHARACTERISTICS: Sour, spicy, cool

ACTIONS: Diaphoretic, antimicrobial, antispasmodic, carminative, emmenagogue, stomachic, febrifuge, nervine, sedative, antiviral, aromatic

RANGE: Introduced in British Columbia, Manitoba to New Brunswick

A native of southern Europe, this perennial now grows all over the world, although here it is mostly found in gardens or old homesteads rather than in the wild. The name Melissa stems from the Greek word for honey, and was probably used because of bees' attraction to it. It grows from 30 to 60 cm. high and has fine hairs; the leaves are opposite, oval, and wrinkled with scalloped edges, and when rubbed give off a lemony scent. The stem is square and branched, the flowers appear in small bunches around the leaf axils and bloom from June to October. The plant dies down in winter but the root is perennial. Harvest in the afternoon in early summer when the aromatic oils are strongest. Best if tinctured fresh.

MEDICINAL USES:

Stress, insomnia, indigestion, wounds, cold sores, hyperthyroidism, tension headaches

- Popular in traditional medicine throughout history, Lemon Balm was once described as a herb that "causeth the mind and heart to become merry and reviveth the heart," and it still holds true as it is one of the most effective at uplifting the spirits and relieving anxiety. Has a tonic effect on the heart, slightly lowering blood pressure and easing tension, depression, and palpitations. Promotes relaxation and helps calm the mind, ease muscle spasms, and when combined with other herbs, will help sleep due to its calming effect.
- Soothes upset stomach especially where there is anxiety, relieves gas, and promotes appetite. Drink a tea before meals to help digestion.
- Used by Indigenous Peoples in preparations for colds, fever, and chills; it induces perspiration.
- Antiviral, it is used in ointments to prevent and relieve cold sores, herpes lesions. Heals open wounds and ulcers and stops bleeding.
- Leaves steeped in wine were once used to relieve insect bites and stings.
- A mild carminative, it settles a nervous stomach and reduces colic in babies. Its antispasmodic and nervine properties make it effective for tension headaches and menstrual cramps when there is stress involved.
- Often used by herbalists for hyperthyroid conditions and Graves' disease.
- Improves cognitive function and clears the mind, both in healthy people and those with dementia.

OTHER USES: Can be used in pesto, or as a flavouring for soups, beverages, or salads. Makes an effective bug spray.

INFUSION: 1 tsp.–1 tbsp. herb in 1 cup boiling water, steep covered for 15–20 minutes.

TINCTURE: Fresh plant 1:2 in 50–75% alcohol, dried 1:5 in 30–50% alcohol, take 1–2 ml. as needed.

CALMING TEA:

- 4 parts Lemon Balm
- 3 parts Chamomile
- 2 parts Skullcap
- 1 part Motherwort
- Use 2–3 tsp. to 1 cup boiling water. Steep for 10 minutes.

COMBINATIONS: With Fennel and Chamomile for a colicky baby, taken before breastfeeding. For hyperthyroidism, add Bugleweed and Motherwort. For herpes lesions, combine with Licorice and St. John's Wort and use in a compress or salve. To calm stress, use with Motherwort or Skullcap and to promote sleep add Valerian, Chamomile, or Hops.

CAUTION: Avoid if you have low thyroid function (hypothyroid). Otherwise, generally considered safe.

LOBELIA

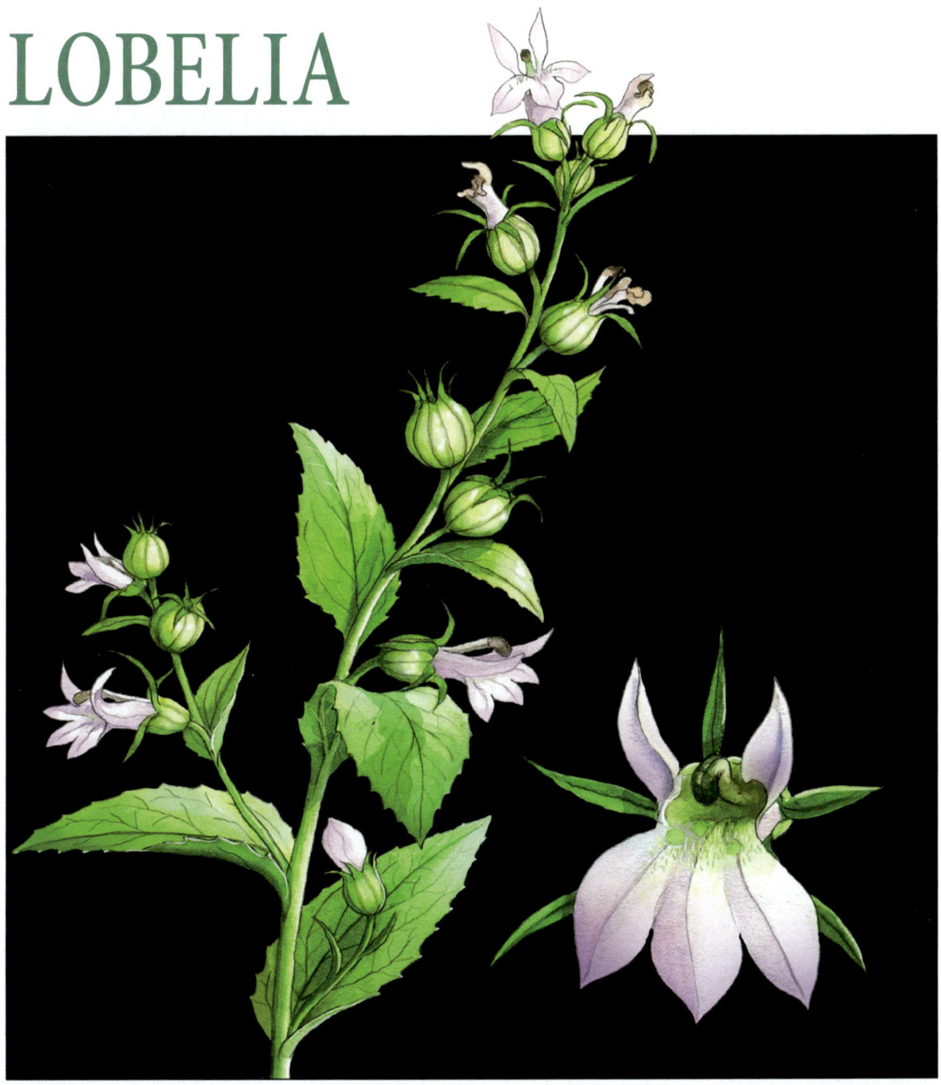

Lobelia inflata

FAMILY: Campanulaceae

OTHER NAMES: Indian Tobacco, Asthma Weed, Puke Weed, Gagwort, *Fr.* Lobélie gonflée

PARTS USED: Leaves, seedpods (twice as potent)

CHARACTERISTICS: Bitter, warming, tingling, drying, pungent

ACTIONS: Antispasmodic, antitussive, anti-asthmatic, diaphoretic, diuretic, expectorant, emetic, respiratory stimulant, mild sedative, relaxing nervine, sialagogue

RANGE: Introduced in British Columbia, native from Ontario to Maritimes

Lobelia is a controversial herb often known by the names Pukeweed or Gagwort, giving us a clue to its powerful emetic properties. However, its real talent lies in its use as an antispasmodic, particularly in cases of asthma or dry, spasmodic coughs. One of the most disputed herbs in the world, it is either feared as being highly toxic and even deadly, or regarded as a miracle herb that can cure even the most hopeless cases. Its use began with Indigenous Peoples of North America, but its popularity in western herbalism started in the 1800s with Samuel Thomson, who claimed it was a "diffusive" that could clear blockages in the life force, arousing or sedating, depending on what was needed. It has a tendency to enhance the effects of other medicines when used in small amounts in compounds, directing them to where they need to go. This is a herb that should not be used by anyone unless they are experienced in its correct and safe use.

An erect annual/biennial that grows 30–60 cm. high, its slightly hairy stem is simple or branched with delicate lavender, pale blue, or white tubular flowers in terminal clusters. Its leaves are alternate, toothed, and lance-shaped. The fruit forms inside a globular "inflated" capsule that splits open when ripe. They should be harvested after these pods have appeared but before they split, and dried for later use. It loses its potency rather quickly once dried. Store out of sunlight.

MEDICINAL USES:

Asthma, dry spasmodic coughs, bronchitis, food poisoning, stings, body aches, stiff neck, smoking addiction, COPD, muscle cramps, tension headaches

- Modern herbalists have found this herb to be one of the most valuable diffusive relaxants available, working on all parts of the body to reduce tension and relax the muscles. This can be particularly valuable in cases of dry, spasmodic coughs, as it stimulates mucous secretion and expectoration, reducing bronchial spasm and dilating bronchial passages. It eases asthma and bronchitis, pneumonia, croup, pleurisy, and whooping cough.
- Diffusive relaxant, it can equalize the circulation of blood, reaching almost every tissue in the body and influencing the nerves and muscles, relieving all types of pain due to muscle spasm. Mild sedative, it slows respiration and lowers arterial pressure and vascular tension.
- Potent emetic, it will induce vomiting if used in too large a dose.
- Once used to quit smoking, it contains lobeline, a nicotine-like substance that is not addictive; however, if used along with tobacco products, Lobelia's toxic effects may be enhanced, so it is not recommended.
- Relatively safe when used topically in the form of liniments or poultices. The fresh stems, leaves and flowers can be mashed and folded into a piece of cheesecloth and placed on the skin with a hot water bottle on top. The herb penetrates into cramped muscles or chest to ease spasms. You can also use dried herbs, moistening with hot water. The herb can also be made into tinctures and added to infused oils to rub on skin without risk of nausea. Be careful to wash hands after applying. Excellent for body aches, stiff muscles, tension headache, menstrual cramps, and coughs.

ACID TINCTURE: Put 3–4 tbsp. dried herb mix (leaves, flowers, small percentage of seedpods) in a mason jar, add 2 tbsp. raw, organic apple cider vinegar and ½ cup vodka. Cover and macerate in a dark place for 3–6 weeks. Strain into dropper jar and label. Start with 1 drop and titrate up from there for next dose until desired effect is achieved, stop if nausea occurs. Do not exceed 10 drops per day.

COMBINATIONS: Equal parts Lobelia tincture, Cramp Bark tincture, and Almond oil make a good massage oil for chest constriction, muscle cramps, and tension headaches. May be combined with Skullcap for mental tension, or Wild Yam for abdominal congestion.

CAUTION: Contraindicated for use with heart disease, wet coughs with heavy phlegm, low vitality, pregnancy and lactation, inflammatory bowel, or tobacco sensitivity. Side effects may include nausea, extreme vomiting in too-large doses, diarrhea, tremors, rapid heartbeat, mental confusion, and dizziness. Begin with low doses and increase slowly as long as it's tolerated. Do not exceed 1 ml. at a time. Internal use should be only under care of a professional.

MARSHMALLOW

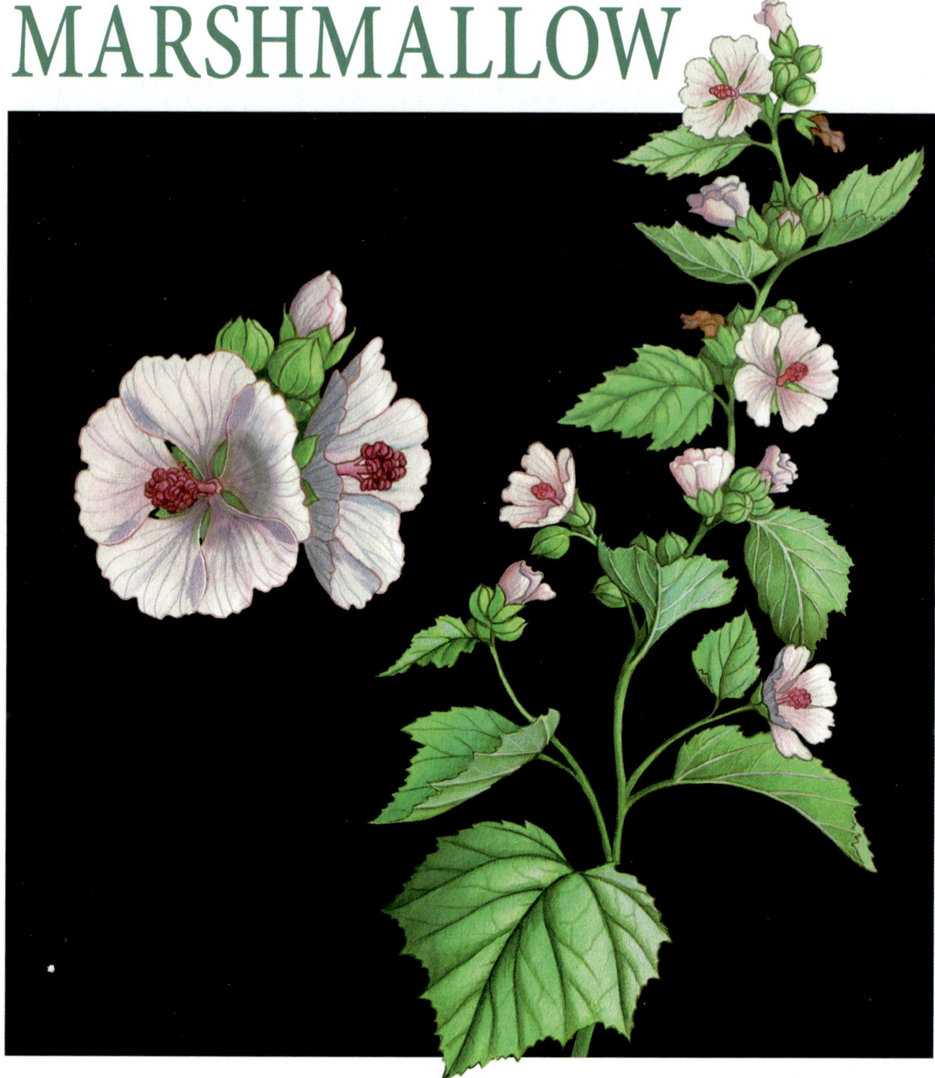

Althaea officinalis

FAMILY: Malvaceae

OTHER NAMES: White mallow, *Fr.* Guimauve

PARTS USED: Leaf, flowers, root

CHARACTERISTICS: Cool, moist, sweet

ACTIONS: Demulcent, alterative, diuretic, vulnerary, mild laxative, emollient, expectorant, antibacterial, anti-inflammatory, antioxidant, carminative

RANGE: Introduced Ontario and Quebec

This tall perennial has been used for centuries all over the world as a vegetable, but is also one of the most treasured healing herbs available. The treats we buy today with the same name no longer contain any trace of the plant, but in the early 1800s in France, there was a confection called Paté de Guimauve, which was a spongy square made from the plant's gooey root sap along with whipped egg whites and sugar that eventually evolved into our modern campfire treat.

The erect stems can be up to 1.5 m. tall, with alternate, irregular-toothed leaves that are soft and velvety on both sides. The round flowers are pale pink or white with a darker pink centre and 5 petals. The roots are white and mucilaginous, tasting somewhat like parsnip. It typically thrives in damp places, such as marshes—as its name suggests—but is now almost exclusively grown in the dry soil of cultivated gardens. Plants should be at least 2 years old before using as medicine. Flowers are best used just as they are coming into bloom in mid to late summer. Leaves should be picked on a dry day and the root should be harvested in the fall.

MEDICINAL USES:

Soothes mucous membranes of digestive, urinary, and respiratory tracts; reduces skin inflammation

- The compounds in Marshmallow are ideal for soothing irritation and inflammation. The root contains 10–30% mucilage and forms a coating on tissues to soothe, cool, and moisturize. Often added to warmer, more active herbs to moderate their harshness and make them easier to take. Best when taken in a lukewarm decoction, as alcohol and temperatures over 60°C reduce its effectiveness.
- Because of its mucilaginous properties, an infusion made from the leaves can help relieve a dry cough, asthma, and bronchitis, as well as soothing the mucous membranes of the throat and mouth, forming a protective layer over inflamed tissue. The flowers can also be used to make a cough syrup.
- A cold decoction of the root eases heartburn, indigestion, ulcers, and since the mucilage reaches the colon, it can help with ulcerative colitis and Crohn's disease. Mix with peppermint or Ginger for a soothing tea.
- The root is also good if taken as a decoction at the first sign of cystitis to speed healing.
- A peeled root may be used as a chew stick for teething infants.
- Powdered dry or crushed fresh roots can be used externally in a warm poultice for skin irritations, boils, burns, sores, and minor wounds; reduces inflammation and speeds healing. Added to creams or salves to treat eczema or contact dermatitis. Fresh leaves may be applied to bee stings. A warm poultice can reduce breast engorgement in lactating women.

COLD DECOCTION: Soak 2 tbsp. Marshmallow root (fresh or dried) in cold water for half an hour, then peel and cut into small pieces. Let peeled root stand in the water for another 2 hours. Sweeten mixture with honey and drink lukewarm. Good for coughs, indigestion.

CAUTION: Marshmallow tends to coat the stomach lining, so it may interfere with absorption of other herbs or drugs. Best taken several hours before or after taking other medications. May decrease blood sugar. Talk to a doctor before taking if you have diabetes.

MAYAPPLE

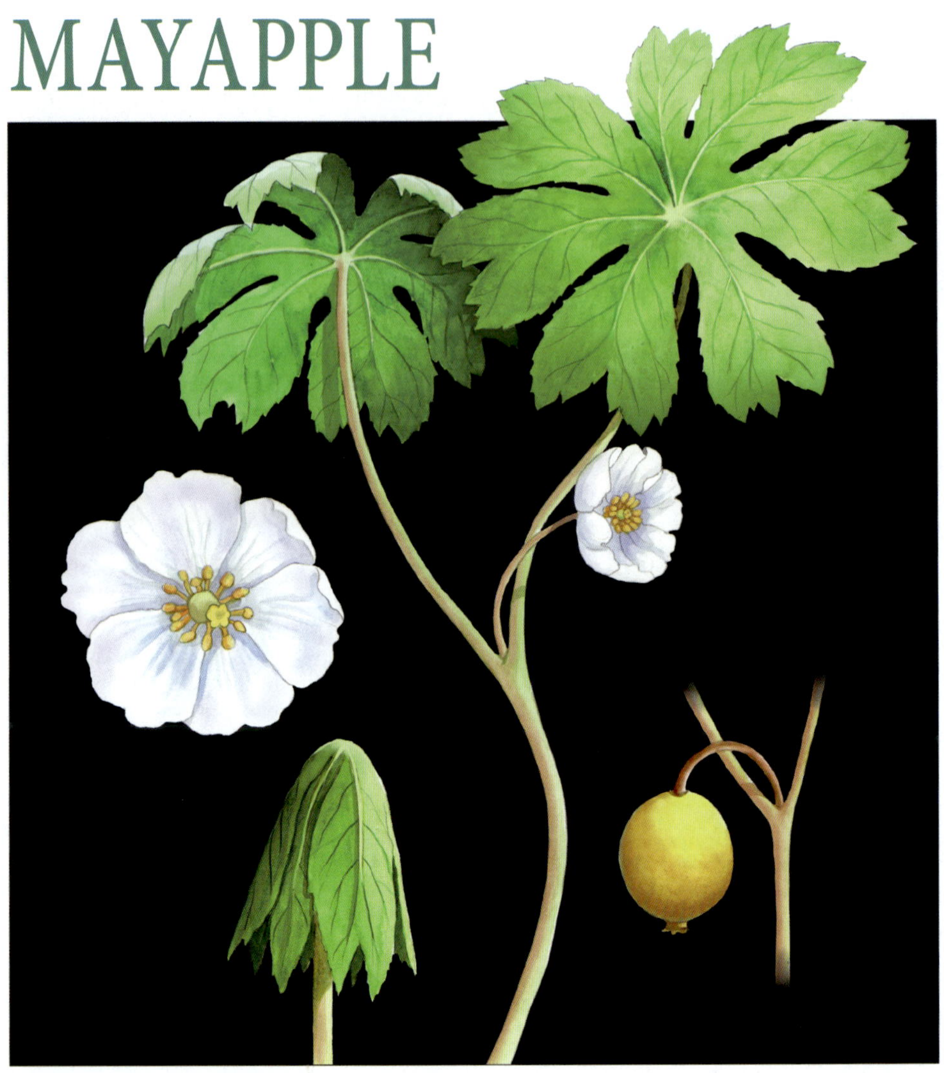

Podophyllum peltatum

FAMILY: Berberidaceae

OTHER NAMES: Wild Mandrake, Indian Apple, *Fr.* Pomme de mai

PARTS USED: Rhizome

ACTIONS: Antiviral, diuretic, laxative, purgative, emetic, anthelmintic, cholagogue, immunosuppressive, antioxidant, antispasmodic, antibacterial, antifungal, anticancer

RANGE: Native to Ontario, Quebec, Nova Scotia

The root was in common use by many Indigenous Peoples long before European settlers arrived in North America, despite its reputation as a powerful purgative, emetic, and even deadly poison. Easily recognized by its distinctive umbrella-like foliage, this perennial forms low-growing, dense colonies in meadows and woods and along roadsides. At first the leaves resemble a closed umbrella, only unfolding when it reaches a height of 30–45 cm. Its smooth stem is branched and its two deeply lobed leaves each spread to 15–20 cm. across. The single white or pinkish flower with yellow centre looks similar to an apple blossom, has a distinctive pungent odour, and grows out from the axil of the leaves. It is about 5 cm. in diameter with 6–9 waxy petals and typically blooms in May. The fruit, a single egg-shaped berry about 5 cm. long, matures in August, turning from green to yellow when ripe. Highly sought after by foragers for its sweet aroma and lemony flavour, but wildlife love them too so you'll have to beat them to it. The ripe fruit is the only edible part, the rest of the plant including the unripe fruit is highly toxic.

MEDICINAL USES:

Rheumatism, liver and gall bladder problems, genital warts, snakebites, skin diseases, cancer

- It has a rich history of traditional use by Indigenous Peoples for rheumatic pain, digestive problems, hemorrhoids, headaches, deafness, whooping cough, cholera, pneumonia, genital warts, worms, and snakebites, but it was used with a great deal of respect and care, and should not be used by anyone without the training to do so safely.

OTHER USES:

- Ripe fruit is used to make jams and jellies or added to beverages.
- The root soaked in water was used for sprouting corn or to kill potato bugs.

RESEARCH: This plant has recently sparked interest from pharmacologists and medical researchers because of its anti-inflammatory, antimicrobial, and immunosuppressive effects and ability to inhibit viral and cellular DNA replication, and subsequently its potential in treating various diseases like cancer and viral infections. The most active ingredient in Mayapple or *Podophyllum* resin is podophyllotoxin, a lignan with anticancer properties that has lead to developing new drugs like etoposide to treat testicular cancer, COVID-19, and small-cell lung cancer, and has been proven effective in the treatment of a range of other cancers such as non-Hodgkin lymphoma, leukemia, and various types of genital cancers. *Podophyllum* is also useful in treating herpes type 1 virus, genital warts, HPV, and measles, as its compounds limit the ability of the virus cells to replicate. There is undoubtably a great deal of potential in this plant, but continued research is essential to explore its benefits while paying special attention to using it safely and preserving sustainability.

CAUTION: All parts of the plant are toxic, particularly the roots and unripe fruit. Contains podophyllotoxin, which interferes with cell division and can cause nausea, vomiting, diarrhea, abdominal pain, confusion, hallucinations, seizures, liver damage, and even death. Its toxins can be absorbed by the skin particularly when applied to broad areas or in excessive doses. Wear gloves when handling and do not plant where exposed to children or animals. As with any herb containing toxic compounds, there is a fine line between a poison and an effective medicine. Should only be used under strict supervision of a healthcare professional.

MEADOWSWEET

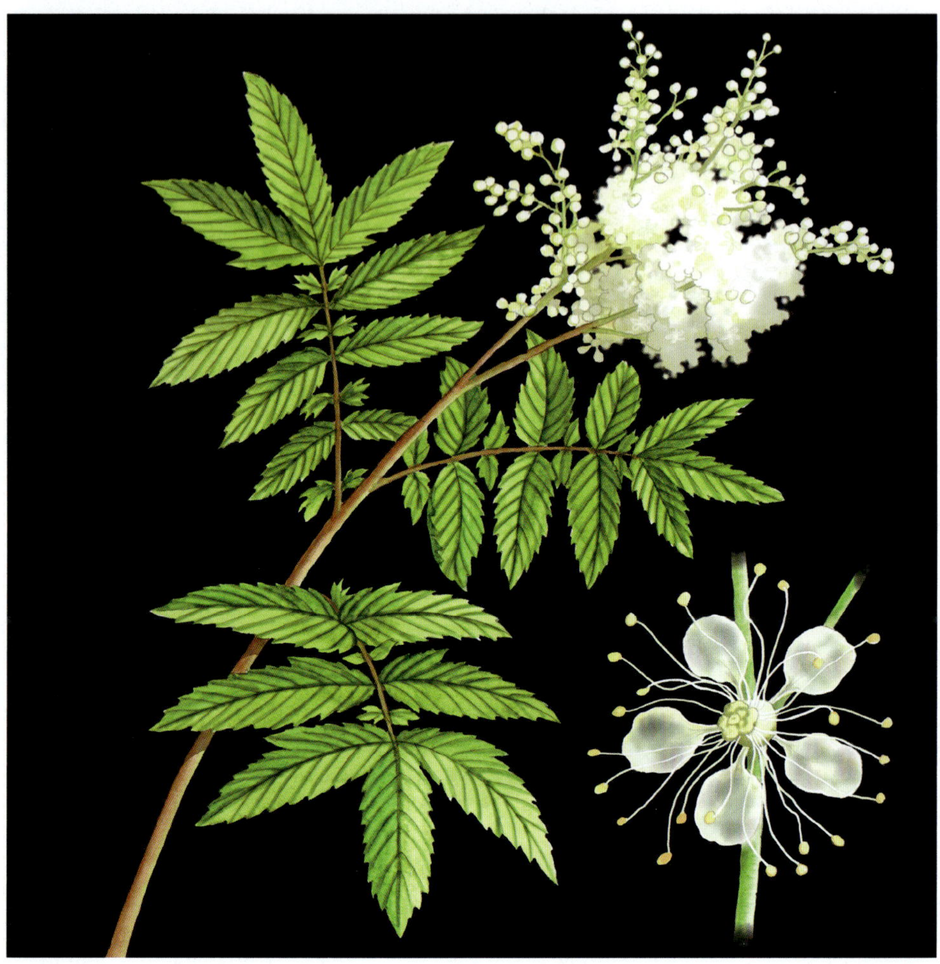

Filipendula ulmaria

FAMILY: Rosaceae

OTHER NAMES: Queen of the Meadow, Lady of the Meadow, Meadwort, *Fr.* Reine des prés

PARTS USED: Whole plant, especially flowering tops

CHARACTERISTICS: Sweet, slightly bitter, cooling, drying

ACTIONS: Antioxidant, anti-inflammatory, antispasmodic, analgesic, antibacterial, aromatic, anticoagulant, astringent, diaphoretic, diuretic

RANGE: Introduced in British Columbia, Ontario, Quebec, New Brunswick, Nova Scotia, Prince Edward Island, Newfoundland and Labrador

This perennial, native to Europe and Western Asia, has a history of use as a medicinal plant dating back to the fourteenth century. Renowned for the sweet aroma of its flower clusters, it was often added to bridal bouquets to bring joy and blessings to the bride, and was popular in love spells, potions, and enhancing psychic abilities. It is usually found in moist areas along riverbanks, in meadows and forests. Growing 0.9–1.8 m. high, its erect stems are furrowed and reddish to purple in colour, terminated by a delicate creamy white flower cluster or cyme. Top leaves are compound and serrated, with up to 5 pairs of leaflets and a 3-lobed leaflet at the tip, dark green on upper side and downy underneath. Flowers bloom from June through to September. Dry quickly to prevent mold from forming, preferably in an oven at a low temperature.

MEDICINAL USES:

Liver disorders, heartburn, flatulence, cystitis, gastritis, diarrhea, pain, arthritis

- An effective digestive aid, it soothes and protects the liver and membranes of the upper digestive tract and stomach lining. Reduces acidity, heals ulcers and heartburn, helps with GERD, acid reflux, gastritis, and its astringency makes it useful in treating diarrhea, especially in children.
- Flowering tops contain salicylic acid, the active component in aspirin that eases pain and reduces inflammation, but does not irritate the stomach like aspirin does. Helps relieve colds, headaches, arthritis, gout, muscle pain.
- Has demonstrated antimicrobial and antifungal activity against many pathogens, including candida, E. coli, and salmonella.
- May improve blood circulation.

INFUSION: ½–1½ tsp. dried herb in 1 cup boiling water (covered). Drink 3 times a day. (May take 6–8 hours to take effect)

TINCTURE: Fresh leaf and flower 1:2, 95% alcohol; dried leaf and flower 1:5, 50% alcohol, 30–60 drops, up to 3 times a day.

COMBINATIONS: With Slippery Elm, Licorice, and Aloe Vera for stomach complaints.

RESEARCH: Contains coumarin, tannins, salicylates, flavonoids, and terpenoids, which treat inflammatory diseases and act as antioxidants to fight tissue damage caused by free radicals. An extract was shown to have a considerable impact on decreasing colorectal tumours in rats and reducing tumour size and metastasis in Lewis lung carcinoma and vaginal and cervical cancers in mice. There have been no significant studies to date on humans.

CAUTION: Large doses may cause nausea and vomiting. Contains coumarin, which in high doses may prevent blood from clotting. Avoid if taking anti-coagulants or if you have a blood disorder. Generally considered safe in small or moderate doses. Not recommended for children under 18 or people with asthma.

MILK THISTLE

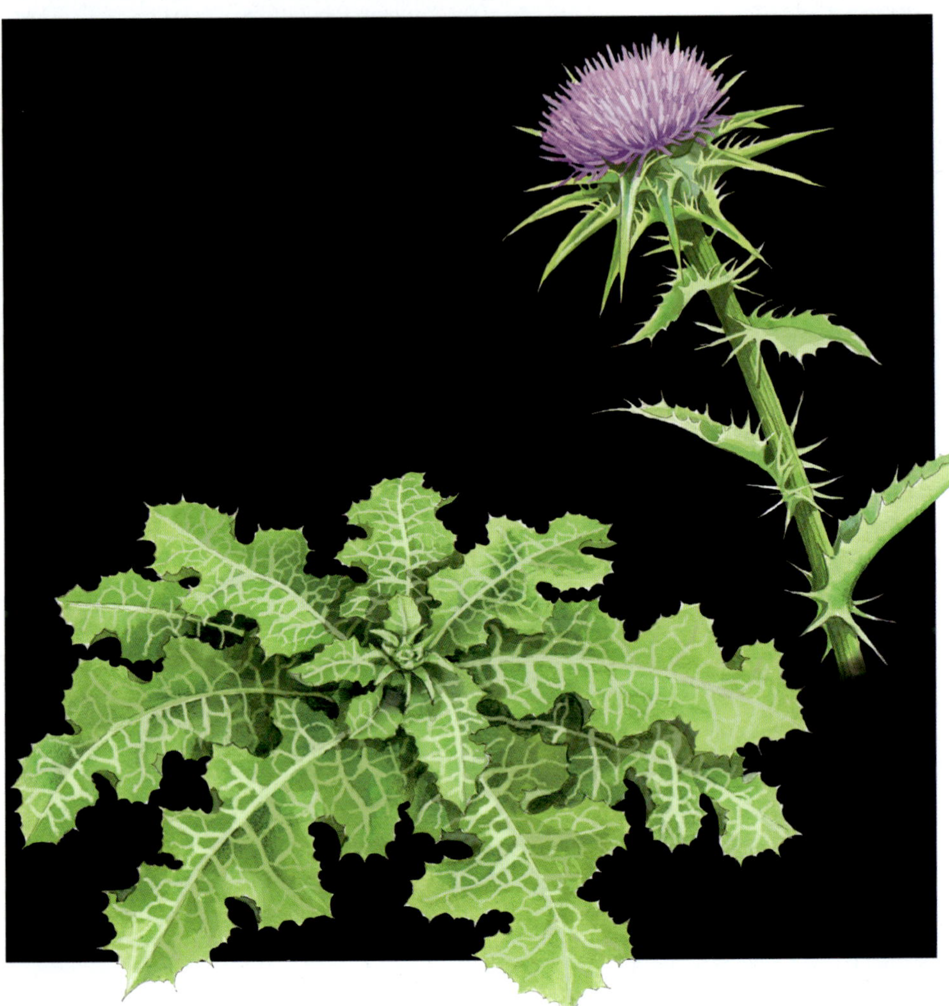

Silybum marianum

FAMILY: Asteraceae

OTHER NAMES: St. Mary's Thistle, *Fr.* Chardon-marie

PARTS USED: Seeds, leaves, root

CHARACTERISTICS: Aromatic, sweet, warm, bitter

ACTIONS: Antioxidant, anti-inflammatory, astringent, cholagogue, diaphoretic, diuretic, galactagogue, demulcent, hepatoprotective

RANGE: Introduced in British Columbia, Alberta, Saskatchewan, Ontario, Quebec, New Brunswick, and Nova Scotia

Milk Thistle, or St. Mary's Thistle, has been used for thousands of years throughout Europe and the Middle East as a liver remedy. Large and distinctive, its spiny leaves are marbled with white veins that were said to be the milk of the Virgin Mary, hence it its name. It can grow up to 1.5 m. tall, and its magenta-coloured flowers appear at the top of the stems from April to October. Spiny bracts surround the flowers and give them a star-like appearance. It's considered a noxious weed in some areas, as it can be toxic to cattle and sheep, especially when grown in nitrate-rich soil. It should be harvested only from organic areas that have not been used for farmland or treated with pesticides. Should not be confused with Blessed Thistle (*Cnicus benedictus*), which is a different species from the same family, and has red or yellow flowers and different medicinal properties.

MEDICINAL USES:

Liver, spleen and kidney congestion, mushroom poisoning, alcohol and drug abuse, low milk production

- One of the best liver remedies available, it contains silymarin, which has been studied extensively for its anti-inflammatory and antioxidant activity and free radical scavenging. Proven to be effective at regenerating liver cells and protecting them from toxins. Its antioxidants increase the resiliency of liver cells, it stimulates bile production, relieves congestion in the liver, reduces inflammation in the gallbladder, and assists digestion of fats.
- Commonly used in cases of liver disease, fatty liver, cirrhosis, hepatitis, and indigestion. Prevents toxic substances from damaging liver cells and helps to expel them, making it effective in alcohol and drug abuse cases. It repairs damage from junk food, chemical pollution, or other threats to normal liver function and promotes more effective detoxification. Can reduce the toxicity of Amanita mushroom poisoning.
- Helps to repair and regenerate protein enzymes and DNA in kidney cells.
- Enhances the flow of breast milk.

OTHER USES:

- All parts are edible, however the thorns need to be removed from each leaf.
- 1–2 tsp. ground seeds per day may be added to smoothies. Reduce dose if it causes diarrhea.

DECOCTION: 1–2½ tsp. dried seeds in 1 cup boiling water, simmer 15–20 minutes. Drink up to 3 times a day.

TINCTURE: Seeds 1:3 in 70% alcohol, ½–1 tsp. up to 4 times a day. Dosage will depend on the severity of the condition. Consult a professional for more severe liver problems.

COMBINATIONS: May be used with Celandine, Dandelion root, Barberry, Burdock root, and Golden Seal for liver support.

CAUTION: Generally safe, but use only organic seed from a reputable dealer. May interfere with some medications, consult your healthcare provider.

MILKWEED, PLEURISY ROOT

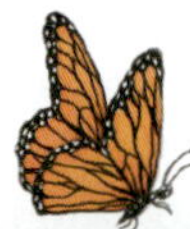

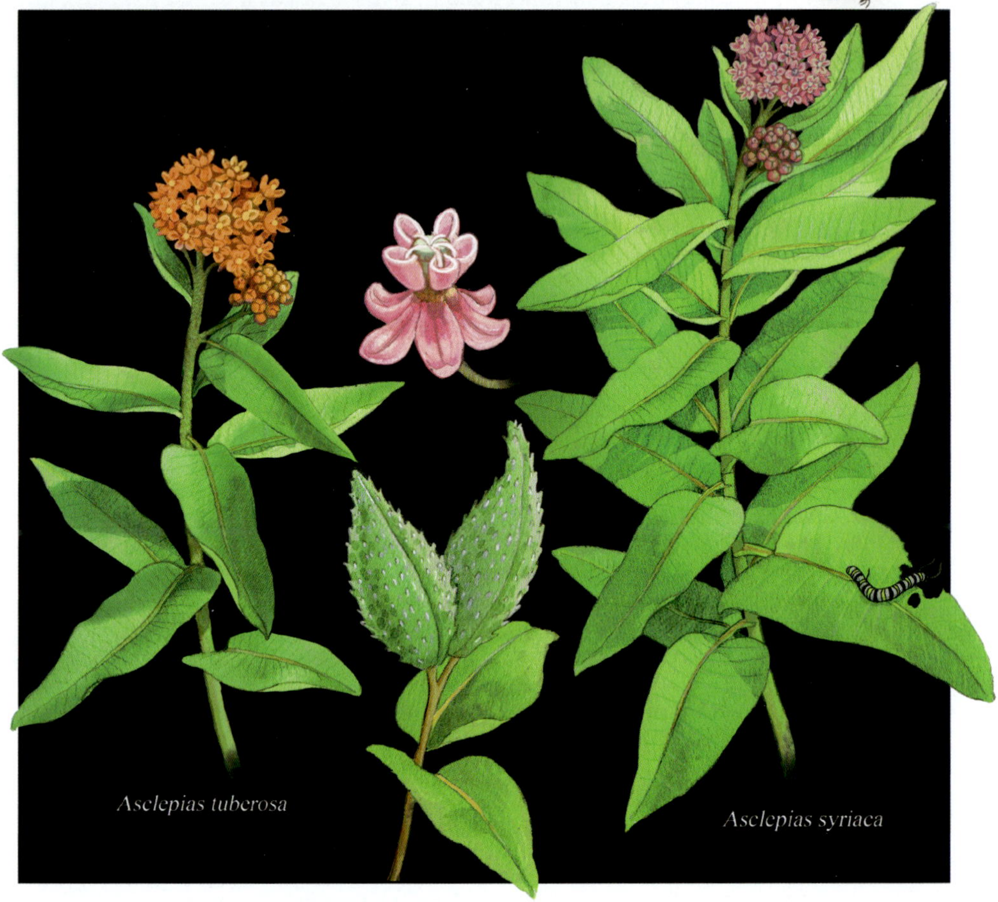

Asclepias tuberosa

Asclepias syriaca

Asclepias syriaca (Common Milkweed)
Asclepias tuberosa (Pleurisy Root)

FAMILY: Apocynaceae

OTHER NAMES: *A. syriaca:* Common Silkweed, Cottonweed, *Fr.* Herbe à la ouate, Cochons de lait; *A. tuberosa:* Butterflyweed, Orange Milkweed, *Fr.* Asclépiade tubéreuse

PARTS USED: Whole plant

ACTIONS: Diuretic, anodyne, emetic, purgative, alterative, tonic, diaphoretic, expectorant (roots also emmenagogue)

RANGE: *A. syriaca:* Native from Saskatchewan to Nova Scotia, introduced in Prince Edward Island and Newfoundland and Labrador; *A. tuberosa:* Native to Ontario, Quebec, New Brunswick, Nova Scotia, Newfoundland and Labrador

These colourful perennials are known for their attractiveness to monarch butterflies, whose caterpillars eat only the leaves and who lay their eggs on the plant. Chemicals in the plant make the insect distasteful to predators, so it protects it as well. The plant was once eradicated from many places due to its toxicity to farm animals, until it was discovered that the butterflies were dependant on it and were being eradicated as well. It grows in clumps beside roadways, waste places, and abandoned farms, 1–2 m. in height with an erect hairy stem and lance-shaped alternate leaves that are smooth on top and velvety underneath. Its showy composite flowers bloom from July through September in flat flower clusters at the top of the stem. They are followed by the growth of fleshy seed pods which are about 5–12 cm. long, grey-green and warty with prickles, and contain a wad of feathery down and flat brown seeds arranged in overlapping rows. The tough roots are collected in the fall after the second year of growth and are used either fresh or dried. Unlike its cousin Milkweed, Pleurisy Root does not have the milky sap and both can be toxic to humans, so it must be used with caution.

MEDICINAL USES:

Coughs, pleurisy, lower respiratory tract infections, indigestion, warts, insect bites, fever

- Despite its toxicity, both Indigenous Peoples and European settlers considered the fresh or dried root of this plant a valuable medicine, particularly for coughs and chest congestion, and if used in moderation it can be an effective remedy. It relaxes the bronchioles, reduces coughing and spasms, and liquifies mucus in the lungs, making it easier to cough up. Its antispasmodic, tonic, and anti-inflammatory actions are useful for pleurisy, bronchitis, asthma, whooping cough, and dry coughs where there is a build-up of thick mucus.
- To remove warts, the fresh milky sap of *A. syriaca* can be applied several times a day over a few weeks until the wart disappears. The plant can also be used as a poultice on eczema, burns, sores, bruises, and wounds, and warmed cooked stems ease the pain of arthritis.
- Strong diaphoretic, it induces sweating to bring down a fever, and stimulates circulation to the extremities. Particularly useful in eruptive diseases like chickenpox and measles.
- A tea made from the leaves can relieve indigestion, colic, or gas.
- Powdered root was used externally for venereal diseases, hemorrhoids, and snakebites.

OTHER USES:

- The young shoots (up to 20 cm. high) and young leaves before the flower buds form, the flower buds and soft seedpods (about 2.5 cm. long) are all edible if properly cooked. Place in boiling water, cook for 10 minutes, drain, rinse, and boil another pot of water, then place plant material in the freshly boiled water and cook again for 10 minutes. Do not use older plant parts, as they contain more toxins.
- Because of the strength of the stem fibres they have been used by various Indigenous groups to make cords and rope and weaving cloth.
- Silky tufts on the seeds are used to stuff pillows and clothing.

COLD INFUSION: Dried root, 1 tsp. in 1 cup water, infuse 4–8 hours, take ⅛–⅓ cup, up to 3 times a day.

TINCTURE: Dried root, 1:5, 50% alcohol, 1–5 ml. 3 times a day. Do not exceed 20 ml. per week.

COMBINATIONS: With Lobelia tincture in small doses for dry, constricted cough. For sinus congestion, combine with Eyebright and Chamomile. For fevers, may be used with Ginger or Yarrow.

RESEARCH: Research has shown that the seeds show promise in managing blood glucose levels, and could one day be used as a natural alternative for regulating diabetes, but so far there have been no human trials.

CAUTION: Milkweed species contain cardiac glycosides that are toxic to humans and animals, however the root is relatively safe. Do not use if you have a heart condition or high blood pressure or are on heart or hormone medications. Avoid if pregnant or breastfeeding. Older leaves are poisonous if consumed, may cause vomiting and diarrhea, muscle weakness, rapid weak pulse, or difficulty breathing in large doses. Consult your health care provider if you have ulcers or hiatus hernia due to emetic effects. Sap may cause dermatitis or eye irritation, wash hands thoroughly after use.

MINT

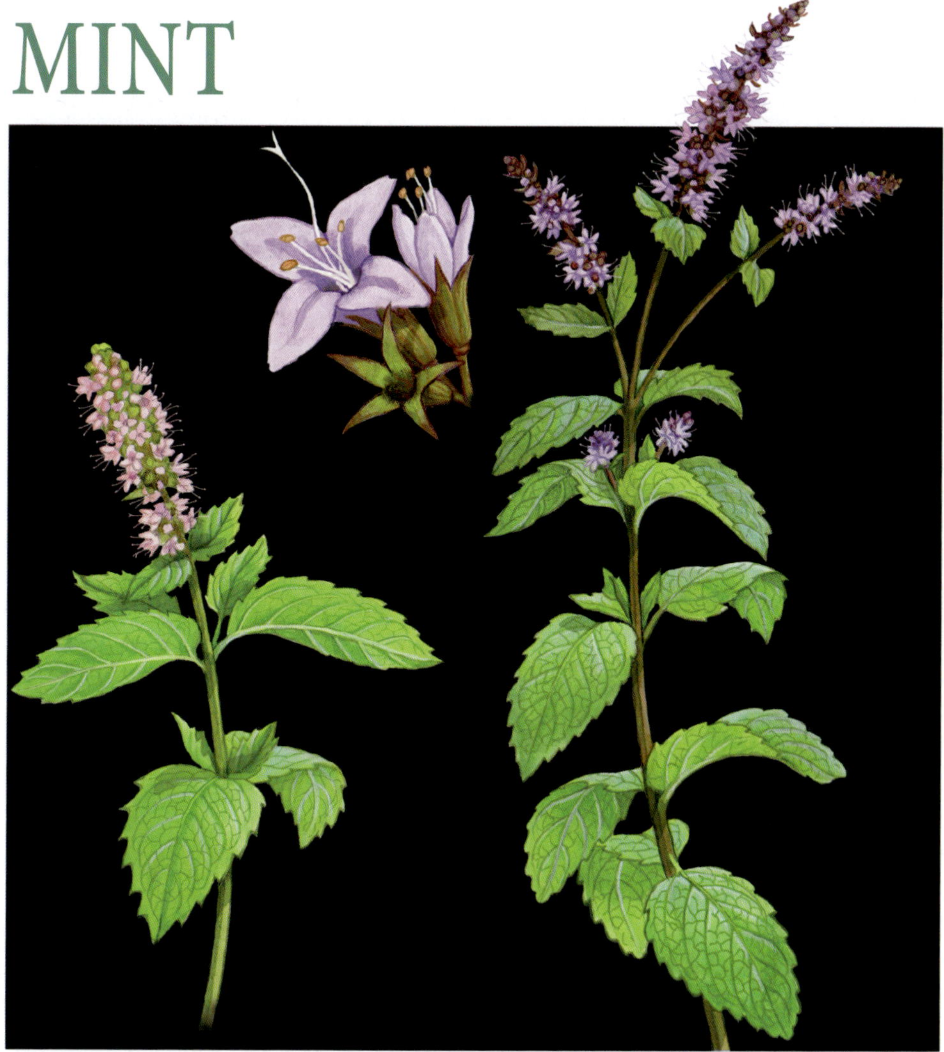

Mentha x piperita, Mentha spicata

FAMILY: Lamiaceae

OTHER NAMES: *M. x piperita:* Peppermint, *Fr.* Menthe poivrée; *M. spicata:* Spearmint, *Fr.* Menthe à épis

PARTS USED: Whole plant

CHARACTERISTICS: Cool, pungent, drying, aromatic

ACTIONS: Carminative, antispasmodic, antiviral, antibacterial, antioxidant, antihistamine, analgesic, aromatic, diaphoretic, antiemetic, nervine, antimicrobial, emmenagogue, relaxant, stimulant, antipruritic, anti-inflammatory, antifungal, anticancer

RANGE: *M. x piperita* introduced in British Columbia, Ontario, Quebec, New Brunswick, Nova Scotia, Prince Edward Island; *M. spicata* introduced across all provinces except Saskatchewan and Newfoundland and Labrador

Mint is a well-known invasive perennial easily identified by its familiar cooling aroma and taste. There are hundreds of varieties, but the two most popular are probably Peppermint (*M. x piperata*), a hybrid between Spearmint and Watermint and the one usually used in herbal medicine; and Spearmint (*M. spicata*), although many others grow wild throughout Canada. They are visually similar but with a slightly different taste and odour. Both grow up to just under 1 m. tall, with square stems and runners that spread quickly if not confined. They prefer damp, moist soils and have toothed, oblong leaves. The flowers are pink, mauve, or white, and grow in spikes throughout the summer. Harvest when the plants are in bloom and have the most flavour.

MEDICINAL USES:

Indigestion, upper respiratory ailments, colds and flu, sore muscles

- Mint has been used for thousands of years, particularly as a remedy for indigestion and other digestive tract disorders. It has a mildly sedative, analgesic, and antispasmodic action and cools inflammation, effectively soothing stomach upsets. The tea can relieve heartburn, nervous stomach, bloating, gastritis, and symptoms associated with overeating, stimulating digestive juices, and easing cramps. The aromatic essential oils help calm morning sickness and ease spasms associated with vomiting, and a drop or two on a sugar cube can relieve colic in children. Enteric coated peppermint oil can sometimes be more effective for IBS, Crohn's, or other intestinal issues, as it bypasses the digestive enzymes of the stomach. A few drops of oil mixed into Vaseline and rubbed under the nose can relieve sinus congestion.
- A hot infusion, usually combined with Elder flower, is effective at reducing fevers through sweating, and its vapours help decongest lungs and sinuses during colds and flu. Essential oils can be rubbed on the chest for upper respiratory congestion, on the temples to relieve headaches, or to soothe achy muscles.
- Spearmint, unlike Peppermint, is also diuretic and may be used in a warm infusion to reduce inflammation of a urinary tract infection.
- Topically, the essential oil is analgesic and can be useful in inflammatory skin conditions. Cools allergic itching, hot flashes, and neuralgic pain. May relieve nipple pain from breastfeeding.

OTHER USES:

- Leaves were once scattered around the house to repel vermin and rid the place of foul odours.
- Flavouring in toothpaste, candies, and beverages.

INFUSION: For colds and flu, place 2 tbsp. each of Peppermint and Elder flowers in a pot, pour in 3 cups of boiling water, cover and keep warm on low (do not boil) for 15 minutes. Strain and give ¼ cup every hour, keeping the rest covered and warm, until the patient is sweating. For digestion, use a standard infusion.

COMBINATIONS: May be used with Chamomile, Fennel, Ginger root, Caraway, Licorice root, or Marshmallow root for indigestion. With Boneset, Yarrow, or Elder flower for colds, flu, and fevers.

CAUTION: Avoid using more than 1–3 drops of Peppermint oil at a time, as it is highly concentrated and should be mixed with a carrier oil, especially in young children. May cause dermatitis in some people. Avoid taking internally if breastfeeding, as it may dry up milk. Avoid if you have GERD, as it may worsen symptoms.

MOTHERWORT

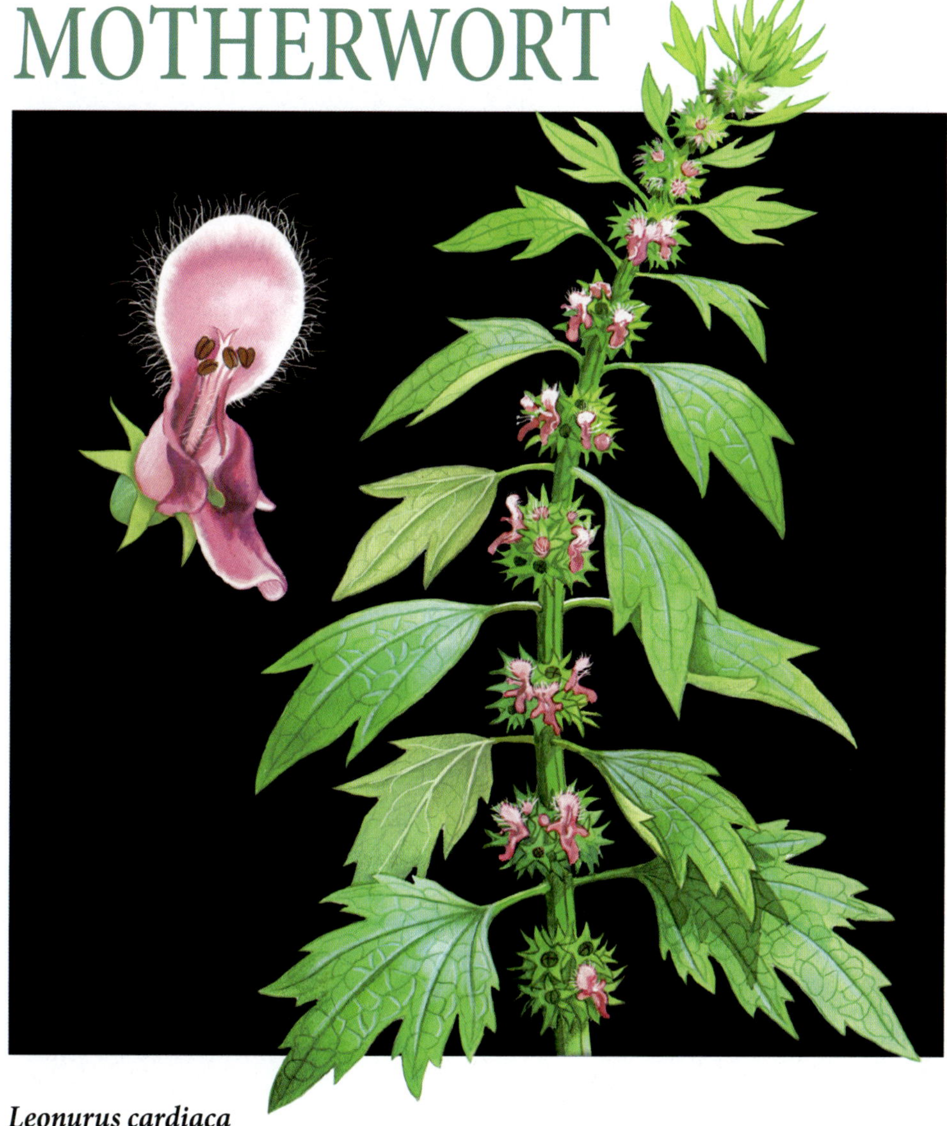

Leonurus cardiaca

FAMILY: Lamiaceae

OTHER NAMES: Lion's Tail, Heartwort, *Fr.* Agripaume

PARTS USED: Leaves and flowers

CHARACTERISTICS: Bitter, spicy, cool, pungent, dry

ACTIONS: Analgesic, sedative, emmenagogue, antispasmodic, cardiac tonic, hypotensive, nervine, diuretic, carminative, astringent, anti-inflammatory, aperient, febrifuge, diaphoretic, antidepressant, uterine tonic

RANGE: Introduced in all provinces except Newfoundland and Labrador

Motherwort is a perennial plant native to continental Europe. It has been grown since medieval times for its effectiveness in dealing with anxiety and "female disorders" (which then would have included anything from childbirth, menopause, menstruation, and "hysteria"), and even to promote longevity. It thrives in humus-rich soil and bright sun and can be cultivated from seeds or by root propagation in spring or fall. The erect, square stems are up to 1.5 m. tall, and are often red and slightly hairy. The leaves are opposite and have 3–5 pointed lobes, also slightly hairy, and greyish on the underside. The 3-lobed flowers appear in July or August and are pink or purplish, hairy, and grow in clusters at the leaf axils which become sharp and spiny after the flowers die. Motherwort may be collected when it blooms, before the seeds are formed, and dried for later use. Make sure to leave part of the stalk so as not to kill the plant.

MEDICINAL USES:

Menstrual problems, anxiety, palpitations, angina, menopausal symptoms

- As its name suggests, Motherwort is a classic remedy for women's problems, particularly for pain and menstrual disorders. It is classed as a uterine tonic, but when there is tension or anxiety, not just in women but in men as well, it also acts as a cardiac tonic, and helps release tension trapped in the chest that often leads to other problems like palpitations and angina. It reduces tension in the diaphragm, and helps to release emotional stress and relax breathing.
- Brings on suppressed menstruation, especially when there is anxiety or emotional distress. Relieves blood congestion, cramps, painful periods. Tonifies and relaxes.
- Tones the heart, eases palpitations, angina, tachycardia, and hypertension. Improves blood circulation and suppresses inflammation and oxidative stress. Can be useful for a racing heart in hyperthyroidism.
- Helps to improve mood and ease anxiety, grieving, or heartbreak. Eases migraines.
- Strengthens the uterus, preparing it for childbirth. Should only be taken before becoming pregnant as it can cause miscarriage. Can restore strength after childbirth as well. Use only under supervision of a professional.
- Aids hot flashes and other menopausal symptoms.

TINCTURE: Fresh plant 1:2, 60% alcohol, dried plant 1:5, 60% alcohol. Take 10–20 drops, increase until effect is felt, up to 60 drops, 4 times a day.

INFUSION: Dried herb, ½–1 tsp. in 1 cup boiling water. Drink as needed.

COMBINATIONS: May be used with Bugleweed and Lemon Balm to reduce cardiac symptoms of hyperthyroidism. Combined with Hawthorn, Skullcap, or Valerian, it may prevent and treat atherosclerosis, ease anxiety, and strengthen the heart.

CAUTION: Do not use during pregnancy, except during or after childbirth, and under supervision of a professional. Do not use if you have heavy menstrual bleeding or blood clotting disorders or are taking anti-coagulants.

MUGWORT

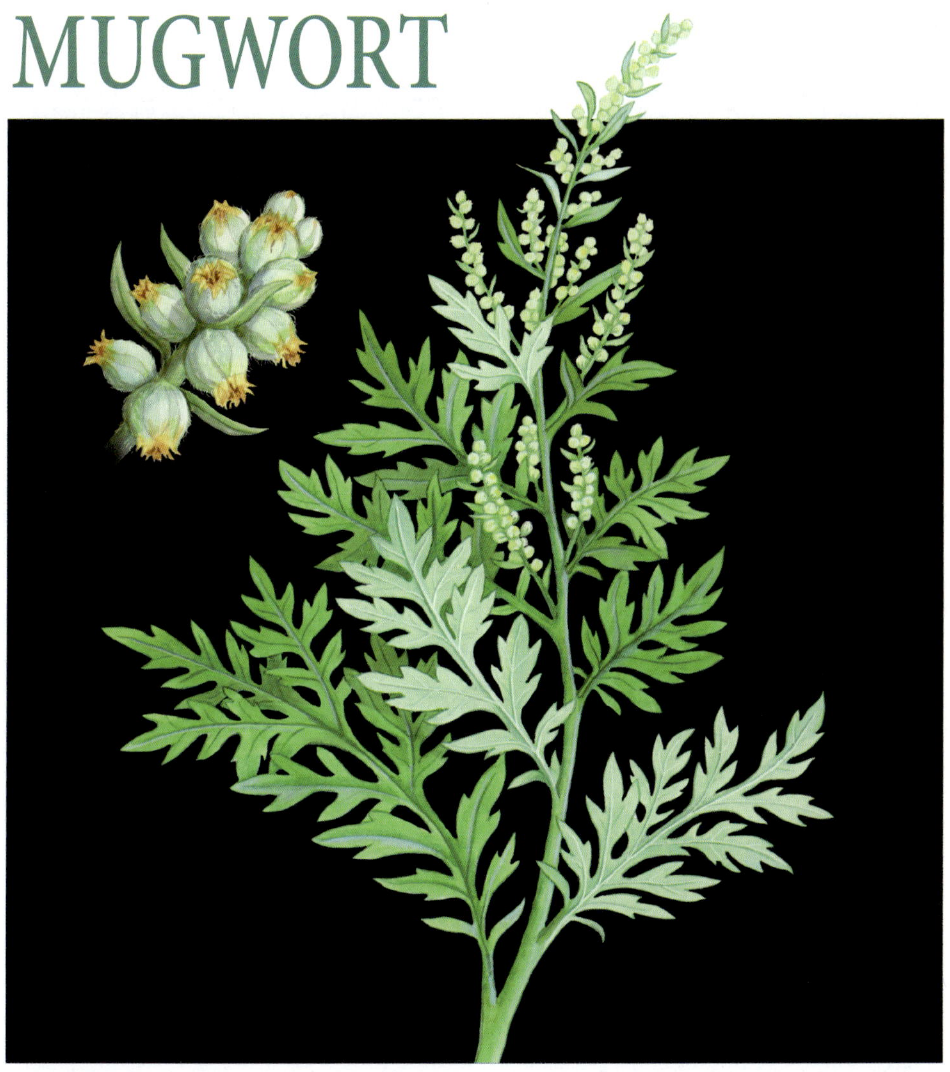

Artemisia vulgaris

FAMILY: Asteraceae

OTHER NAMES: Moxa, Felon Herb, St. John's Plant, *Fr.* Herbe Saint Jean, Armoise commune

PARTS USED: Leaves and roots

CHARACTERISTICS: Bitter, acrid, slightly warm, aromatic, astringent

ACTIONS: Cholagogue, vermifuge, emmenagogue, haemostatic, antispasmodic, diuretic, diaphoretic, mild narcotic, nervine, bitter tonic, carminative, alterative, hepatic, stimulant, stomachic, uterine tonic, anti-inflammatory

RANGE: Introduced across all Canadian provinces

Mugwort has had a long history of magic and protection in many parts of the world, especially for its influence on dreams. Native to Europe, Asia, and Africa, it has now spread to most of North America and is part of many Indigenous traditions and folklore. Growing up to 1.5 m. tall, it has green to purplish stems with smooth, pinnate leaves that are pointed, deeply cut, dark green on top and woolly and silvery-coloured underneath. Flowers are cottony and yellowish-green or reddish-brown in small oval heads growing on long terminal spikes.

It can easily be mistaken for Wormwood (*Artemisia absinthium*), which looks similar and has many similar medicinal properties, but there are a few differences. Wormwood has a very bitter taste, is more silvery in colour, and is aromatic and quite bushy. Its flowers are larger and yellow when in bloom. By contrast, Mugwort has very little scent, is only slightly bitter, and is taller and more slender. The leaves and flowers should be collected just before blooming, usually in August. Cut the top third of the plant and hang to dry. The roots can be harvested in the fall and dried whole.

MEDICINAL USES:

Painful or irregular periods, anxiety, digestive disorders, liver congestion

- Known for its ability to move blood and tone tissues, it is particularly effective in relieving stagnation in both the digestive and female reproductive systems. Its bitter quality works to stimulate appetite and aid sluggishness, and its estrogenic effects also help regulate menstruation and move stagnant blood. Some claim it even helps move stagnant energy, helping the patient get past stuck issues.
- A mild emmenagogue, it relieves painful periods and scanty bleeding, normalizing menstruation and reducing PMS.
- Reduces digestive discomfort, acidity, gas, and bloating, stimulating appetite and aiding sluggishness. It promotes the secretion of bile, which aids in the digestion of fats and reduces constipation while toning the digestive tract.
- Its mild nervine action helps ease tension and anxiety, promoting relaxation and sleep.
- May be effective at reducing inflammation and cholesterol build-up in the cardiovascular system, reducing high blood pressure, but more research is needed to support this claim.
- Used in acupuncture for centuries, moxibustion, or burning a stick of dried, ground mugwort over acupuncture points, helps to enhance treatments. Particularly effective when treating pain in the knee joints.
- Oil of Mugwort used topically can relieve deep muscle pain, especially when combined with other oils like St. John's Wort.

FOLKLORE: A lot of lore surrounds this herb. In ancient China and Japan, it was hung in doorways to keep disease out, and similarly used throughout Europe to ward off evil spirits. Travellers carried it on their persons to keep away wild animals and stuffed it in their shoes to alleviate fatigue. Mugwort tea was often consumed before divinations, as it was thought to be a visionary herb. Some Indigenous Peoples use a Mugwort smudge to purify the air. Leaves placed under a pillow may produce lucid and colourful dreams.

TINCTURE: Dried herb, 1:5, 50% alcohol, 2–4 ml. per day.

INFUSION: Mix 1 tsp. dried or fresh herb in 1 cup boiling water; steep for 10 minutes. Add honey if desired.

CAUTION: May cause miscarriage; do not use if pregnant or breastfeeding. Not recommended for use by women who have heavy periods. May cause allergic reactions. Do not exceed recommended dosages or use for an extended period of time. Pain and spasms are symptoms of overdose.

MULLEIN

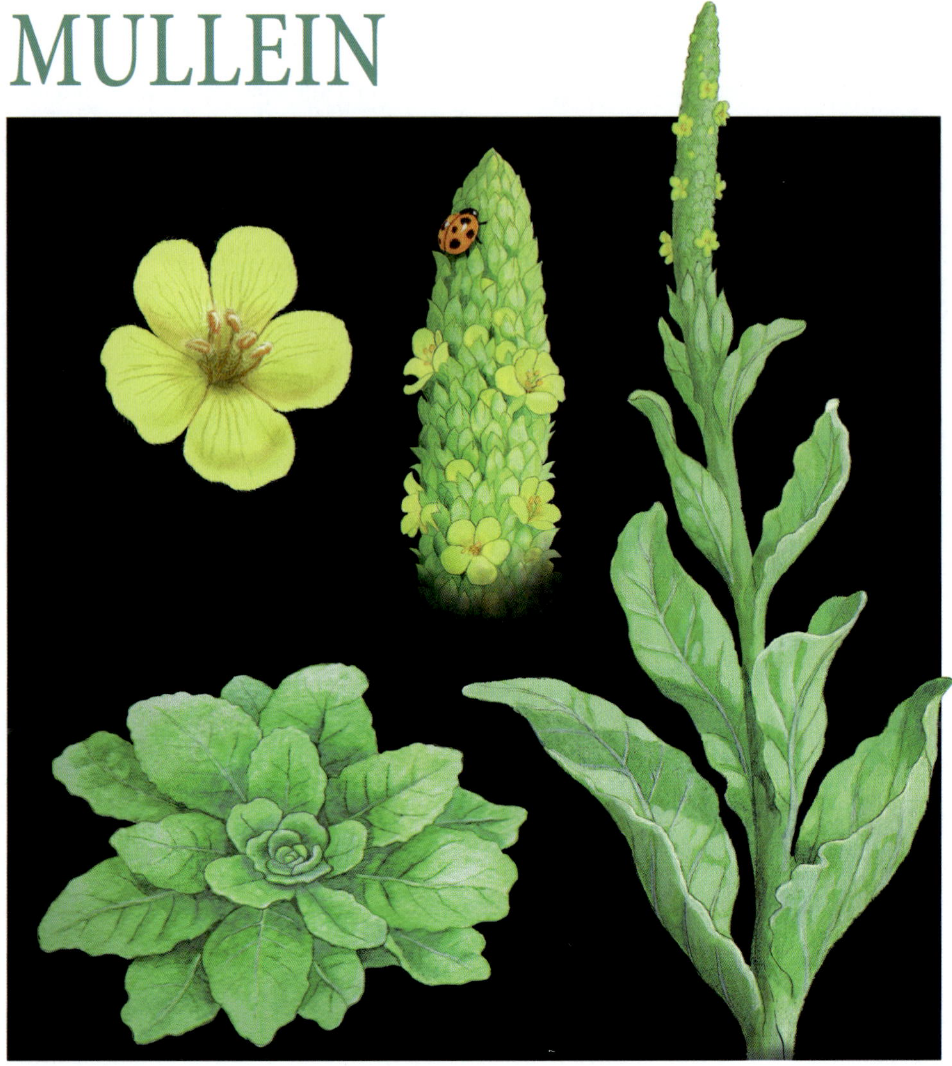

Verbascum thapsus

FAMILY: Scrophulariaceae

OTHER NAMES: Great Mullein, Torches, Flannel Plant, Candlewort, Candlewick, *Fr.* Molène vulgare, Bonhomme, Tabac du diable, Bouillon blanc

PARTS USED: Leaves, roots, and flowers

CHARACTERISTICS: Cool, bitter, sweet, drying, astringent

ACTIONS: Antiseptic, antiviral, antifungal, astringent, analgesic, antioxidant, anti-inflammatory, demulcent, emollient, expectorant, vulnerary, antispasmodic, antimicrobial

RANGE: Introduced across Canada

Mullein is a hard plant to miss as it often grows to a height of 1.5–1.8 m. During the first season of growth, only a rosette of soft, hairy leaves up to 38 cm. long appears, then the following spring a hairy stalk emerges from the centre, with leaves joined to the stalk becoming smaller toward the top. The top becomes a flower spike, usually about 30–60 cm., with flowers blooming randomly along the stalk. The flowers are composed of 5 petals, about 2.5 cm. in diameter. They should be harvested and dried quickly and carefully so as not to bruise the delicate petals since this will diminish their efficacy. Take only a few leaves so as not to kill the plant.

MEDICINAL USES:

Chest colds, bronchitis, asthma, earaches, and eczema

- Primarily used to reduce inflammation in the respiratory tract due to infections. Contains mucilage to soothe tissues and saponins that stimulate the lining of the respiratory tract to loosen stuck phlegm. Works well with bronchitis where there is a hard, dry cough with soreness, as well as chest colds, asthma, and laryngitis. Used by Indigenous Peoples to treat tuberculosis in the mid 1900s.
- Fresh leaves work externally as a poultice to ease pain, bruising, itching, and heal slow-healing wounds, burns, rashes, tumours, and hemorrhoids. Also used topically to ease pain from arthritis, swelling, or broken bones.
- Oil made by macerating flowers in olive oil is quite effective in relieving earache or eczema in the ear and to soften ear wax, making it easier to remove. Can be used to treat gum and mouth ulcers, or massaged into the scalp to condition hair and keep it free from dandruff.
- Some Indigenous Peoples smoke the leaves to treat asthma, or steep them in water and inhale the vapours.
- An extract from the roots can relieve toothache pain.

OTHER USES:
- Used in cosmetics to soften the skin.
- The leaves were once stuffed in shoes to keep feet warm.
- A yellow dye can be made from the flowers.
- Also used as a hair rinse.

FOLKLORE: The stem stripped of leaves and dipped in tallow was used as a torch and to protect against enchantment. Smoked leaves were believed to clear the air of negative energies and often used in witches' ceremonies. The leaves were even carried to prevent conception.

INFUSION: Dried leaves, 2 tbsp. in 1 cup boiling water, steep 10–15 minutes, strain through a fine sieve to remove tiny hairs. Drink 3–4 times a day. Add honey if desired.

TINCTURE: Dried leaf 1:3 in 50% alcohol, 1–2 ml. every few hours as needed.

EAR OIL: For earaches, or eczema in the ear, cut blooms into small pieces, place in a small glass jar, cover with organic extra virgin olive oil. Mix well and mash with wooden spoon. Add a few drops of vitamin E oil. Cover and shake. Put in a dark place and macerate for 6 weeks, shaking often. Strain well and pour into dark coloured jar. Store at room temperature. To use place 2–3 drops in ear 2–3 times a day.

COMBINATIONS: With Coltsfoot, Marshmallow, Thyme, or Licorice root for painful coughs, Elecampane for deep lung congestion.

CAUTION: Preparations using leaves and taken internally should be strained through a fine cloth or sieve to remove tiny hairs that can be irritant to the digestive tract. Not recommended during pregnancy or if taking anti-diabetic or diuretic medications.

MUSTARD

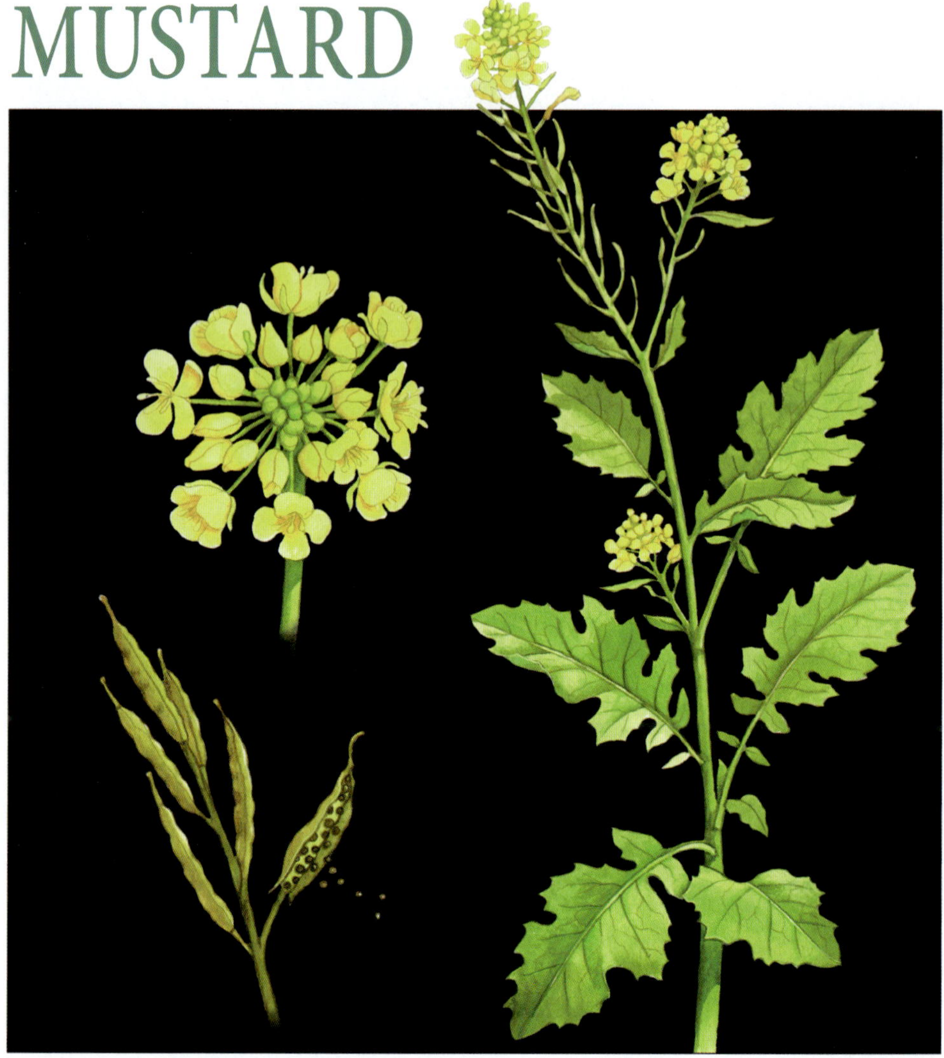

Brassica nigra (Black Mustard)
Sinapis alba (White Mustard)

FAMILY: Brassicaceae

OTHER NAMES: *Fr.* Moutarde

PARTS USED: Seeds, leaves, oil

CHARACTERISTICS: Warm, pungent

ACTIONS: Rubifacient, irritant, stimulant, diuretic, emetic, carminative, tonic, diaphoretic, vasodilator, febrifuge, expectorant, demulcent, antioxidant, anti-inflammatory, antimicrobial

RANGE: *M. nigra* introduced from British Columbia to Newfoundland and Labrador; *M. alba* introduced, the Yukon, British Columbia to the Maritimes

This common spice is a native plant of Europe, but is now often cultivated across North America, although it has escaped farms and is also growing wild just about everywhere. There are dozens of mustard species worldwide, and it is not only one of the oldest medicinal plants, but has also been used as a vegetable for hundreds of years. It is an erect annual that grows up to 1 m. in height. Its lower leaves are bristly and coarsely lobed, and the upper leaves are lance-shaped and hairless. The flowers of both Black and White Mustard species are yellow with 4 rounded petals arranged in the shape of a cross, Black being slightly smaller. The fruit of the 2 plants is quite different. The White variety grows horizontally and is hairy, roundish, and swollen, with 4–6 seeds, which are larger than the Black and have a sword-shaped beak at the tip. The short-beaked Black Mustard pod is smooth, erect, and flattened, with 10–12 small dark-red or black seeds. The black Mustard plant is stronger in flavour and pungency, and is more effective medicinally than the White variety. The young plants (before flowering) are nutritious, good in salads, and have a slightly pungent flavour.

MEDICINAL USES:

Chest congestion, arthritis, muscular or skeletal pain, athlete's foot, dyspepsia, fevers

- The spicy taste of Mustard seeds and young leaves warms and stimulates the movement of fluids throughout the body, breaking down congestion, thinning mucus in the lungs and sinuses, increasing blood flow in the extremities, and improving digestion by stimulating digestive enzymes. The leaves are rich in vitamins and minerals, the seeds contain glucosinolates, volatile oils that give it the hot, pungent flavour and act as a decongestant and antimicrobial.
- Infusion of ground seed relieves coughs and cold symptoms, bronchitis, sinus infections and fevers, warming and encouraging blood flow to the extremities to produce sweating and release heat and toxins. May be used as a gargle for sore throats.
- Tea or tincture can relieve bloating, stomachache, or colic.
- Mustard plaster placed on the chest can relieve congestion in the lungs in pneumonia, pleurisy, or bronchitis by drawing blood from the site of inflammation to the surface. Also works for sinus infections, neuralgia, muscular or skeletal pain, and spasms.
- Bruised seeds mixed in warm water makes a nice footbath to help to get rid of a cold or dispel a headache. Soak for 10 minutes. Increases circulation.
- 1 tbsp. dry mustard added to a cup of tepid water acts as an effective emetic. A teaspoon dissolved in boiling water will cure hiccups.
- In diluted form, the oil can be used as a liniment for aching muscles or arthritic joints, and is said to stimulate hair growth.
- A few drops of mustard oil in a footbath can treat athlete's foot.
- Greens eaten raw or steamed can reduce cholesterol and provide magnesium and calcium, which are beneficial to menopausal women.
- Seeds are antioxidant and anti-inflammatory, beneficial for people with cardiovascular problems or cancer.

INFUSION: 1 tsp. ground seed in 1 cup boiling water, infuse 5 minutes.

TINCTURE: ⅓ cup crushed seeds in 8 oz mason jar, fill with 50% alcohol. Steep 4–6 weeks, strain, take 1 dropper in water.

MUSTARD PLASTER: Mix 1 tbsp. dry yellow mustard with 1–2 tbsp. flour; mix in enough warm water to make a thick paste. Spread between two pieces of soft flannel, and place on chest until it becomes warm, around 10 minutes, less for children. Attention: Mustard plasters left on the skin for too long can cause blisters. Don't leave for more than 15 minutes.

FOOT BATH: Add 2 tsp. crushed seeds per 3.5 cups of hot water, soak feet for 20 minutes.

CAUTION: Not recommended for people with gastrointestinal ulcers, hyperacidity, or inflammatory kidney disorders. Don't use oil or tinctures undiluted, as they can cause blisters. Do not use for more than 2 weeks. Do not leave plasters on skin for more than 15 minutes or place near the eyes. Avoid using while breastfeeding or on children under six years. Avoid if you have hypothyroidism.

OAK

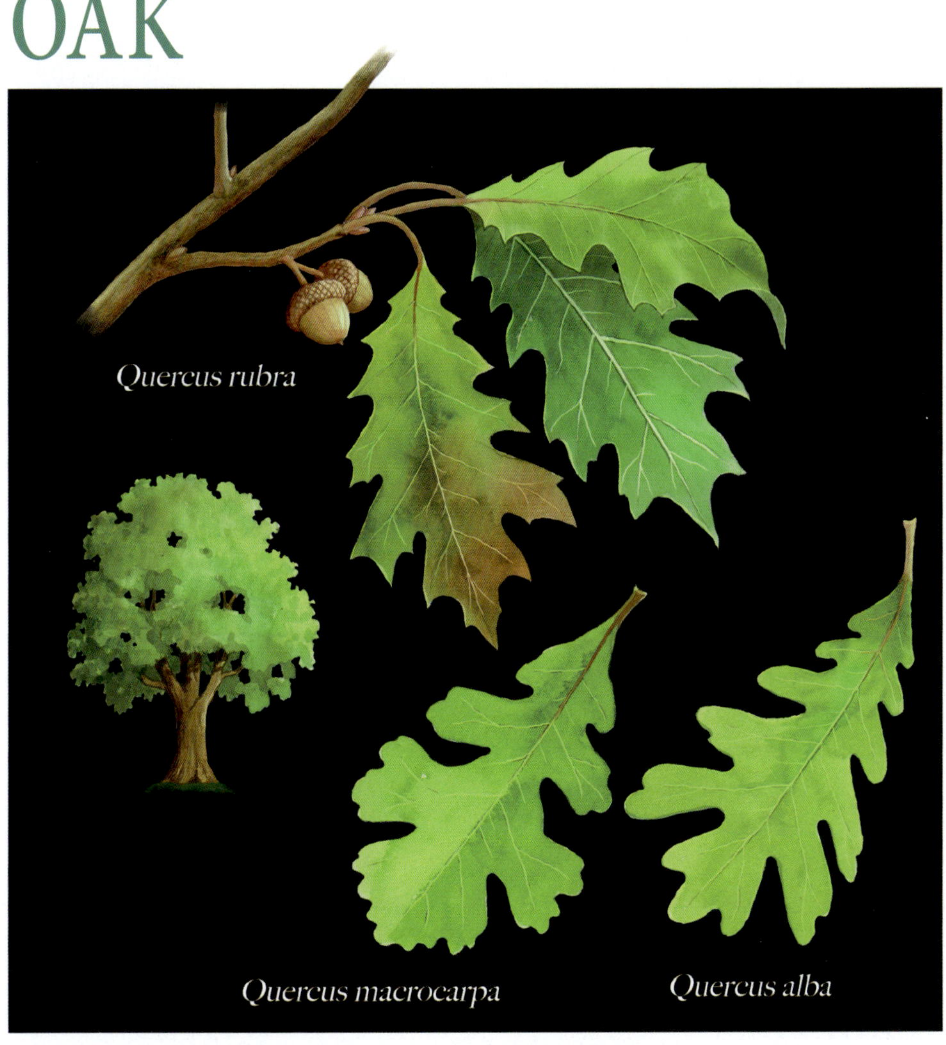

Quercus alba; Quercus rubra; Quercus macrocarpa

FAMILY: Fagaceae

OTHER NAMES: *Q. alba:* Northern White Oak, *Fr.* Chêne blanc; *Q. rubra:* Northern Red Oak, *Fr.* Chêne rouge; *Q. macrocarpa:* Bur Oak, *Fr.* Chêne à gros fruits

PARTS USED: Inner bark, fruit, leaves, galls

CHARACTERISTICS: Bitter, astringent

ACTIONS: Antiseptic, antioxidant, antimicrobial, anti-inflammatory, astringent, hemostatic, hepatoprotective, tonic

RANGE: *Q. alba* native to Quebec, Ontario; *Q. rubra* native from Ontario to Maritimes; *Q. macrocarpa* native from Alberta to New Brunswick

The Oak tree has for many centuries been a symbol of strength, power, and ancient wisdom, its roots reaching deep into the earth and providing a connection between the heavens and the underworld. Comprising more than six hundred species worldwide, some living to be a thousand years old, they can reach up to a height of 100 m., depending on the species. They tend to prefer full sun, have low flammability, and their wood can last for hundreds of years so is often used for construction. Indigenous Peoples have long used the acorns as a food source and have many medicinal uses for its bark. The Northern White Oak, which is most often used for medicine, has leaves with 5–9 rounded lobes and turns dark red in the fall, its dried leaves usually remaining on the tree over the winter months. Inner bark is best collected from smaller branches so as not to harm the tree. Gather in the spring from trees 10–25 years old and dry for later use.

MEDICINAL USES:

Coughs, diarrhea, intermittent fevers, bleeding gums, skin sores, hemorrhoids, leukorrhea, varicose veins

- Bark is rich in tannins, which tightens and tones lax tissues and dries dampness. Used traditionally in a decoction as an expectorant for damp coughs, congested sinuses, intermittent fevers, colds, and asthma.
- Its astringency is also useful in treating diarrhea, leukorrhea, prolapsed uterus, hemorrhoids, menorrhagia, and varicose veins. It may be used both topically and internally.
- Makes a good wash or gargle for sore mouth, bleeding gums, loose teeth, sore throat.
- Topically, a decoction is used for skin eruptions, sores, burns, rashes, chapped skin, and muscular pains.

OTHER USES:

- Bark used to tan leather, yields a reddish-brown dye, important lumber source.
- Beverages aged in Oak barrels prolong storage life and enhance flavour.
- Acorns may be used as an important food source, however they must be treated to leach out the tannic acid. There are several methods to make flour, some use cold water and some boil the nuts. The cold-water method tends to preserve the starch better, but takes a long time, typically 7–10 days. For the hot-water method, examine acorns for wormholes, discard along with caps, roast acorns in oven at 250°F for ½ hour. Break open the shell; to leach out tannins boil 5–10 minutes, pour off cloudy water from the top, and repeat 5 or 6 times until nuts have no more bitterness. Strain well, dehydrate in low oven or food dehydrator, then grind into flour.

DECOCTION: Cut off a small branch, peel off outer bark, and chop 1 tsp. of the inner bark into 2.5 cups of water, boil 15–20 minutes. Strain and cool, sip frequently throughout the day for diarrhea, drink plenty of fluids. May also be used as a wash or for other internal problems.

COMBINATIONS: With Violet leaf and Plantain to tighten gums. With Witch Hazel, Calendula, Chamomile, or Rose in creams or lotions.

RESEARCH: Studies have found that a wood extract from *Quercus robur* (English Oak), available in a commercial product known as Robuvit, is effective in enhancing energy capacity in chronic fatigue patients and those suffering from burnout, liver or renal insufficiency, mild heart failure, PTSD, and fatigue after surgery. Phenolic compounds, triterpenoids, and flavonoids have been found to have anti-inflammatory, hepatoprotective, antidiabetic, and anticancer effects, but more research is needed to study the safety and efficiency of these properties.

CAUTION: Generally considered safe if taken for 3–4 days or applied topically for 2–3 weeks. Avoid use if suffering from eczema, constipation, liver, or kidney problems, or if pregnant or breastfeeding.

OLD MAN'S BEARD

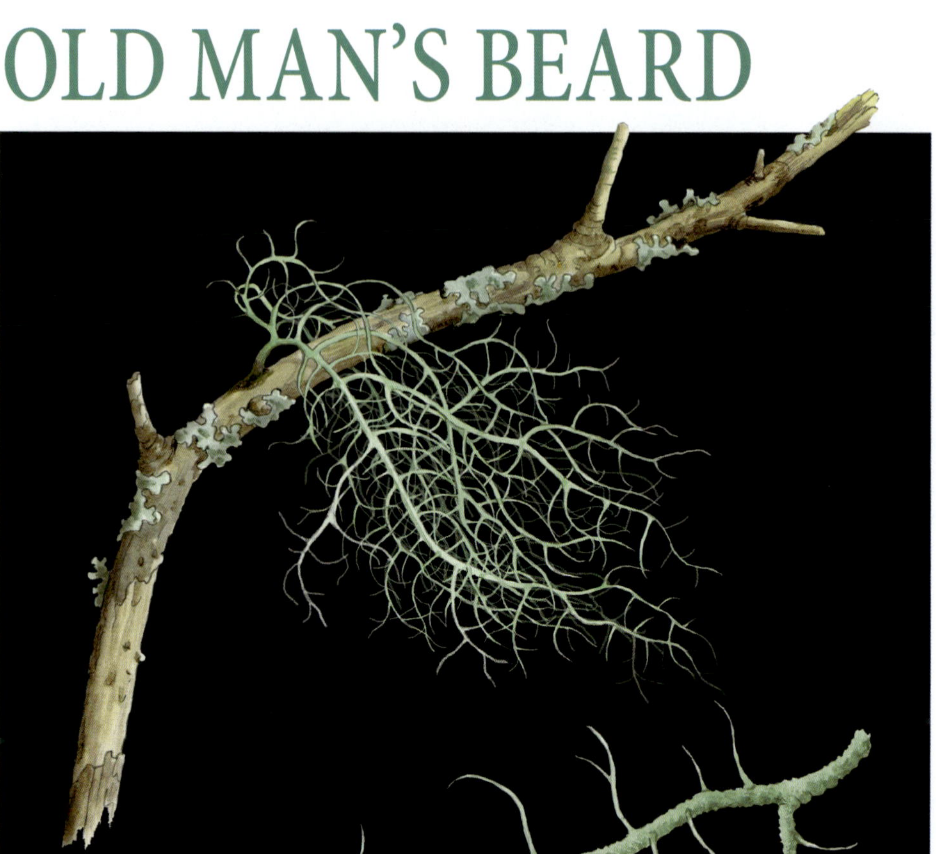

Usnea barbata
U. longissima

FAMILY: Parmeliaceae

OTHER NAMES: Usnea, Beard Lichen, Witches Hair, *Fr.* Usnée barbue

PARTS USED: Whole lichen

CHARACTERISTICS: Bitter, dry, cool

ACTIONS: Antibacterial, antiviral, antifungal, astringent, styptic, tonic, vulnerary, antimicrobial, antipyretic, anti-inflammatory, immune tonic, antioxidant

RANGE: *U. barbata* native across Canada; *U. longissima* native to British Columbia, Ontario to Newfoundland and Labrador

Usnea, or Old Man's Beard, is a greenish-grey lichen, an organism that has a symbiotic relationship between algae and fungi. It grows on the branches of older trees, often ones that are sick or dying, and can be distinguished from other similar-looking lichens by a white elastic thread (fungus) running through the middle that is revealed by gently pulling apart a filament (algae). There are hundreds of species, and it has been used for centuries worldwide as a powerful antimicrobial—that is, it is effective against a wide range of pathogens. *U. barbata* can grow up to 20 cm. long, *U. longissima* much longer, and since it is very slow growing it should be harvested from dead or fallen branches to avoid over-harvesting. Choose a clean location as it easily absorbs heavy metals and pollution from the environment. Store in a dry place, chop finely before using.

MEDICINAL USES:

Bacterial, viral, and fungal infections, wounds, gastric ulcers, burns

- Used on a wide range of diseases, and as it can kill pathogens without disrupting most gut flora, it is a valuable prevention and treatment for many infections, both viral and bacterial. Effective against gram-positive bacteria like *Streptococcus* and *Staphylococcus*, as well as pneumonia, upper respiratory tract infections, and urinary tract infections, but unlike most antibiotics, it won't kill off healthy gut bacteria. Combats common viral infections such as herpes and Epstein–Barr. It works through the mucous membranes to fight lung and bronchial infections, often with yellow or green phlegm and fevers.
- Effective against fungal infections, both topically and internally, like candida, athlete's foot, and ringworm, although lifestyle and diet modifications should be made in order to completely eradicate them, as they are usually hard to get rid of.
- May be useful in treatment for gastric ulcers and shows potential as a possible cancer treatment, particularly oral cancer.
- May be applied topically as a powder or diluted tincture for skin infections or acne, eczema, wounds, or burns. A diluted tincture works well as a throat or nasal spray.

FOLKLORE: It is seen by many Indigenous Peoples of North America as having a sacred relationship with the trees, helping them fight off infection.

TINCTURE: Dried chopped herb 1:5, Everclear alcohol, macerate 2–4 weeks, strain and measure the alcohol. To make a dual extraction, place the Usnea plant material in a small crockpot and add twice the amount of filtered water as alcohol. Heat on lowest setting and cook until it has reduced by half, about 24 hours. Strain and combine water extraction with the alcohol extraction, bottle and label. Take 1–4 ml. in a little water.

CAUTION: May cause liver toxicity or gastrointestinal irritation in large doses or if used over a prolonged period of time due to presence of usnic acid. Not recommended during pregnancy or breastfeeding. May cause skin irritation when used topically in some people.

OREGON GRAPE

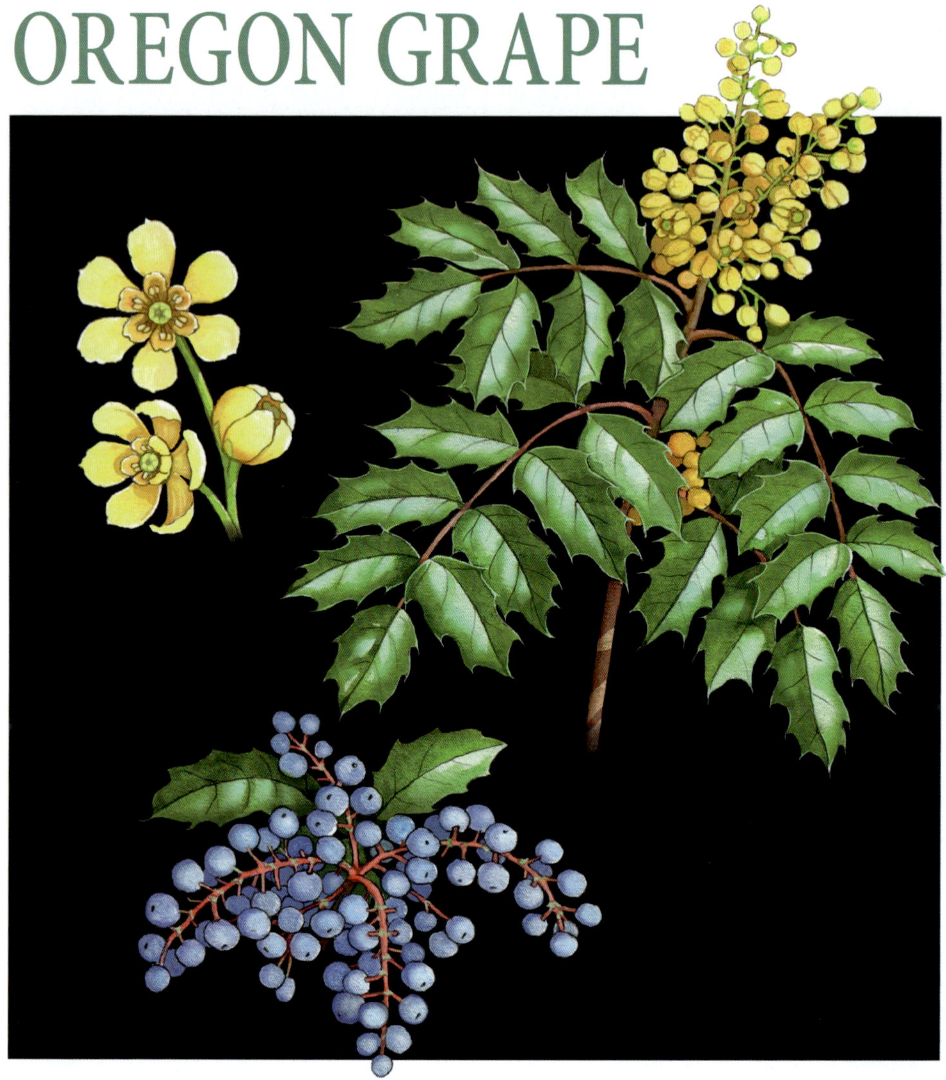

Mahonia aquifolium

FAMILY: Berberidaceae

OTHER NAMES: Mountain Grape, Holly-leaved Barberry, *Fr.* Faux-houx, Mahonia

PARTS USED: Root/rhizome, stem bark

CHARACTERISTICS: Root: bitter, drying, cooling; berries: tart

ACTIONS: Alterative, analgesic, anti-inflammatory, anticatarrhal, antiemetic, antimicrobial, cholagogue, blood tonic, diuretic, tonic, slightly stimulating, hepatic, antibiotic, depurative, antifungal

RANGE: Native to British Columbia and Alberta, introduced in Ontario and Quebec

An ornamental evergreen shrub that typically grows in mountainous country in altitudes of up to 2,000 m., Oregon Grape belongs to the Barberry family, known for its bitter alkaloid berberine. Growing 2–3 m. tall, it has shiny leaves that look similar to Holly; but unlike Holly, they are pinnately arranged, with 5–11 ovate leaflets. Dark green on top and lighter underneath, they have spiny tips on the toothed edges and turn reddish in the fall. The yellow, scented flowers bloom in early spring in terminal clusters, then in summer the dark blue berries appear, covered in a dusty coating. They are somewhat bitter, very sour and unpalatable, but edible, and may be made into jams or jellies. The bark of stems, roots, and rhizomes is bright yellow when you scrape off the surface, and should be collected in late fall or early spring, paying special attention to not kill the plant, taking only a small part of the root or stem. Chop up while fresh and dry for future use.

MEDICINAL USES:

Digestive weakness, lack of appetite, skin diseases, bacterial dysentery, infected wounds

- Used both internally and externally, it is both anti-inflammatory and antibacterial, and contains a bitter alkaloid called berberine that stimulates the digestive system, cleanses toxins from the body, and improves acute and chronic inflammatory skin conditions and infections.
- A bitter liver and gallbladder tonic, it stimulates the digestion and bile flow, improving liver function and purifying the blood of toxins. This action also helps loss of appetite, gastritis, digestive weakness, IBS, and diarrhea, and improves absorption of nutrients. Root is antibacterial and can treat enteric infections like bacterial dysentery.
- Noted for its effectiveness at treating skin diseases, both topically and internally. Strongly anti-inflammatory, it calms and cools pain and itching. In psoriasis it slows skin cell renewal, reducing lesions, and can reduce the size of eczema patches when applied to the skin. Treats localized skin infections and wounds, acne, and candida infections in the mouth and vagina. May also be used internally to improve the skin, as it cleanses toxins and clears stagnation from the liver; however, it is also necessary to improve the diet and eliminate unhealthy food to allow the digestive system to heal and become more effective.
- When used alongside antibiotic treatments, it helps to decrease bacterial resistance to antibiotics, making them more effective against certain bacteria.
- Fruit is a gentle laxative.
- Infusion may be used as a gargle for sore throats.
- Indicated for any abnormal discharges, phlegm, catarrh, leukorrhea, or candida where there is heat and inflammation.

OTHER USES:

- Yellow dye made from bark and roots, dark green and purple dyes from the fruit.
- Berries are tart but can be made into jams or jellies.

DECOCTION: 1 tsp. dried root per 1 cup water, simmer 5–20 minutes to extract the medicinal compounds. The longer you simmer it, the more bitter it gets, so for digestive problems taken internally, use a milder decoction, but for topical applications it can be stronger.

TINCTURE: Dried root 1:5 in 40% alcohol, take 10–60 drops up to 3 times a day.

COMBINATIONS: Cascara Sagrada for chronic constipation, Pipsissewa for hepatitis, jaundice and arthritis. Licorice root should not be used in combinations as it nullifies the effects of Oregon Grape root.

RESEARCH: Studies found that five out of seven studies on people with psoriasis had a significant improvement from application of a commercially available cream containing Oregon Grape, and one study on eczema showed it to be more effective than the placebo. In vitro data shows that whole-plant extracts were also effective against fungal infections like athlete's foot, ringworm, and candida overgrowth, but there have been no human trials. May improve insulin sensitivity and blood sugar management, and could possibly lower cholesterol levels, but there are very few human studies to date.

CAUTION: Avoid use for more than 2 weeks. Not recommended for children or pregnant or lactating women. Avoid in hyperthyroidism. High doses may cause vomiting, low blood pressure, reduced heart rate, lethargy, skin and eye irritation, kidney infection. Consult a professional if taking heart or diabetes medications.

PACIFIC MADRONE

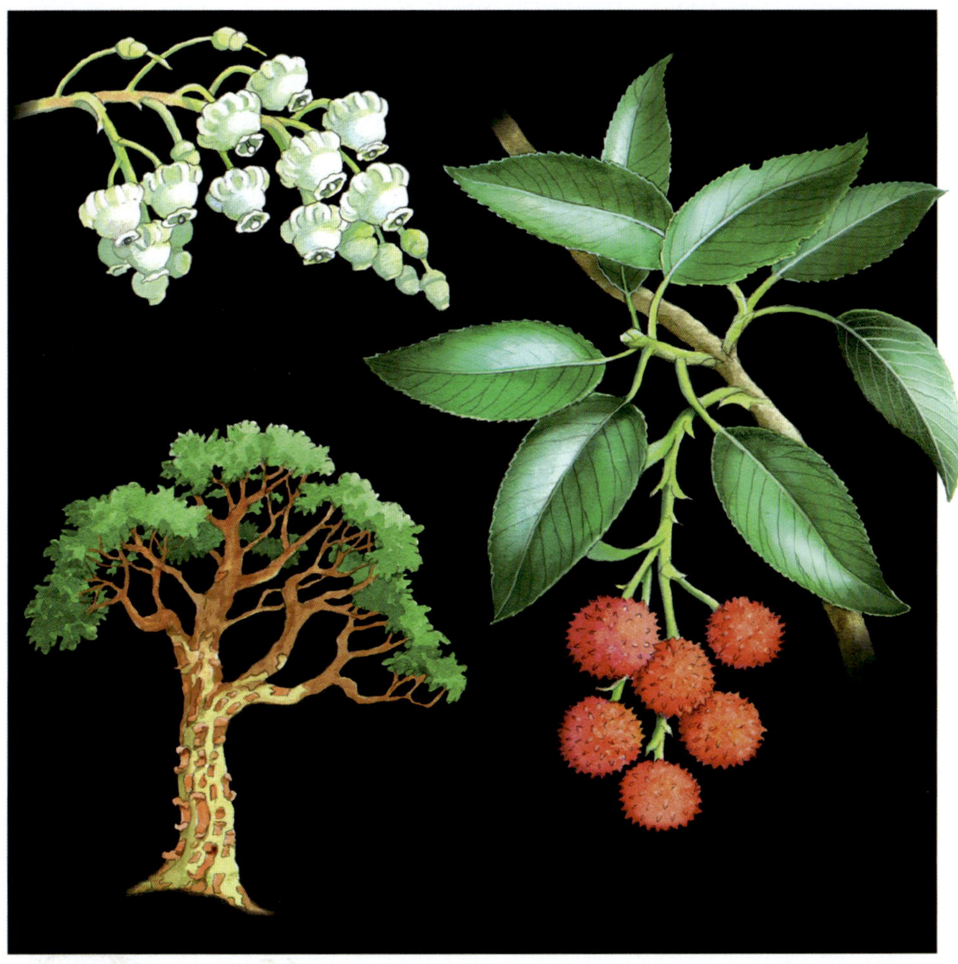

Arbutus menziesii

FAMILY: Ericaceae

OTHER NAMES: Madrona, Pacific Arbutus, *Fr.* Arbousier d'Amérique

PARTS USED: Leaves, bark

CHARACTERISTICS: Spicy, pungent

ACTIONS: Stomachic, vulnerary, astringent, antioxidant, anti-inflammatory, antibacterial

RANGE: Native to southern British Columbia coastline

The Pacific Madrone or Arbutus is found growing near sea level in the extreme southwest of British Columbia. Preferring dry, open, well-drained forests along the coastline, it is the only broad-leaved evergreen tree in Canada. Easily recognizable by its thin, papery, reddish-brown bark that peels off in curls and strips exposing its smooth green or silvery wood underneath, it can grow up to 30 m. tall, although it's typically shorter. It is known to rely on forest fires to open up the understorey, reducing competition so it can re-sprout from an underground burl, even after being destroyed aboveground. Its thick, glossy leaves are alternate and oval shaped, with finely toothed or smooth edges, and turn from dark green to red-orange in the second year, falling off once the second year's growth has appeared. Its fragrant, urn-shaped flowers bloom from April to May and are designed to attract bees, growing in terminal drooping clusters. The red berry that appears later in the summer and into the fall has a bumpy surface with hooked barbs that cling to passersby. Its astringent and mealy taste is not usually found palatable by humans, although wildlife love them, and they are sometimes used to make cider or jellies. Harvest leaf clusters from branch tips from mid-spring to fall, berries should be fully red before picking. Dry and store for future use.

MEDICINAL USES:

Bladder infections, stomachache, sore throat, skin inflammations, vaginal yeast infections, colds, rheumatism

- Bark and leaves contain tannins that make an astringent decoction useful in treating bladder infections, stomachaches, cramps, colds, and sore throats. Leaves may be chewed for the same ailments.
- An infusion of the bark can be used for skin ailments such as impetigo, sores, burns, and cuts. Reduces redness and leaves skin soft and smooth, closing the pores. A cup of infusion can be added to a sitz bath for vaginal inflammation and yeast infections.
- Astringent and antimicrobial properties of bark and leaves help tighten gums and reduce inflammation in the mouth.

OTHER USES:

- Tannins in bark used as a preservative for wood and ropes, tanning leather, and as a source of brown dye.
- Bark dried and ground to use as a spice, having a taste somewhere between cinnamon and mushrooms with a hint of fruitiness.
- Dried berries can be ground into powder as a spice or sugar substitute, or strung into necklaces. Berries can also be made into cider or used as bait for fishing.

TINCTURE: Dried 1:5, 50% alcohol, 30–60 drops in 1 cup of water, up to 3 times a day.

INFUSION: Standard infusion, ⅓–½ cup up to 3 times a day.

CAUTION: Not for use during pregnancy. Restrict internal use to 4–6 days.

PARTRIDGEBERRY

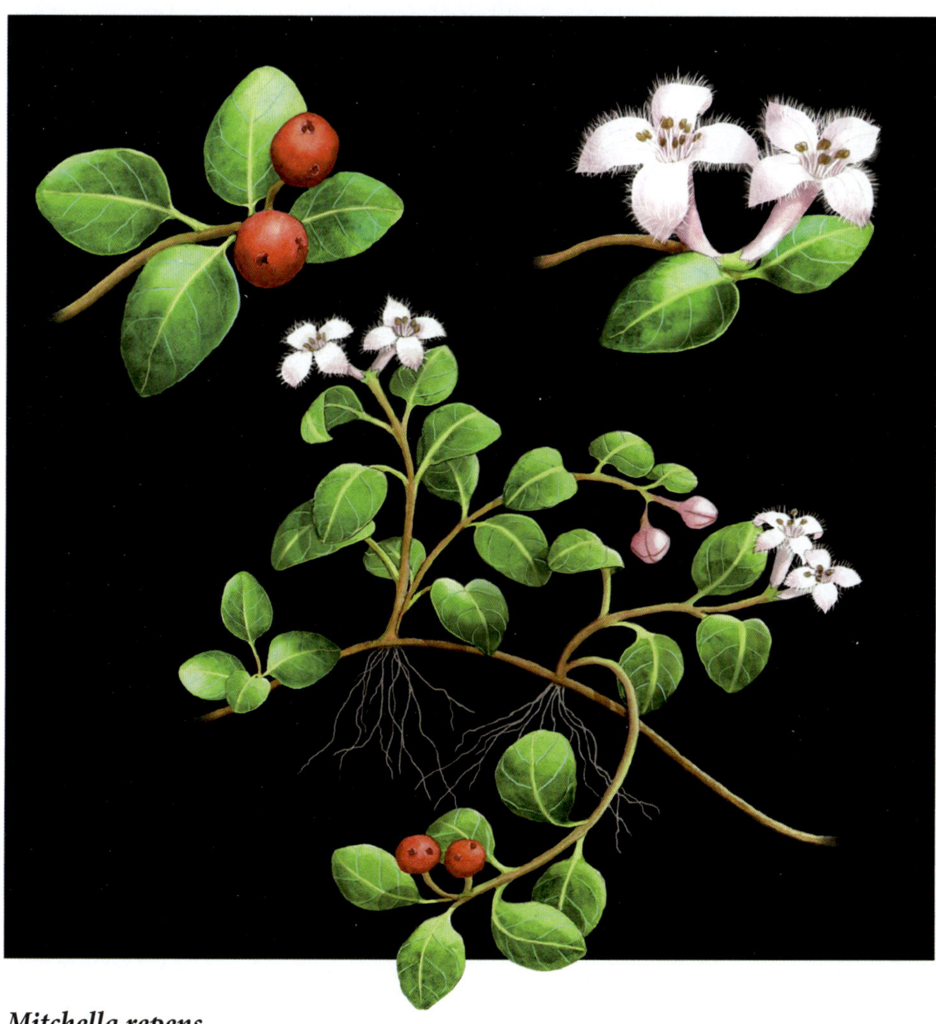

Mitchella repens

FAMILY: Rubiaceae

OTHER NAMES: Two-Eyed Berry, Running Fox, *Fr.* Mitchella rampante, Pain de perdrix

PARTS USED: Leaves, stems, berries

CHARACTERISTICS: Cooling, drying, bitter

ACTIONS: Astringent, anti-inflammatory, antioxidant, diuretic, parturient, sedative, uterine tonic, styptic

RANGE: Native from Ontario to Newfoundland and Labrador

Partridgeberry is a small, woody evergreen perennial that forms mats about 5 cm. high along the forest floors, with trailing stems that extend 15–30 cm., rooting at the nodes. The dark green, shiny leaves are opposite and ovate with a yellowish midrib, and in late spring a pair of white or pinkish fragrant, funnel-shaped flowers appear, with 4 hairy petals. These flowers must both be pollinated to produce one round, red berry in the fall, formed by the fusion of their 2 ovaries, so that each berry has 2 red indentations on its surface, which distinguishes it from similar plants, specifically Teaberry or Wintergreen (*Gaultheria procumbens*). The fruit are edible but tasteless and seedy, not to be confused with *Vaccinium vitis-idaea,* commonly called Partridgeberry as well but a relative of the cranberry with very different medicinal properties. Harvest only the growing tips, leaving the roots intact, as it is becoming rare in some places.

MEDICINAL USES:

Menorrhagia, amenorrhea, dysmenorrhea, childbirth, diarrhea, urinary tract infection, hemorrhoids

- Traditionally used by Indigenous Peoples as a woman's herb or uterine tonic, particularly to aid in childbirth and help labour pains and sore nipples, but also to ease menstrual cramps, heavy bleeding, and leukorrhea. The Abenaki also apply mashed leaves and stems externally for swellings, and the Iroquois use an infusion of bark and roots for back pain. Has been used by some herbalists in formulas to prevent miscarriage, however it should be used with caution for this purpose and only under supervision of a professional.
- Diuretic and astringent properties make it useful in decoctions internally to help urinary tract infections, diarrhea, inflammatory bowel, insomnia, rheumatic pain, and fluid retention, and externally as a compress or paste to ease pain, hemorrhoids, and skin irritations.

OTHER USES: Berries are rich in vitamins A, B, and C as well as minerals.

DECOCTION: 1 tsp. dried or 2 tsp. fresh finely chopped herb in 1 cup water, simmer 20 minutes, and strain. Take 3 times a day.

TINCTURE: Fresh 1:2 or dried 1:4 in 60% alcohol, 1–4 ml. 3 times a day.

CAUTION: Avoid use in first or second trimester of pregnancy as it may cause miscarriage. If used to tone the uterus, stop using 3 months before conception.

PENNYROYAL

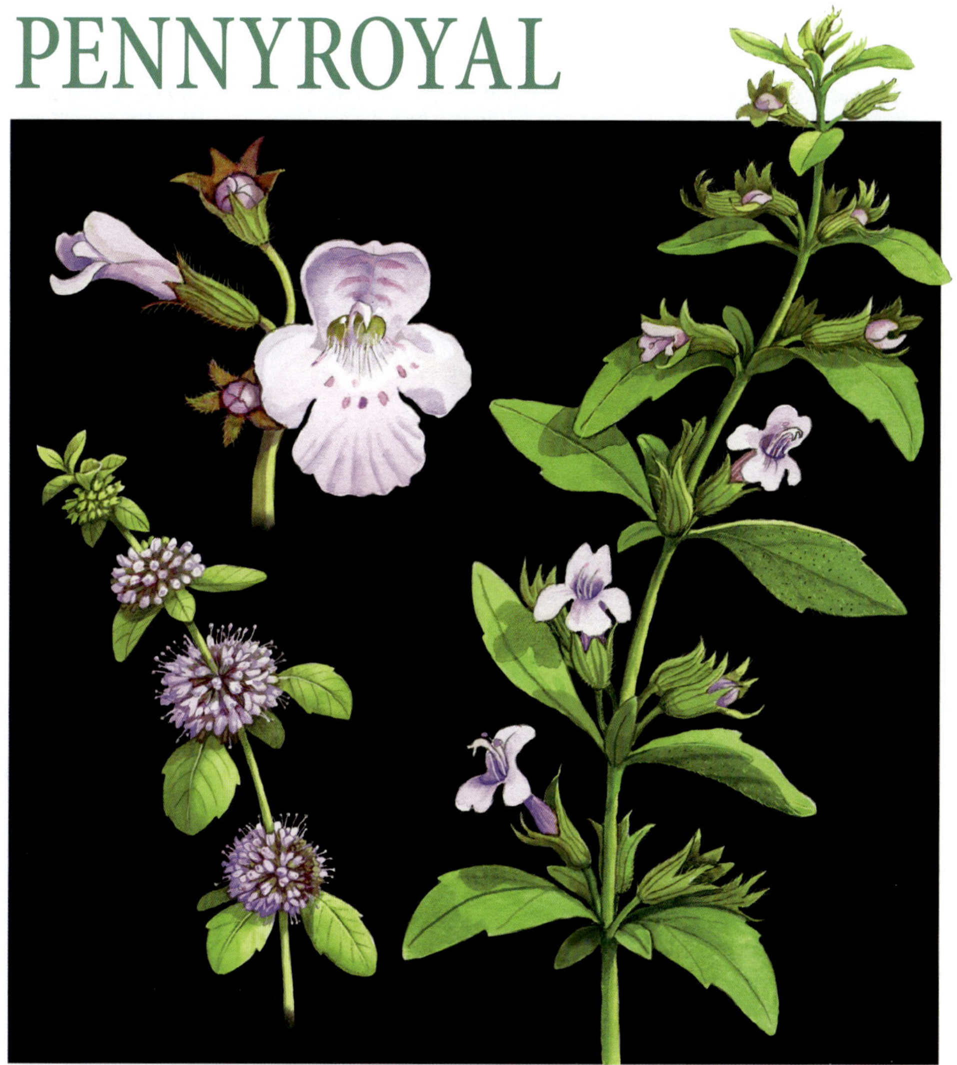

Hedeoma pulegioides
Mentha pulegium

FAMILY: Lamiaceae or Labiatae

OTHER NAMES: *H. pulegioides:* American Pennyroyal, False Pennyroyal, Tickweed, Mosquito Plant, *Fr.* Hédéoma faux-pouliot; *M. pulegium:* European Pennyroyal, *Fr.* Menthe pouliot

PARTS USED: Leaves

CHARACTERISTICS: Spicy, bitter, cool

ACTIONS: Diaphoretic, diuretic, emmenagogue, carminative, antispasmodic, mild sedative

RANGE: *H. pulegioides* native to Ontario, Quebec, New Brunswick, Nova Scotia; *M. pulegium* introduced in British Columbia

Our native Pennyroyal is very similar in properties to the European Pennyroyal, *Mentha pulegium*, but the latter only appears in BC, where it was introduced with the first settlers. Both varieties belong to the Mint family and smell much like it, and have an erect, square branching stem 15–30 cm. high. The leaves are lance-shaped, often with a few teeth, around 1.3 cm. long and hairy on the underside. Flowers are tubular, small and blue to mauve in colour, with 5 lobes, and appear from June to September. It can be found in fields and along roadsides and should be gathered before flowering and dried for later use.

MEDICINAL USES:

Digestive complaints, amenorrhea, fevers

- Historically this herb was used to relax spasms, relieve cramps and menstrual pain especially from chills or nervous shock, and bring on menstruation. Will strengthen uterine contractions during labour, and was once used in large doses along with Brewer's Yeast as an abortifacient. However, doing so may damage the mother's liver and even cause death, so it is strongly discouraged.
- Eases flatulence, nausea, intestinal cramps, and colic. Added to formulas to prevent griping.
- For colds and flu where the skin is hot with no sweat, a hot infusion promotes sweating and breaks up fever. Helps with phlegm, spasmodic coughs, and respiratory infections.
- Soothes sore gums, mouth sores, and toothaches.
- Externally, an infusion is used as a wash for itching, rashes, eruptions, and repelling insects.
- Used for centuries by Indigenous Peoples for coughs and whooping cough, colds and fevers, digestive disorders, menstrual problems, and toothaches. However, internal use is strongly discouraged due to toxicity.

OTHER USES: Leaves can be used in pet's bedding to repel fleas, or wrapped in a dog's bandana before walking through wooded areas.

INFUSION: 1 tsp. dried herb in 1 cup of hot (not boiling) water. Infuse covered 10–15 minutes. Drink 3 tbsp. every 1 or 2 hours.

CAUTION: Contains pulegone, a strong toxin that can cause liver or kidney failure when taken in large doses. Do not use Pennyroyal essential oil externally unless well diluted with vegetable oil and do not take internally. Do not give even a weak infusion to infants or children. Abortive, do not take if pregnant or breastfeeding. Avoid if taking iron supplements as it reduces effectiveness.

PIPSISSEWA

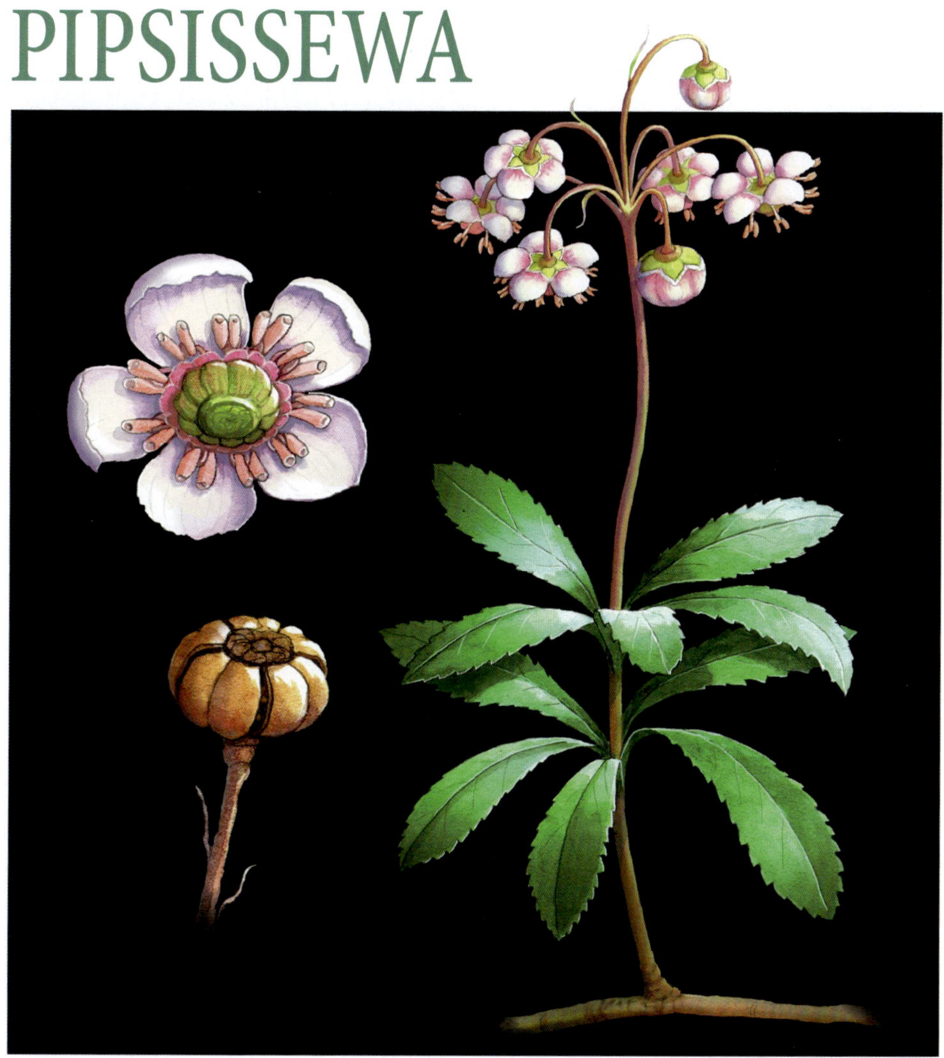

Chimaphila umbellata

FAMILY: Ericaceae

OTHER NAMES: Prince's Pine, Winter Green, Butter Winter, Ground Holly, *Fr.* Chimaphile à ombelles, Herbe à clef, Pyrole en ombelle

PARTS USED: Leaves

CHARACTERISTICS: Sweet, slightly bitter, warming

ACTIONS: Alterative, antibacterial, antioxidant, antifungal, astringent, diuretic, diaphoretic, rubefacient, stimulant, tonic

RANGE: Native across Canada, except Nunavut

Pipsissewa is a small perennial evergreen found growing in well-drained coniferous forests and woodlands of low to middle elevations throughout Canada. Shade-tolerant and in need of a specific mycorrhizal association in order to thrive, it is not easy to grow and has become rare in certain parts of the country due to overharvesting. The name Pipsissewa comes from the Cree word meaning "break into small pieces," referring to its ability to break up kidney stones. It grows to a height of 10–25 cm., and has creeping yellow rhizomes with several erect stems and shiny, dark-green toothed leaves that appear to grow in whorls around it. There are usually 5–7 white, pink, or purplish 5-petalled flowers that are nodding, waxy and fragrant, growing in a loose terminal cluster. They appear from July to August, and the fruit, an erect dark-brown capsule with five sections, remains, eventually cracking open to disperse its seeds. The upper leaves may be harvested before flowering, but be careful not to over-harvest. Leave the roots intact and avoid trampling the surrounding soil. Dry carefully, preferably in a dehydrator, in order to retain the green colour and its medicinal properties.

MEDICINAL USES:

Bladder and kidney disorders, rheumatism, gout

- Contains hydroquinone, which helps disinfect the urinary tract and ease the symptoms of cystitis and urethritis and break up bladder or kidney stones. Its mild diuretic, antiseptic, and anti-inflammatory actions make it safe to use for acute infections with internal heat, with no irritating side effects. Tones and strengthens the bladder, helps with incontinence and bedwetting. Its anti-inflammatory and diuretic actions also remove toxins, helping to relieve pain from arthritis, rheumatism, or gout.
- Used by some Indigenous Peoples for colds, coughs, fevers, arthritis, bladder infections, stones, stomachaches, rheumatism, and back pain.
- Decoction or compresses or warm, fresh leaves can be applied topically to relieve pain from arthritis, swellings in feet and legs, and backaches. Helps heal sores, insect bites, and skin ulcers.

OTHER USES: Flavouring for candies, soft drinks.

TINCTURE: Fresh 1:2, dried 1:5, in 50% alcohol. Take 20–40 drops up to 4 times a day. For kidney stones, take 5–10 drops every 3 hours.

INFUSION: Mix 1–3 tsp. dried leaf with 1 cup boiling water, infuse 10–15 minutes. Take ½–1 cup, 2–3 times a day.

COMBINATIONS: Some Indigenous Peoples combined Pipsissewa with Mullein to relieve bedwetting in children. Use with Agrimony and Corn Silk for bladder infections. Combine with False Unicorn Root and Partridgeberry for leukorrhea.

CAUTION: Contains hydroquinones, which can be toxic in large doses or over long periods of time. Avoid if pregnant or breastfeeding due to lack of research.

PITCHER PLANT

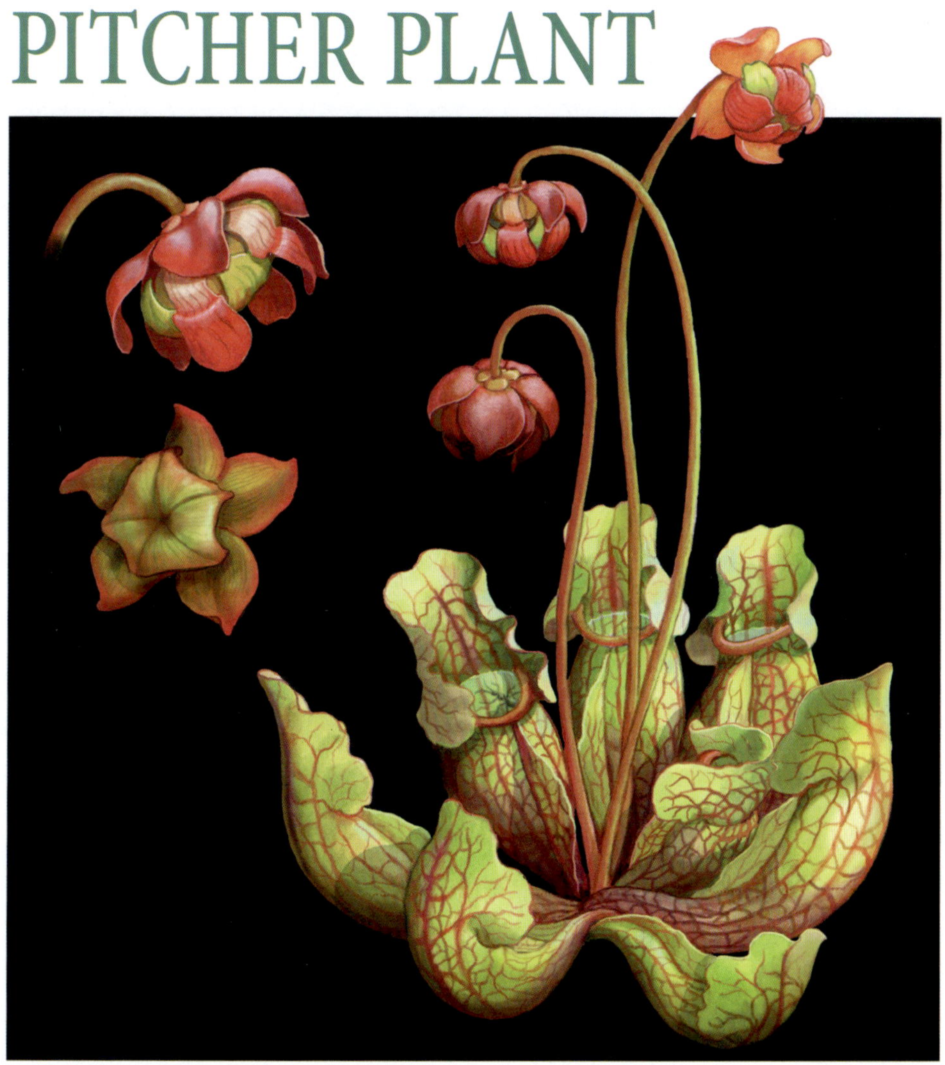

Sarracenia purpurea

FAMILY: Sarraceniaceae

OTHER NAMES: Eve's Cups, Flycatcher, Fly-trap, Water Cup, *Fr.* Sarracénie pourpre

PARTS USED: Roots, leaves

CHARACTERISTICS: Bitter, cooling

ACTIONS: Diuretic, hepatic, stimulating tonic, laxative, stomachic, astringent (root), antioxidant, antibacterial, anticancer, antiviral, cardioprotective, hepatoprotective, neuroprotective

RANGE: Native across Canada, except the Yukon

Pitcher Plant is a rather strange and unique carnivorous perennial that can be found in peat bogs and wet meadows throughout most of Canada. Since its habitat is typically nutrient-poor, it has evolved to supplement its diet by trapping insects in its pitcher-like leaves. They fill with rainwater and trap insects and other small creatures inside, due to the downward-pointing hairs inside the tube. The single purple nodding flower, which blooms from May to July, grows atop a leafless stalk 30–60 cm. high. They lose their petals soon after and the fruit, a five-celled seed capsule, persists into the fall, turning from green to red to brown before releasing its seeds. Both leaves and roots are used for medicine, but should not be harvested from the wild as the plant is endangered.

MEDICINAL USES:

Fevers, constipation, indigestion, kidney ailments, diabetes

- This plant has been used traditionally by many Indigenous Peoples to treat a variety of complaints, including diabetes, gynecological problems, indigestion, constipation, and liver and kidney ailments. It was used as a treatment for smallpox and other infectious diseases throughout the nineteenth century, despite the lack of clinical studies proving its effectiveness.
- Contains enzymes which help with slow digestion, bloating, cramps. The root is a mild laxative and stimulates a sluggish liver.
- A mild diuretic, it can help with urinary tract infections.
- Its antibacterial and anti-inflammatory properties make it effective topically for irritated skin and wounds.
- An infusion of dried leaves was used by some Indigenous Peoples to facilitate childbirth.

RESEARCH:

Although very little research has been done on this plant, there have been a few studies showing it has effective anticancer activity, specifically by using the root in an acetone extraction. When combined with the drug 5FU (5 fluorouracil), it enhanced the effectiveness of the drug, indicating that it may have potential for future anticancer chemotherapies. The water extracts did not show antibacterial, antioxidant, or anticancer properties. The leaf extract was also found to have potential as an alternative and complementary treatment for diabetic complications associated with glucose toxicity, but more research is needed.

CAUTION: Avoid if pregnant or breastfeeding, due to lack of research.

PLANTAIN

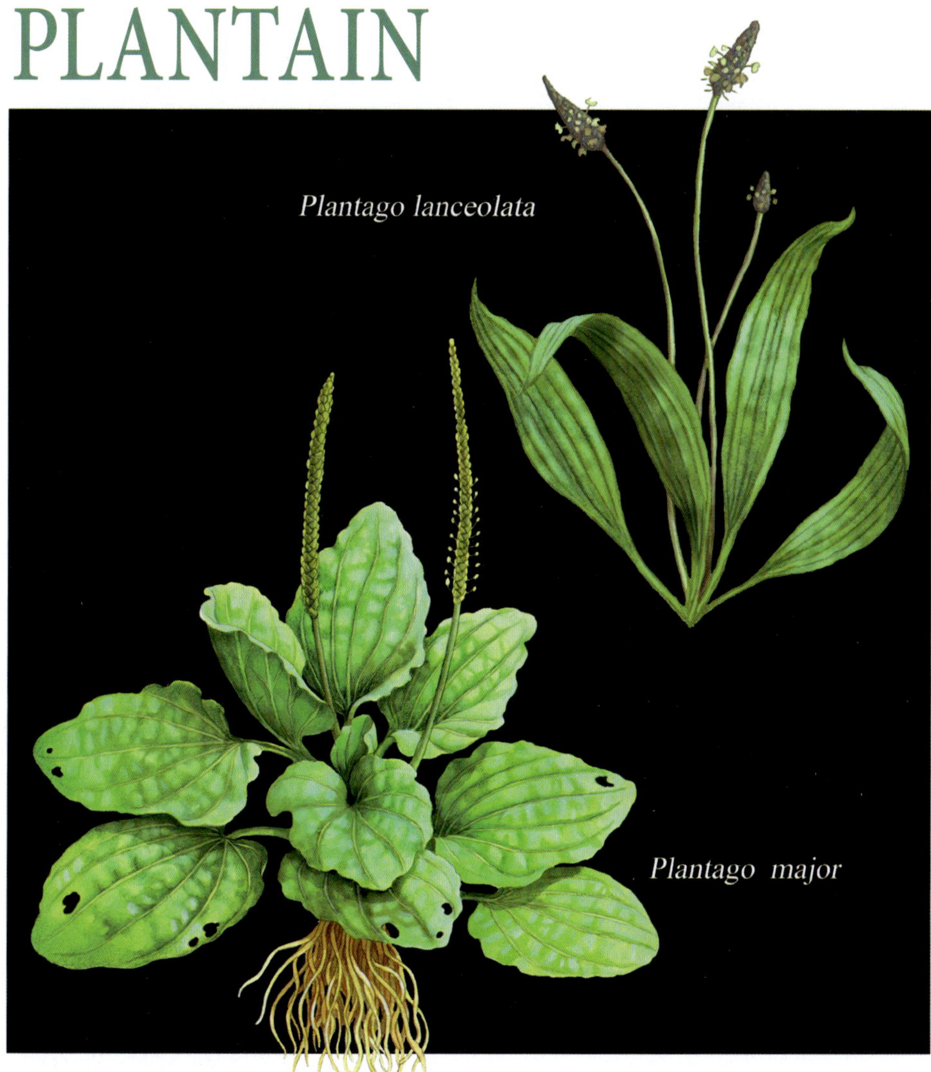

Plantago major
Plantago lanceolata

FAMILY: Plantaginaceae

OTHER NAMES: *P. major*: Broad-leaved Plantain, Common Plantain, *Fr.* Plantain majeur; *P. lanceolata*: Narrow-leaved Plantain, Ribwort, English Plantain, Ribgrass, *Fr.* Plantain lancéolé

PARTS USED: Leaves and seeds

CHARACTERISTICS: Bland, slightly bitter, cool, drying, astringent

ACTIONS: Diuretic, alterative, anti-inflammatory, antioxidant, antifungal, mild laxative, astringent, antimicrobial, antiseptic, hemostatic, vulnerary, demulcent, expectorant, antiviral

RANGE: *P. major* introduced across Canada; *P. lanceolata* introduced across all provinces except Alberta and Saskatchewan

Plantain is one Canada's most common herbs and is seen growing on practically every lawn, roadside, or abandoned lot. Originally from Europe, it was traditionally used on the battlefield to staunch wounds. It will grow virtually anywhere, including paved driveways or in sidewalk cracks, and needs very little sun. It grows close to the ground, with a rosette of ovate, blunt leaves 10–25 cm. long, with long, fibrous ribs. The erect flower spikes are dark green and can be up to 30 cm. long. The Narrow-leaved Plantain (*P. lanceolata*) has narrower leaves and longer-stemmed flower spikes but has much the same medicinal properties as the common variety. The young plants may be eaten in salads in the spring; to preserve for later they should be gathered during flowering throughout the summer and dried quickly as they will tend to discolour rapidly. Use only plants from yards that have never been sprayed with chemicals.

MEDICINAL USES:

Wounds, insect bites, urinary tract infections, digestive tract inflammations, lung infections

- Well-known for its wound-healing properties, both internal and external. Contains mucilage, which makes it soothing and anti-inflammatory; allantoin, which aids healing; tannins, which draw tissues together and dry dampness; and a strong antimicrobial to prevent infections. Common Plantain is perhaps better known for its topical use, whereas Ribwort or Narrow-leaved Plantain is better suited to internal use in cases of lung infections, colds, and diarrhea, but both can be used interchangeably.
- Bruised leaves may be applied directly to stings or insect bites, sunburn, or acne, or used in a salve or ointment; soothes and relieves pain and itching from rashes, hemorrhoids, shingles, Stinging Nettle or Poison Ivy stings, and bed sores.
- Astringent, stops bleeding, promotes healing of exterior wounds. Rich in tannin, which helps draw tissues together.
- Heals urinary tract infections, stems internal bleeding, and eases painful urination.
- Tea brewed from leaves and the seeds, which are high in mucilage, is a folk remedy for colitis, diarrhea, dysentery, and bleeding hemorrhoids. It is also antispasmodic, reducing cramping. Seeds also act as a laxative, its mucilage repairing irritated intestinal membranes. Eases gastric inflammation and ulcers.
- Hot infusion of leaves and seeds can be used as a gentle expectorant for coughs and colds, soothes sore throat. Infusion can be used as a gargle or mouthwash for mouth sores, gum disease.
- Leaves may be heated in warm water and applied to swollen joints or sore muscles.

OTHER USES:

- Cold tea used as a hair rinse for dandruff.
- Once believed to cure rabies and ward off snakes.
- Put on aching feet after a long trek to relieve soreness and fatigue.

INFUSION: 2 heaped tsp. in 1 cup boiling water, steep 10 minutes. Take 3–4 times a day.

TINCTURE: Dried 1:3 in 50% alcohol, 3–8 ml. per day.

HEALING SALVE: Place ½ pound of entire chopped Plantain plant in a non-metallic pan, add ½ cup lard or coconut oil, heat slowly on low heat until it becomes green and wilted, strain, pour into jars, and cool. For use on burns, rashes, bites, and other sores.

COMBINATIONS: With Yarrow and Elder flower for lung infections. With Calendula, Yarrow, Chamomile, or Agrimony for internal bleeding. With Comfrey, Yarrow, or Calendula for external wounds or skin irritation.

PONDEROSA PINE

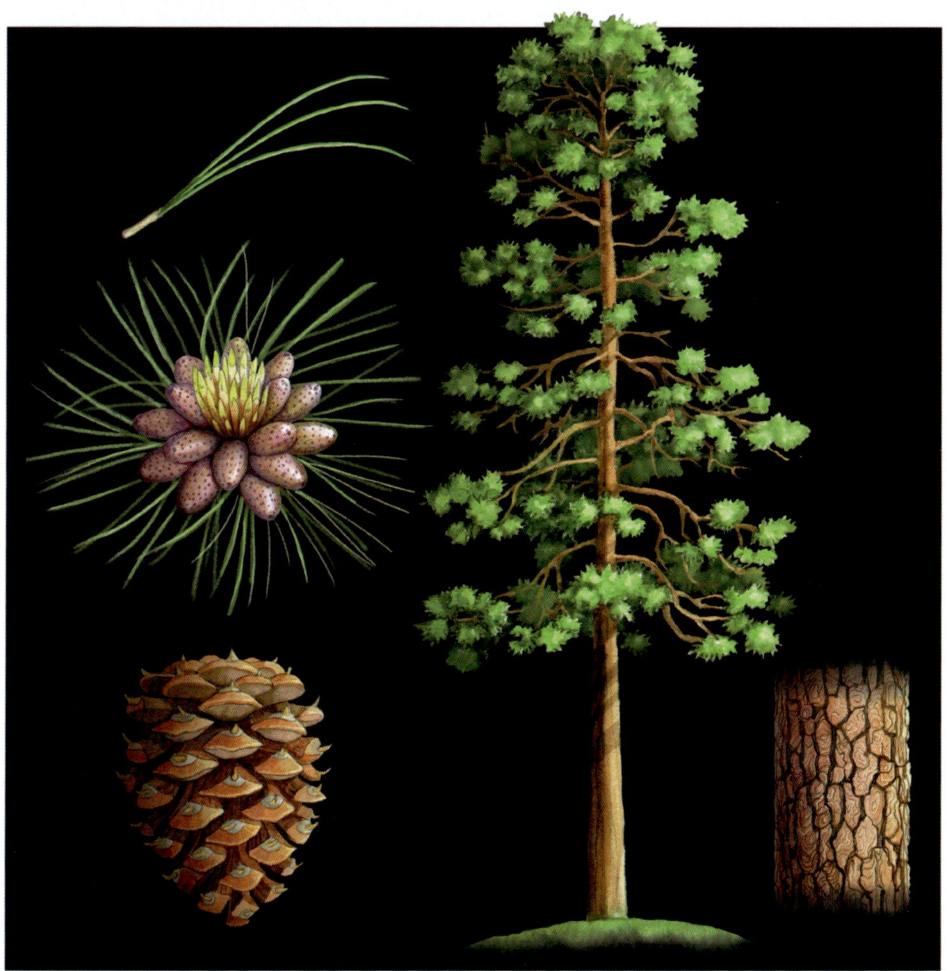

Pinus ponderosa

FAMILY: Pinaceae

OTHER NAMES: Western Yellow Pine, Washoe Pine, Blackjack Pine, *Fr.* Pin ponderosa, Pin lourd

PARTS USED: Inner bark, pitch (resin), needles, seeds, pollen

CHARACTERISTICS: Astringent, pungent, aromatic, warming, drying

ACTIONS: Analgesic, antiseptic, antifungal, diuretic, diaphoretic, expectorant, febrifuge, rubefacient, vulnerary, carminative, antimicrobial, adaptogen, antioxidant

RANGE: Native to British Columbia and southern Alberta

Ponderosa Pine is a majestic, fragrant evergreen revered by the western Indigenous communities for its medicinal properties and its usefulness as building material. The name Ponderosa means "heavy or large" in Latin. With its straight trunk it towers over other trees to a height of 30–40 m. or more and can live up to six hundred years old, its base reaching 1–2 m. in diameter. It is distinguished from other pines by its long, toothed, yellowish-green needles (12–28 cm.) in bundles of three, and its brown or cinnamon-coloured bark that breaks apart easily in pieces resembling a jigsaw puzzle, the dark fissures growing deeper as it ages. Its thick bark makes it particularly resistant to low-intensity forest fires. The cones are egg-shaped with a sharp spike pointing outward at the tip of each scale and contain the seeds, or pine nuts, which are eaten as food. It prefers well-drained soil and is shade intolerant. Its roots extend deep into the earth in search of water. The best time to harvest is in the spring, using the young needles for tea and taking a low-hanging branch for its inner bark, being careful not to strip more than a few square inches off the main trunk, as it can kill the tree. The yellow pollen is harvested from the male cones in the spring; just tap them to see if they are ready. Remove ripe cones and shake into a bowl, then sift out scales. Store in a bottle in the freezer to preserve freshness. Other species of Pine have the same medicinal properties, although Ponderosa Pine is perhaps slightly more potent.

MEDICINAL USES:

Lung or sinus congestion and coughs, joint and muscle pain, fevers, sores or cuts, low energy and immunity, urinary tract infections, indigestion

- Infusion of needles, inner bark, and/or pitch is rich in vitamins A and C. Used traditionally to open sinuses, break up green, sticky phlegm, and increase secretions to help relieve coughs. Improves digestion, relieves gas. May also help with rheumatism or urinary tract infections but do not use if there is kidney inflammation or infection.
- Pitch when slightly warmed to soften, can be chewed for sore throats, coughs.
- Pitch can be used in ointments or salves for sores, boils, or cuts, or to draw out splinters. It will also ease the pain of rheumatism or sore back.
- A decoction of the young branch tips is used for internal bleeding and high fevers.
- Infusion of dried buds can be used as an eyewash.
- Pollen contains phytoandrogens, hormones that mimic the ones naturally occurring in our bodies. They can increase stamina, help with the aging process, decrease inflammation, and improve immunity.

OTHER USES:

- Wood used for construction, building canoes, and in sweat lodges.
- Pitch used to waterproof and preserve wood. Makes a good fire-starter.
- Seeds and inner bark can be dried and ground to add to soups and breads.

TINCTURE: Resin and/or pollen, 1:2, in 95% alcohol. Take 20–60 drops up to 4 times a day. Add honey if desired.

OIL: 1 part resin to 5 parts oil (olive, grapeseed, or almond). Let sit in a warm place for 3 weeks. For salve, add 28 grams of beeswax to warmed infused oil, adjust to desired consistency.

INFUSION: ½ cup young needles and buds added to 1 quart water, boil for 20 minutes. Turn off heat and add some Peppermint leaves. Cover and steep another 15 minutes. Strain and drink hot throughout the day.

CAUTION: Avoid using resins if you have kidney problems. Avoid during pregnancy.

POND LILY

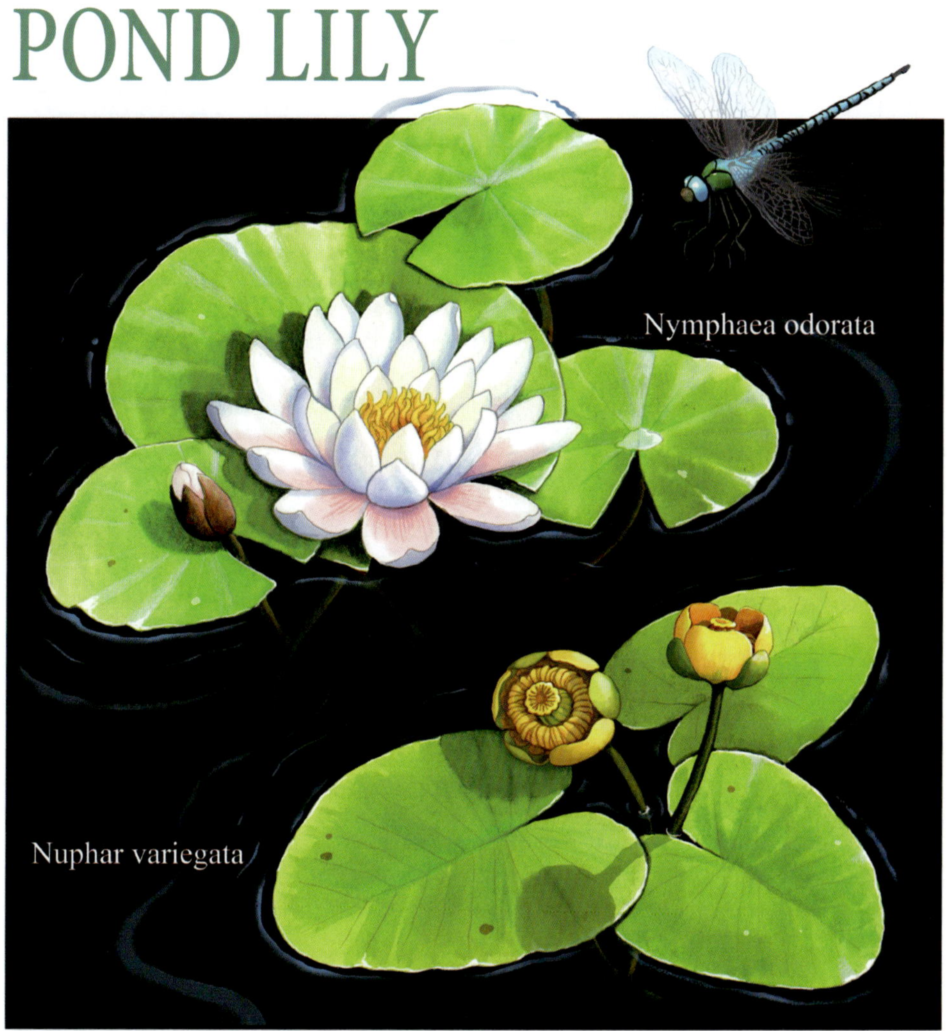

Nuphar variegata, N. lutea
Nymphaea odorata

FAMILY: Nymphaeaceae

OTHER NAMES: *Nuphar variegata:* Yellow Pond Lily, Cow Lily, Bullhead Lily, *Fr.* Grand nénuphar jaune, Pied de cheval; *Nymphaea odorata:* White Water Lily, Fragrant Water Lily, American Water Lily, *Fr.* Nymphéa odorant, Lis d'eau blanc

PARTS USED: Rhizome, flowers, stems

CHARACTERISTICS: Bitter, cool, moistening

ACTIONS: Anaphrodisiac, astringent, demulcent, cardiotonic, antispasmodic, antiscrophulactic, anodyne, sedative, anti-inflammatory

RANGE: *Nuphar variegata* native across Canada except Nunavut; *Nymphaea odorata* introduced in British Columbia, native from Saskatchewan to Newfoundland and Labrador

Water or Pond Lily is a native perennial aquatic plant that grows from an anchor of rootlets buried in the mud of a pond or lake. Its long stem extends upward to the surface, where its flat, waxy, orbicular leaves—dark green on top, purplish underneath, and notched at the base—float on the surface. The large, sweetly scented flowers of the Water variety (*N. odorata*) float on the surface, are around 12 cm. in diameter and are bowl-shaped with many petals. They can be white or pinkish with a yellow centre, and they close up in the evening. The Yellow Pond Lily or Cow Lily (*N. variegata*) has a more oval-shaped leaf that can be up to 35 cm. long and about half as wide, mostly floating on the top. Flowers have 6 yellow sepals that enclose the small petals in a cup shape. They both have similar medicinal properties. Roots can be harvested in the fall when the flowers have died down, and may be dried and ground for later use.

MEDICINAL USES:

Diarrhea, chronic bronchitis, leukorrhea, skin inflammations, boils, mouth infections

- Aside from being a food source, Indigenous Peoples used the mashed roots of these plants for a variety of conditions, primarily as a poultice for sore muscles, arthritis, joint pain, swellings, boils and wounds, bee stings, and generally any inflamed tissues. When mixed with lemon juice it can reduce the appearance of freckles, pimples, and age spots. Contains mucilage, which is anti-inflammatory and softens the skin.
- An infusion of the roots was once used to treat tuberculosis and chronic bronchitis.
- Astringent and demulcent, it has an affinity to the pelvic region, specifically where there is irritation, sharp pain, and heat. Stems excess bleeding and menorrhagia. Helps with leukorrhea, sexually transmitted diseases, testicular inflammation, urinary tract infections, prolapse, cramps, and PMS. The flowers are said to reduce libido and have a tranquilizing effect.
- Eases inflammation in the digestive tract as in Crohn's, IBS, and hemorrhoids. Cools and tones the mucosal lining.
- An infusion of the root may be used as a gargle or mouthwash for inflamed gums, mouth sores, and sore throat.

FOLKLORE: The scientific name derives from the Greek word *numphe*, or "water nymph," and is associated with purity, chastity, or virginity—no doubt due to its anaphrodisiac properties. The Lotus, also a member of the Water Lily family, has been used as a symbol of the Buddha and immortality for thousands of years.

OTHER USES: Flower buds can be cooked as a vegetable; ripe seeds may be ground into meal and used as flour substitute or fried in oil and popped like popcorn.

TINCTURE: Fresh root 1:2 in 95% alcohol, 10–50 drops three times a day.

DECOCTION: 2 tbsp. fresh or dried root, simmer in 2 cups water for 20 minutes. Take ½ cup up to 3 times a day.

CAUTION: Avoid use during pregnancy or breastfeeding. May interfere with drugs affecting the central nervous system (opioids, antidepressants, antipsychotics). Do not consume more than recommended dose. May be poisonous to dogs.

PRICKLY ASH

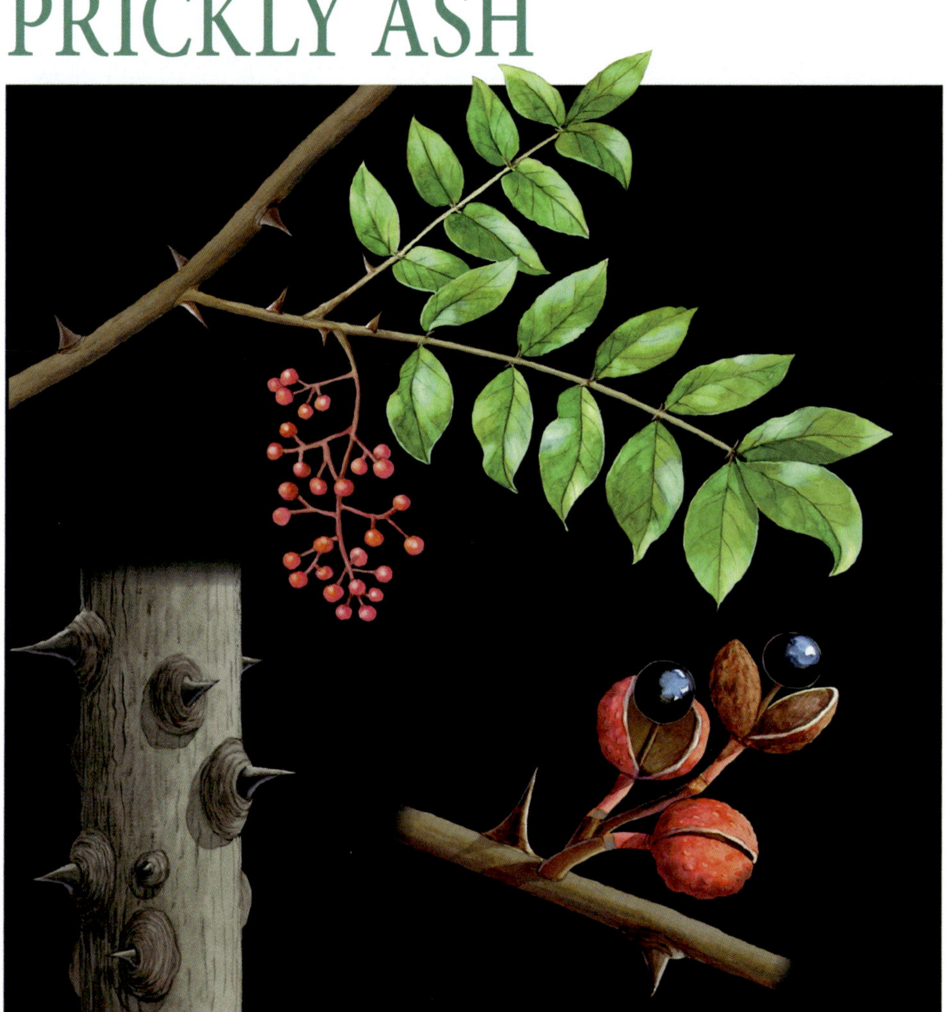

Zanthoxylum americanum

FAMILY: Rutaceae

OTHER NAMES: Toothache Tree, Northern Prickly Ash, *Fr.* Frêne épineux, Clavalier d'Amerique

PARTS USED: Bark and berries

CHARACTERISTICS: Warming, stimulating, bitter, aromatic, drying, numbing

ACTIONS: Antirheumatic, antifungal, antiseptic, antibacterial, anti-inflammatory, antifungal, astringent, diaphoretic, digestive, irritant, rubifacient, sialagogue, stimulant, tonic

RANGE: Native to Ontario and Quebec

Prickly Ash is one of the most effective lymphatic herbs and immune and circulatory stimulants. The bark of this deciduous shrub has been used as medicine by Indigenous Peoples and European settlers for centuries. Its name comes from the arrangement of its leaves, which resembles the Ash tree but is unrelated, and the formidable thorns along its trunk and branches. Growing in thickets typically 2.5–6 m. in height, although it can grow taller, it has alternate leaves composed of 5–11 ovate leaflets that are dark green on top with translucent glands, and lighter green and fuzzy underneath. The greenish-yellow flowers bloom in spring before the leaves emerge, and like the rest of the plant, have an aroma similar to lemon peel. Female flowers form reddish-brown fruit that dry up and open to reveal one shiny black seed. It is a favourite food for the larvae of the giant swallowtail butterfly; they lay their eggs on the underside of the leaves and toxic compounds in the plant protects them from predators. Bark from branches may be stripped in spring and dried for later use. Use gloves to protect the hands from thorns. Berries are safe to eat, but if used as medicine, wait until they open and use only the outer husk.

MEDICINAL USES:

Toothache, coughs, colds, rheumatism, fever, poor circulation, indigestion, skin ulcers, hemorrhoids, fungal infections

- When bark is taken in small amounts, it stimulates the immune system, increases circulation, warming cold hands and feet, and moves the lymphatic system, acting as a tonic. Used for conditions where peripheral circulation is affected, it helps with muscle cramps, Raynaud's syndrome, neuralgia, or varicose veins, improving blood flow and relieving stagnation. Calms inflammation and eases pain.
- Known as the Toothache Tree, it contains alkamides, an immune stimulant that numbs sore gums and produces copious amounts of saliva. Helps improve gum health and tighten loose teeth, although its bitter taste can be off-putting.
- In larger amounts, it works to treat acute digestive disorders, sluggish digestion, diarrhea, constipation. It warms and invigorates. Stimulates appetite.
- Increases blood flow to joints and muscles, relieving pain from arthritis and rheumatism, removing waste more efficiently, and reducing swelling, cramps, and stiffness. May be used as an infused oil or ointment to massage into muscles and joints.
- Diaphoretic action increases blood flow to the skin, increasing perspiration and reducing fevers. Also useful in colds and flu.
- Used topically for skin ulcers, sores and burns, and can be also used internally for eczema, hemorrhoids. Many Indigenous Peoples make an ointment by mixing the ground plant and berries with bear grease.

OTHER USES: Outer husk of fruit can be ground up and used as a lemony-tasting spice.

TINCTURE: Dried berries and bark, 1:5 in 60% alcohol, 1–2 ml. 3 times a day before meals.

DECOCTION: 1–2 tsp. dried berries and bark in 1 cup water, boil 15 minutes. Strain, take 3 times a day.

COMBINATIONS: Add Goldenseal or Ginger for sluggish digestion or candida, Devil's Claw for arthritis, Bayberry or Ginger for circulation, joint pain.

RESEARCH: Research has found that Prickly Ash contains constituents that cause damage to abnormal cells and may prove useful in treating cancer and targeting drug-resistant infectious diseases in the future. Extracts, particularly from the leaf and fruit, also show a broad range of antifungal activity on eleven strains of fungus, including *Candida albicans* and *Aspergillus fumigatus*.

CAUTION: Avoid if pregnant or breastfeeding as it can bring on menstruation. Avoid if you have stomach or intestinal inflammation, ulcers, Crohn's, or IBS. Discontinue if you get hot flashes, acid reflux, or night sweats. Use with caution if taking blood thinners. Do not exceed recommended doses.

PRICKLY LETTUCE

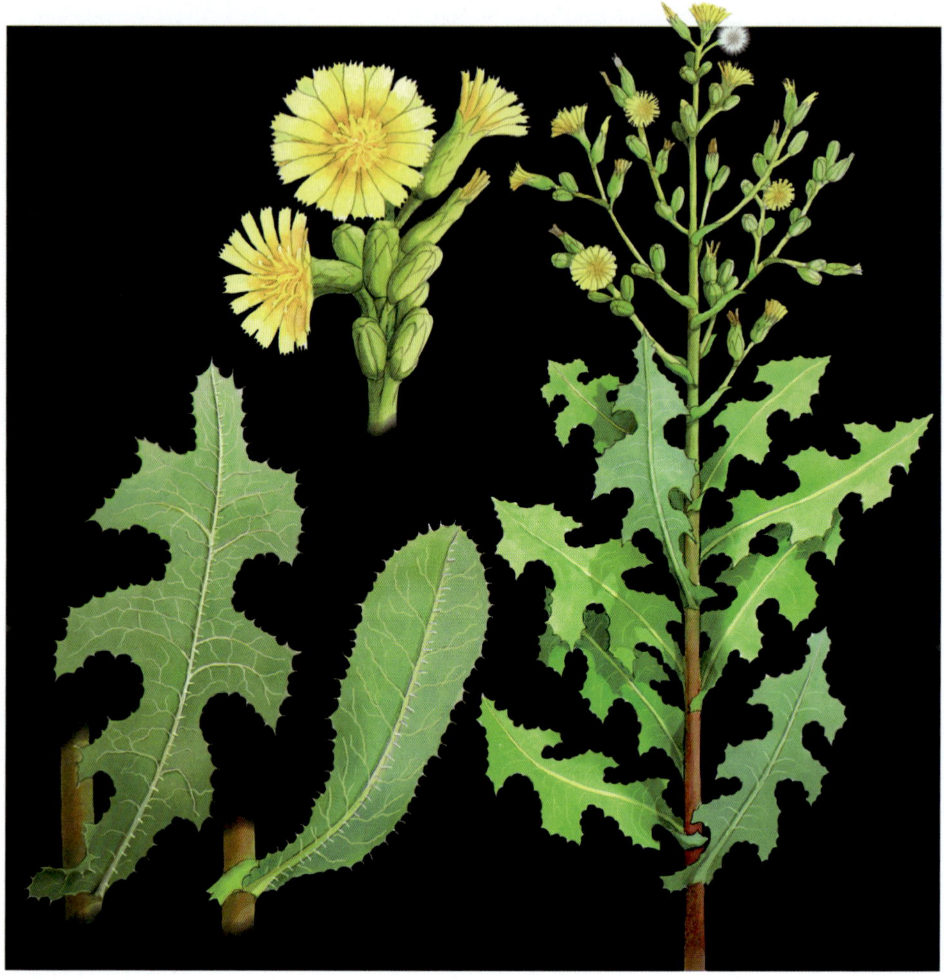

Lactuca serriola

FAMILY: Asteraceae

OTHER NAMES: Compass Plant, China Lettuce, *Fr.* Laitue scariole

PARTS USED: Leaves, dried sap

CHARACTERISTICS: Bitter, cold, salty, moist

ACTIONS: Narcotic, sedative, antispasmodic, expectorant, nervine, diuretic, diaphoretic, anti-inflammatory, laxative

RANGE: Introduced in Northwest Territories, British Columbia to Maritimes

Prickly Lettuce is an annual or biennial herb, originally from Europe, which is related to many different species scattered throughout North America, all having the same or similar properties. It has a smooth stem growing upright from a large white taproot, 30.5 cm. to 2 m. high. Its leaves are prickly along the edges and on the underside mid-vein, and are either lobed or oblong. Both leaves and stems contain a milky latex sap, which oozes out when cut and when dried is often used as a mild narcotic, but contains less than its European cousin *L. virosa* or Wild Lettuce. Basal leaves often twist to face the sun, pointing north and south. The light-yellow composite flowers are similar to a small dandelion and bloom from July to September. It is easily mistaken for Sow Thistle, which has no prickles on the underside vein, but it is also edible. Prickly Lettuce can be found along roadsides and in waste places, and should be gathered in spring or early summer before flowering for teas or salads, but wait until it flowers to collect the sap.

MEDICINAL USES:

Insomnia, anxiety, coughs, colic, headaches, edema, menstrual cramps, pain

- Sap contains lactucin and lactucopicrin, which make it effective as a mild sedative. Historically known as Wild Opium, it was once used as a substitute for opium although it does not contain opiates and the effects are much milder. Should be used in a concentrated tincture for best results. Traditionally used to promote sleep, relieve anxiety and restlessness, and reduce pain.
- Antispasmodic and expectorant, it relieves spasms, colic, and chronic coughs, asthma, and bronchitis when cough is dry and unproductive.
- Diuretic and detoxifying, it removes excess fluid in tissues, reducing edema and swelling in the arms and legs. Promotes sweating.
- Reduces muscle pain and spasms, rheumatism, headaches and migraines. Relieves menstrual cramps and PMS.
- Leaves can be added to salads or lightly steamed.
- Sap may be applied to skin to remove warts.

FOLKLORE: Pagans use Wild Lettuce as incense for divination.

INFUSION: 1–2 tsp. leaves in 1 cup boiling water; infuse 10–15 minutes.

CONCENTRATED TINCTURE (LACTUCARIUM):

- Dry leaves, preferably in a dehydrator, then chop finely in a blender. Weigh, put into a mason jar, then add 4 times that amount of high proof alcohol or Everclear. Leave to extract for several days.
- Place in pan and add water to double the volume. Heat to 180°F for 2 hours, stirring occasionally but keep covered otherwise. Pour through a mesh bag and squeeze out plant material.
- Return liquid to stove and heat to below 180°F, allowing evaporation until it is ⅛ its volume (should look like molasses). This can be dehydrated further in a dehydrator, leaving a substance that can be peeled off and rolled into a ball. To make a tincture, add vodka at 4 times the weight of the extract, dissolving it. In this form it will keep for several years and is easier to take. Start with 1 dropperful and increase up to 2 droppers if needed.

CAUTION: Safe in moderate doses, but large doses may cause nausea, dizziness, or drowsiness. Start with small doses. Not recommended during pregnancy or breastfeeding or if taking other sedatives.

PURPLE LOOSESTRIFE

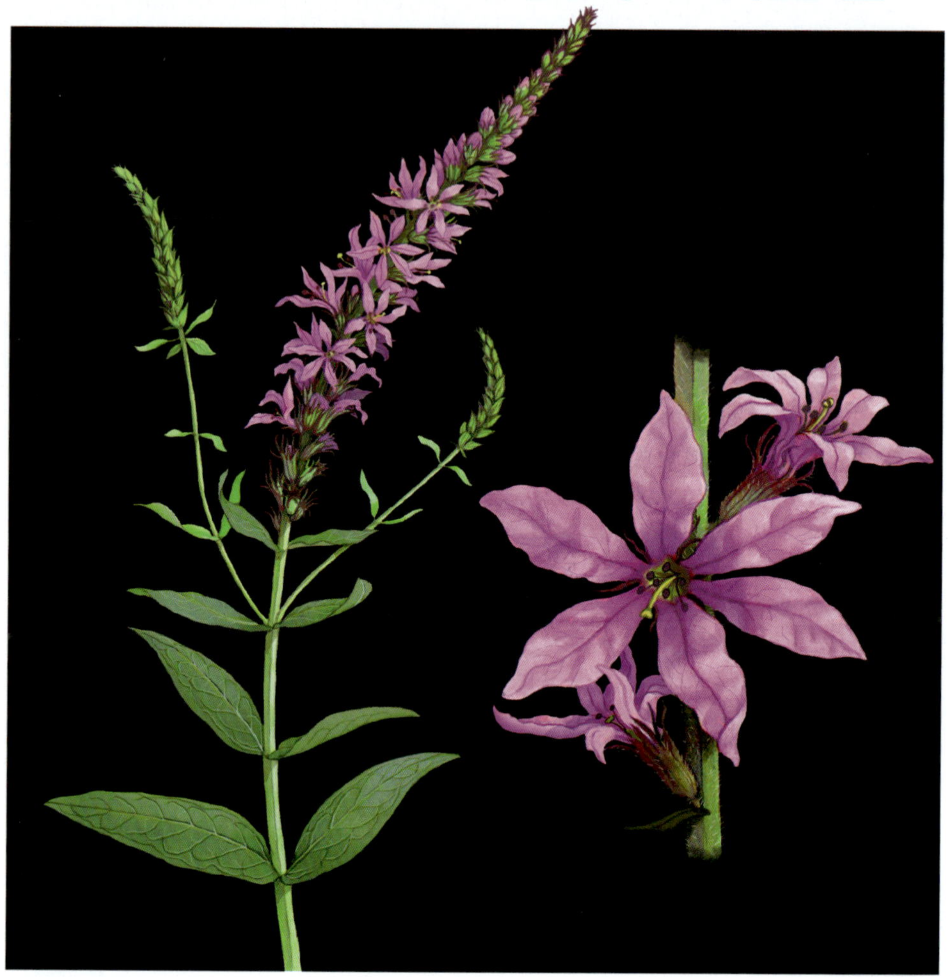

Lythrum salicaria

FAMILY: Lythraceae

OTHER NAMES: Rainbow weed, Purple Willow Herb, Flowering Sally, *Fr.* Salicaire commune

PARTS USED: Aerial

CHARACTERISTICS: Bitter, sour, salty, cool, moist, and drying

ACTIONS: Astringent (leaves and stems), mucilaginous (flowering spikes), antibacterial, antioxidant, antispasmodic, diuretic, demulcent, anti-inflammatory, styptic, tonic, vulnerary, antimicrobial, antifungal

RANGE: Introduced across Canadian provinces

Purple Loosestrife has a bad reputation for being invasive, although it only invades areas laid fallow by human intervention; it usually remains controlled in a natural habitat. However, it can quickly take over wetlands, pushing out native plant species. It is a handsome perennial, growing up to 2.5 m. high, with square or many-sided stems branching toward the top. Leaves are lance-shaped, attach closely to the stem, usually opposite. The taproots are woody with a creeping rhizome. Bright purplish or crimson flowers grow along the top part of the spike from the bottom up, in whorls of 6 or 8 flowers, each composed of a tube with (usually) 6 equal petals and 12 stamens. They produce up to 3 million seeds a year and also reproduce from the rhizomes, so it can spread rapidly, choking out other native plants. It grows mainly in wet, swampy areas, with flowers blooming from July to September. Gather when in full bloom and dry in shade, storing in cloth bags for later use.

MEDICINAL USES:

Chronic diarrhea, leukorrhea, sore dry eyes, fevers, skin inflammation, sores, sinus congestion, gingivitis

- A valuable healing plant since ancient times, Purple Loosestrife contains a balance of tannins or astringency, which tightens and restores tone to tissues, and mucilage, which soothes, lubricates, and eases inflammation. Leaves and stems contain more astringent properties; flower tops are more moistening and mucilaginous.
- Drains fluid from swollen, blocked tissues, strengthening and repairing.
- Used for centuries to heal soldiers with infectious diarrhea, cholera, and dysentery; an excellent remedy for intestinal infections and bleeding, ulcers, and hemorrhoids, restores tone to the digestive tract. Also useful for IBS and leaky gut. A valuable remedy for liver and biliary complaints, helps relieve constipation.
- Astringency actions work topically as a gargle or mouthwash for sore throat, bleeding gums, gingivitis, mouth sores. A weak infusion makes a good eyewash for dry, irritated eyes. A poultice of the leaves will stop a wound from bleeding. Used as a wash for impetigo, eczema, and lupus.
- Commonly used for respiratory problems such as sinus congestion, hay fever, or allergic rhinitis; it drains fluid, shrinks swelling, cools inflammation, and restores tone to the tissues.
- Infusion may be used as a vaginal douche for leukorrhea.

OTHER USES:
- Once used as a hair dye and to drive away insects.
- A decoction may be used to soak wood or rope to prevent rotting.

FOLKLORE: Ancient Greeks hung garlands of Purple Loosestrife around the necks of oxen to help them work better as a team.

TINCTURE: Dried herb 1:5, 30% alcohol, 40–60 drops, 3–4 times a day.

INFUSION: 1–2 tsp. dried herb steeped in 1 cup hot water, 2–3 times a day.

DECOCTION: Place 1–2 tsp. dried herb in 1 cup of hot water; steep 1 hour. Take 1–3 cups per day.

COMBINATIONS: With Usnea for fungal infections, with Stinging Nettle, Goldenrod, Plantain, or Goldenseal for seasonal allergies.

RESEARCH: Studies show high antioxidant, anti-inflammatory, and free-radical–scavenging activity, important in fighting cancer, Alzheimer's, and AIDS, due to high content of phenolic compounds including tannins and flavonoids. Research has confirmed its traditional uses as an antibacterial, specifically against *Candida albicans*, *Staphyllococcus aureus*, and *E. coli,* as well as its antifungal properties, particularly to treat athlete's foot.

PURSLANE

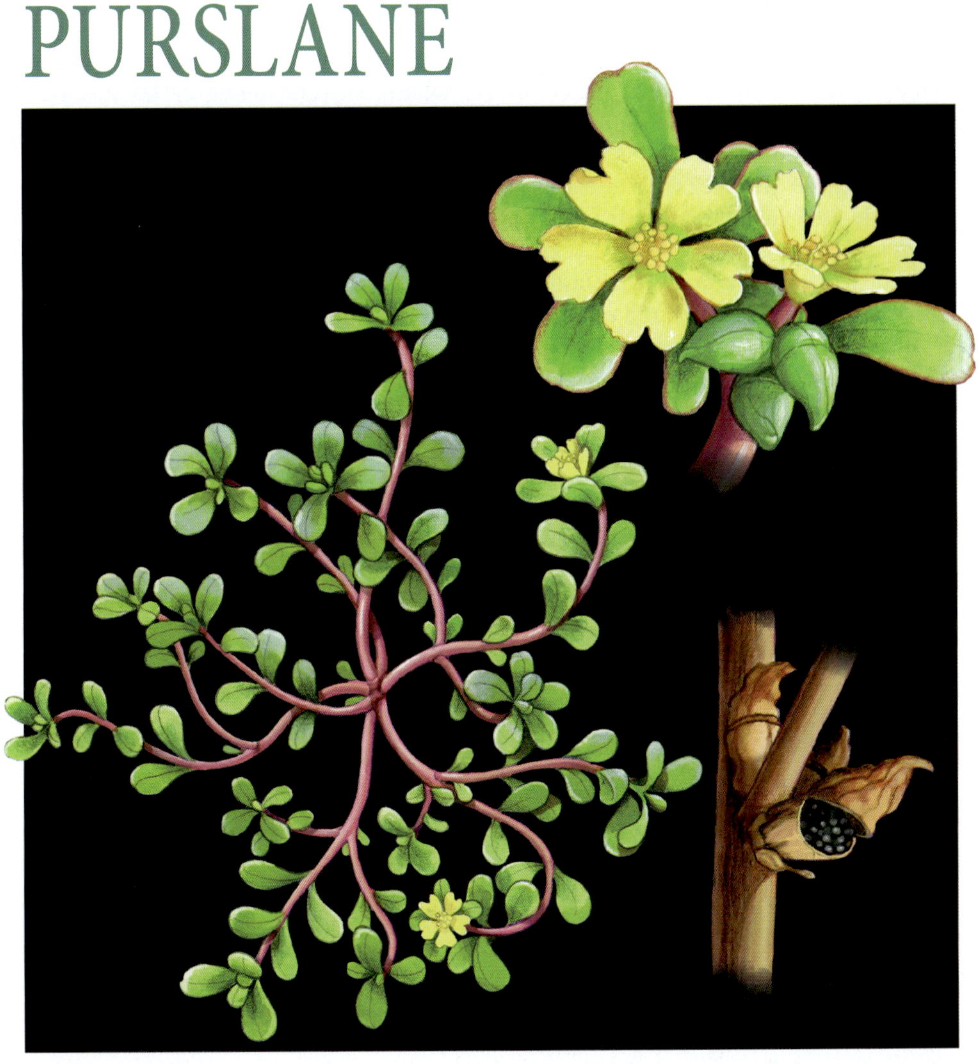

Portulaca oleracea

FAMILY: Portulacaceae

OTHER NAMES: Pigweed, Little Hogweed, *Fr.* Pourpier

PARTS USED: Aerial

CHARACTERISTICS: Sour, salty, moist, cooling

ACTIONS: Antioxidant, anti-inflammatory, antifungal, diuretic, tonic, emollient, relaxant, neuroprotective, hepatoprotective

RANGE: Native from Alberta to Manitoba, introduced in British Columbia, Ontario, Quebec, New Brunswick, Nova Scotia, Prince Edward Island

Purslane is largely ignored in North America and is often pulled out as a weed, but in many countries it is considered a delicacy and is one of the most nutritious herbs available. Reported to have been a common vegetable of the Roman Empire, the succulent stems and leaves have been used for centuries as food and medicine across the globe. Its cylindrical, smooth reddish stems and thick, spatula-shaped, alternate dark green leaves creep along the ground in waste places and gardens. The tiny yellow flowers have 4–6 petals and grow in the leaf rosettes. The tips of the branches are the most tender, but most of the aerial parts can be harvested, preferably in July before the flowers bloom, and in the morning to get a more tangy, sour taste. Best if eaten fresh, but may be dried on a rack or in a dehydrator, or steamed and cooled (don't rinse after steaming as all the minerals will be lost), then vacuum sealed and frozen for later use.

MEDICINAL USES:

High blood pressure, diarrhea, skin problems, osteoporosis

- Described as a powerhouse of nutrition, this innocuous plant is packed full of nutrients, primarily vitamins A, B, C, and E, and many minerals like iron, potassium, magnesium, and calcium. But it is also an excellent source of alpha-linolenic acid, an omega-3 fatty acid that plays an important role in growth, prevention of cardiovascular disease, and maintaining a healthy immune system. It has been shown to be the richest vegetable source, and has 5 times the omega-3 fatty acids as spinach.
- Seeds have been shown to improve the health of people with type 2 diabetes, reducing blood glucose, LDL cholesterol, and triglycerides and helping with weight reduction.
- Rich in antioxidants, it may improve liver function and reduce oxidative stress in the pancreas and ovaries, but more human studies are needed.
- An excellent source of calcium and magnesium, which are essential to bone health and prevention of osteoporosis.
- Used topically as a poultice for burns, scrapes, insect bites, bruises, and sore eyes. It cools, soothes irritation, and promotes healing.
- Rich in mucilage, it cools excess heat in the digestive tract, eases diarrhea and dysentery, and stems bleeding.

OTHER USES:
- As a food, it can be eaten raw, cooked in soups, or stir-fried, pickled, or juiced.
- If using in a tea, steep until cooled to extract the mucilage.

FOLKLORE: Was once strewn around the bed to ward off evil spirits.

CAUTION: Avoid if pregnant or breastfeeding, or if you have kidney disease or stones. Contains oxalates that can irritate the kidneys if eaten in large amounts.

QUEEN ANNE'S LACE

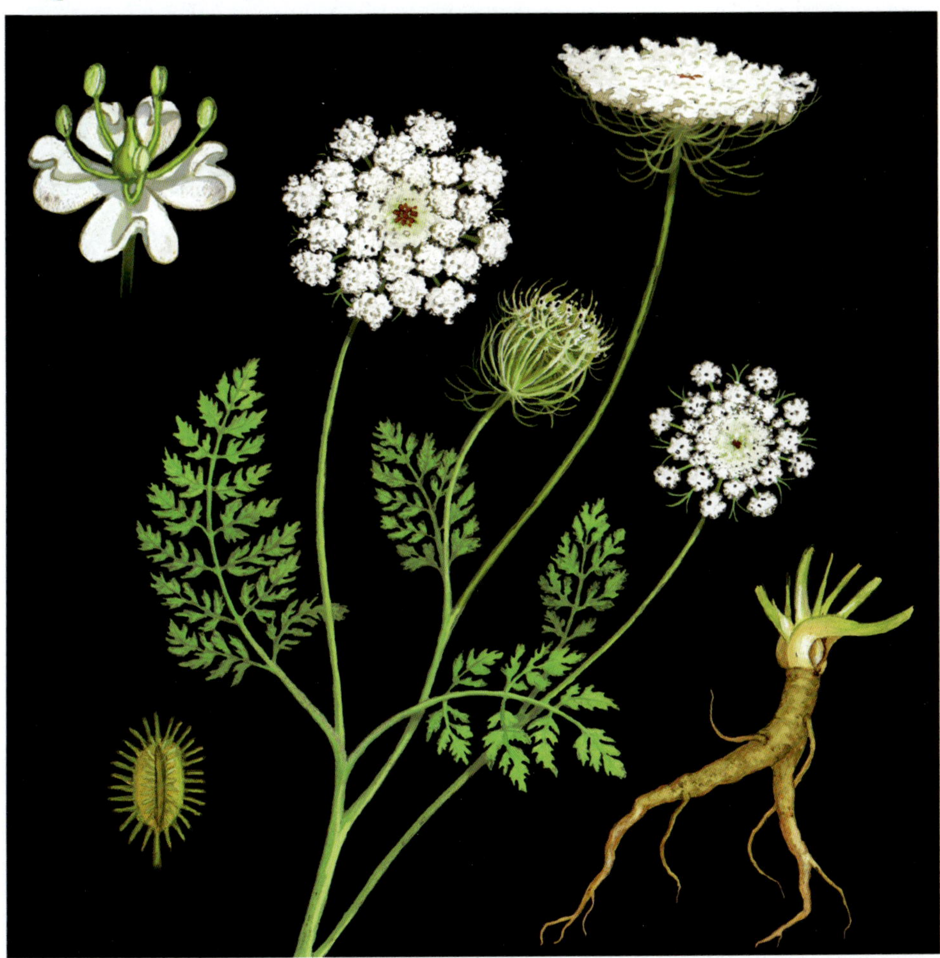

Daucus carota

FAMILY: Apiaceae

OTHER NAMES: Wild Carrot, Bee's Nest, Bird's Nest, *Fr.* Carotte sauvage

PARTS USED: Root, leaves, and seeds

CHARACTERISTICS: Bitter

ACTIONS: Diuretic, antioxidant, antimicrobial, hypotensive, anti-inflammatory, analgesic, purgative, vermifuge, anthelmintic, carminative, antilithic, antifungal, emmenagogue

RANGE: Introduced across all provinces

Queen Anne's Lace, a direct descendant of our garden carrot, is a biennial herb found along roadsides and fields throughout most of southern Canada during the summer months. A native of southern Europe, its stems are up to 90 cm. high, erect and branched, with finely dissected, fern-like leaves. Flowers are densely clustered white umbels radiating from the central stalk with a tiny purple or pink flower in the centre. As the seeds ripen, the umbels contract and curve inwards, forming a nest-like appearance, hence the name Bird's Nest. The large taproot is whitish and bitter and smells like carrot. It is harvested in late summer and should be cut longitudinally and dried or the tender smaller roots may be eaten fresh in the spring. The plant should be picked in July before it has gone to seed as the seeds are more potent when collected just before they are fully mature. Rub them between your hands to remove the tiny hairs. Be careful to properly identify this plant, as there are several in this family that look alike, particularly Poison Hemlock (*Conium maculatum*), which should not even be touched. Its stems are smooth with purplish spots, there is no central red flower, and it is normally taller, whereas the stem of Queen Anne's Lace is hairy with no purple spots (remember, the Queen has hairy legs!) and the flowers have a distinct umbrella-like shape. Of course you can always smell the root to be sure, but if there's any doubt, wear gloves.

MEDICINAL USES:

Urinary antiseptic, kidney stones, gout, rheumatism, relief of flatulence and colic, diuretic for edema, birth control

- Highly valued for its effectiveness as a diuretic, it is useful for relieving chronic kidney problems, stones, and bladder infections. By removing extra water and uric acid from the body, it can help with weight loss, gout, and edema.
- An infusion of the leaves and seeds can help with digestion, to ease flatulence, and settle the stomach.
- The seeds are known to stimulate the pituitary gland, which in turn stimulates the sex hormones to bring on menstruation. It has been used to prevent conception, although when use is stopped, it may increase chances of conceiving as it tones the uterus. Reduces heavy flow and helps with endometriosis.
- The root is slightly bitter but edible, and is rich in vitamin A. It can be used in a poultice to ease the pain of skin ulcers, or in infusions as a mild laxative, or to expel kidney stones.
- It has been used widely by Indigenous Peoples for pimples, paleness, lack of appetite, to expel intestinal worms, and as a poultice to reduce swelling and soothe sores. An infusion of the blossoms is used to treat diabetes.
- Recent studies using primarily the root show promise in treating several types of cancer, Alzheimer's, cardiovascular disease, and hair loss.

OTHER USES:

- Seeds contain an essential oil used in anti-wrinkle cream.
- A decoction of the seeds and root make a good insecticide.
- Seeds and root can also be used as flavouring for soups and stews.

FOLKLORE: The tiny red flower in the centre is apparently how Queen Anne's Lace got its name, since Queen Anne, according to legend, pricked her finger while making lace. The flower was once believed to cure epilepsy.

INFUSION: Pour 1 cup of boiling water onto 1 tsp. of dried leaves or bruised seeds, infuse 10–15 min. Drink 3 times a day.

TINCTURE: Dried herb 1:5, 60% alcohol, 20–60 drops twice a day.

CAUTION: Avoid if pregnant or breastfeeding. May affect blood pressure, stop use 2 weeks before or after surgery. Consult a professional if you have serious kidney problems.

RASPBERRY

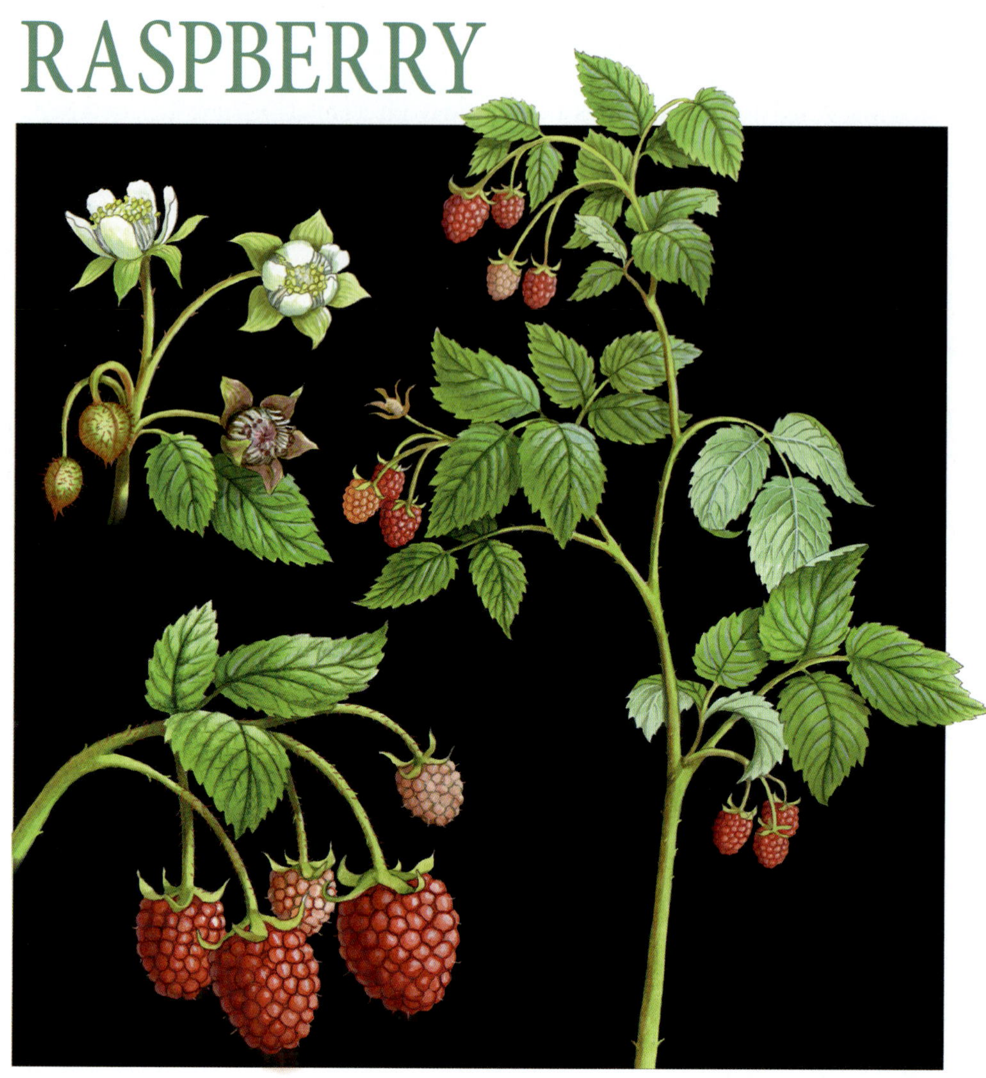

Rubus idaeus

FAMILY: Rosaceae

OTHER NAMES: *Fr.* Framboise

PARTS USED: Leaf, fruit, root

CHARACTERISTICS: Mild, bitter, cool, drying

ACTIONS: Astringent, anti-inflammatory, hemostatic, alterative, parturient, anti-emetic, uterine tonic, antimicrobial, antioxidant, carminative, diuretic, sedative, styptic, vulnerary

RANGE: Native across Canada

The sweet red fruit of the raspberry plant is well-known to most North Americans, but few know of the plant's use as an herbal remedy. A member of the Rose family, Raspberry has creeping perennial roots and grows up to 1.8 m. high. It's easily identified by its tangle of bristly vines along roadsides and fields. Its compound leaves are alternate and pointed, with 3 to 7 toothed leaflets. The small white or pinkish 5-petalled flowers bloom in June or July, and are followed by clusters of bright red berries, which usually appear in July or August. The leaves should be harvested on a dry day in early summer and dried quickly to prevent mould from forming on the leaves.

MEDICINAL USES:

Helps birthing process, fever, diarrhea, colds, incontinence, menorrhagia, sore throat

- The berries are high in vitamins B and C, and both berries and leaves are rich in magnesium, potassium, iron, and calcium, as well as many trace minerals, making it an excellent source of nutrients and a blood tonic. Known for its ability to balance hormones, it not only tones the uterus, but its astringent qualities strengthen and repair tissues.
- A wonderful uterine tonic, the leaf tea has been used for centuries by women to strengthen the muscles of the uterus, facilitate delivery, prevent miscarriage, and reduce excessive menstrual bleeding. Encourages milk production, tones the uterus after delivery, and has been used to treat fibroids, endometriosis, and heavy, painful, or irregular periods.
- Infusion of leaves and root are used as a mouthwash or gargle for sore throat, tonsillitis, gingivitis, and mouth sores.
- Reduces fevers, sore throat, cold symptoms, and diarrhea.
- Nourishes the blood; replenishes iron and other minerals.
- Leaves are crushed and used in an infusion by the Mi'kmaq to relieve stomach upset and prevent vomiting. Roots are used to treat diarrhea, and bark tea relieves stomachaches.
- Applied topically to wounds, a leaf poultice speeds the healing process and prevents infection. A strong tea can soothe sunburn, eczema, and rashes, and when used as a mouthwash, it can improve gingivitis.

INFUSION: Dried or fresh leaf, 2 heaped tsp. in 1 cup boiling water, use as needed.

TINCTURE: Dried 1:5, 50% alcohol, 1 dropper 2–3 times a day.

COMBINATIONS: With Lady's Mantle for weakened uterus, with Shepherd's Purse or Cramp Bark for heavy, painful periods, with Flax seeds for constipation, or with Yarrow for leaky gut.

RESEARCH: Studies on pregnant women who consumed Raspberry leaf had shorter labours, with less complications than a control group and a significant reduction in incidences of caesarian deliveries.

CAUTION: Avoid in the first 6 months of pregnancy, otherwise considered safe.

RED ALDER

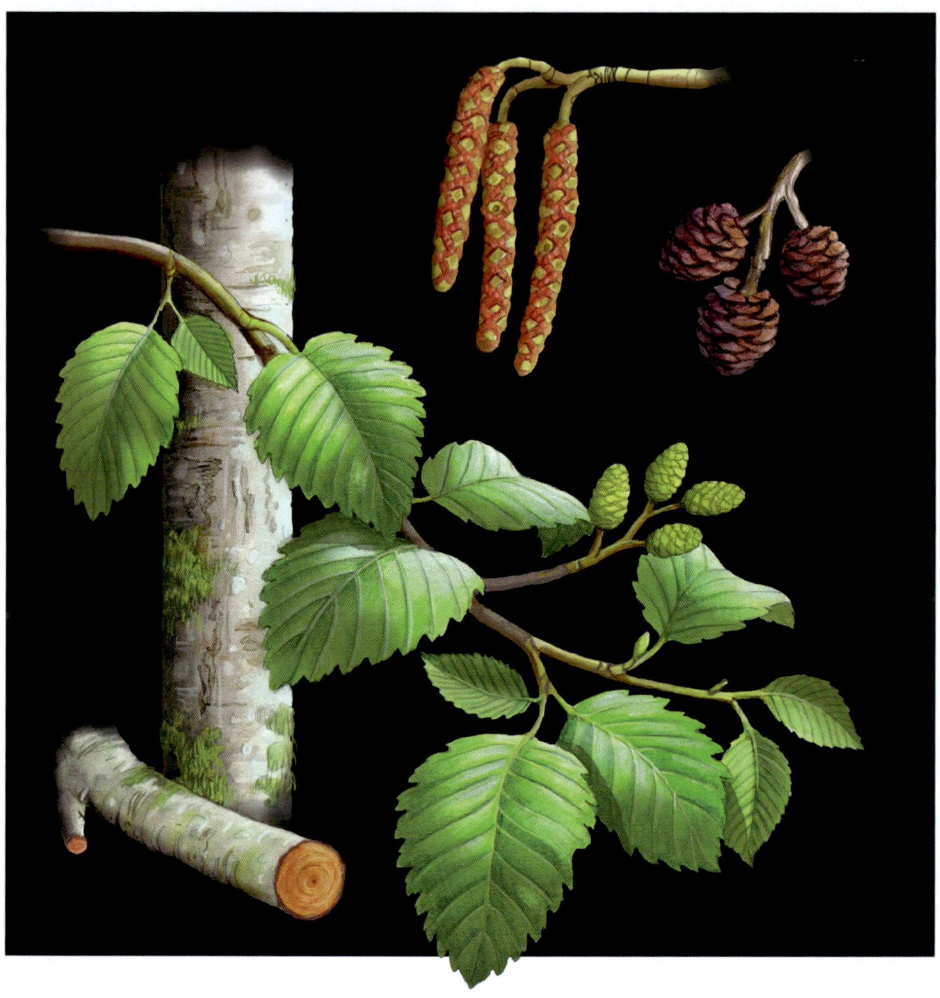

Alnus rubra

FAMILY: Betulaceae

OTHER NAMES: Oregon Alder, Western Alder, *Fr.* Aulne rouge

PARTS USED: Inner bark, catkins, leaves, buds

CHARACTERISTICS: Bitter, cold, dry, stimulating

ACTIONS: Alterative, anti-inflammatory, antioxidant, astringent, antimicrobial, cathartic, febrifuge, hemostatic, hepatoprotective, emetic, stomachic, tonic, vulnerary, antiviral

RANGE: Native to west coast of British Columbia

Indigenous Peoples have used the dried inner bark of this deciduous tree as food and medicine for many years. Native to North America and a member of the birch family, it grows up to 25 m. tall, with thin grey or whitish bark often spotted with white patches of lichens or moss. When scraped or cut the inner bark turns a rusty red colour, hence its name. The leaves are alternate, toothed, and slightly lobed. The underside has rusty patches and soft hairs, and the entire leaf turns yellow in the fall. Male flowers or catkins open before leaves and grow in long, hanging clusters. Female catkins, small and cone-like, grow on the same branch. Near the coast of British Columbia and Alaska it grows mainly on cool, moist slopes; inland, often next to rivers and wetlands. Other Alder species have similar properties, but Red Alder is the most commonly used. Gather bark in early spring or late autumn, no more than a 3–4-inch strip to avoid killing the tree. Dry before using.

MEDICINAL USES:

Pain and headaches, skin problems, digestive sluggishness, hepatitis, diarrhea, lymphatic disorders

- Dried Red Alder bark has been used by Indigenous Peoples for many years to relieve pain, congestion, eliminate toxins, and give a sense of grounding. The tree cleanses impurities from water systems, and also cleanses our blood and lymph, getting things moving. Contains salicylic acid, which acts like aspirin to relieve pain and cool inflammation. Astringency action tightens and tones tissue, and antimicrobial action fights infection.
- Decoction of bark relieves pain from headaches, rheumatism.
- Alder's bitterness can help support liver function and aid digestion, relieving bloating from overeating. Stimulates gastric juices, aids bowel function, and increases bile flow. Tonic action can heal mucous membranes in the digestive tract, decreasing leaky gut, ulcerative colitis, diarrhea, constipation, and intestinal bleeding. Inhibits *Helicobacter pylori,* heals and prevents recurrence of gastric ulcers.
- Can be used both internally and externally for skin problems like eczema, boils, premenstrual and teen acne, poison oak or ivy, insect bites, scabies, or lice. Helps many chronic or cyclic skin conditions, stops bleeding, and heals wounds. Inner bark can be ground and used as a poultice or in decoction.
- Decoction useful as a mouthwash or gargle for sore throats, gum disease, and thrush.
- Traditionally used for tuberculosis, scrofula, and enlarged lymph nodes. Increases flow of lymph, relieving congestion and colds.
- Used in sitz bath for hemorrhoids and anal fissures.
- Oil infused with buds can be massaged into sore muscles, arthritic joints, sprains, or to ease backache.

OTHER USES:

- Ground inner bark added to soups and bread, catkins high in protein but bitter; used only as survival food.
- Reddish-brown dye made from bark.
- Wood used for furniture.
- Helps control erosion and replaces nitrogen in nutrient-poor soil.

TINCTURE: Dried bark and catkins 1:5, 50% alcohol, up to 35 drops 2–4 times a day.

DECOCTION: Simmer 1 tsp. dried bark in 1¼ cups water for 10–15 minutes. Let steep for 1 hour, take up to ⅓ cup 4 times a day.

COMBINATIONS: With Gentian, Chamomile or Oregon Grape for digestion, constipation with diarrhea, or oral infections. With Calendula, Red Root, or Chickweed for swollen glands or lymphatic congestion.

CAUTION: Avoid use internally if allergic to aspirin. Use only dried inner bark internally; fresh bark is emetic.

RED CEDAR

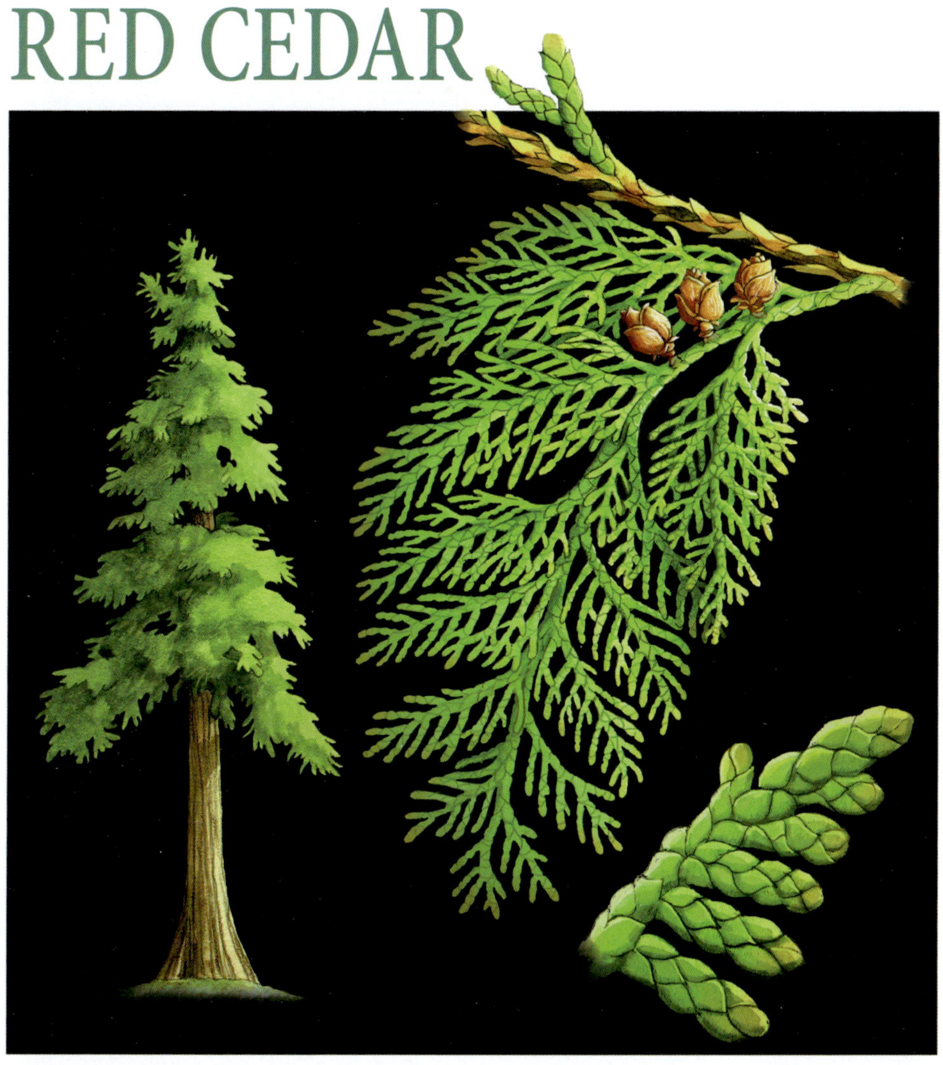

Thuja plicata

FAMILY: Cupressaceae

OTHER NAMES: Western Red Cedar, *Fr.* Cèdre de l'Ouest, Thuya géant

PARTS USED: Inner bark, fresh or dried leaves

CHARACTERISTICS: Bitter, pungent, aromatic, warming, drying

ACTIONS: Anti-inflammatory, antibacterial, antioxidant, astringent, alterative, antifungal, diuretic, diaphoretic, stimulant, antiviral, antimicrobial

RANGE: Native to British Columbia and Alberta

The Western Red Cedar has long been considered an important plant to many Indigenous Peoples, holding a sacred place as a symbol of cleansing, protection, and healing. It seems to have an uncanny ability to counteract negative energy. Older trees have been known to reach over 1000 years of age and can often reach a height of 60 m. and a diameter of 3–5.7 m.; however, overharvesting of trees has left old-growth cedar forests endangered and rare. Its thin, reddish-brown bark is easily peeled off in strips, and the straight trunks flare at the base. The fragrant, fan-shaped groupings of leaves are evergreen, and its name *plicata*, meaning "plait" or "braid," describes the placement of the leaves on its branches. The inconspicuous pollen cones are located at the tips of the twigs. The seed cones grow to 1–2 cm. with thin, leathery scales, each one bearing one or two winged seeds. Only harvest from freshly fallen branches, as this species is endangered. Hang branches to dry, then chop finely before using. Western Red Cedar and Eastern Red Cedar should not be confused, as the latter is actually a variety of Juniper and found only in Eastern Canada.

MEDICINAL USES:

Respiratory tract infections, fevers, colds, kidney problems, rheumatism, skin problems, delayed menstruation, diarrhea, warts

- This tree has a long history of medicinal use among the coastal Indigenous Peoples, particularly for its antimicrobial and antifungal properties. It also improves circulation and stimulates the white blood cells to increase immunity and fight off infection. Essential oils inhibit bacterial and fungal growth. However, due to its potential toxicity, it should be used sparingly if taken internally.
- Hot infusion, steam, or tincture of inner bark and/or leaves helps relieve upper respiratory conditions, fevers, coughs, bronchitis; add honey if desired. Good where there is excessive mucous. Stimulates the immune system to fight infection.
- Cold infusion or tincture targets infections in the kidneys and urinary tract.
- Dries oozing skin conditions such as poison oak, eczema, or fungal infections. Oil, salve or tincture can be applied to skin to remove warts. Should be applied 2–3 times a day for a couple of weeks until the wart disappears.
- Stimulant properties help relieve sluggishness in digestive, respiratory, urinary, and reproductive systems. A decoction of the bark will induce menstruation.
- Soft pounded bark used to bind open wounds, heal sores, and reduce swelling.
- Decoction from boughs used to help dandruff. Green buds may be chewed to relieve toothache.
- Poultice from crushed bough tips mixed with oil may be applied to the back for coughs, back pain, or rheumatism.

OTHER USES:

- Dried ground inner bark added to flour for making breads.
- Bark used by Indigenous Peoples to make baskets, shredded to make rope and clothing.
- Wood resists decay, often up to a hundred years. Used for building and making canoes, totem poles.
- Offered to sacred fire during sweat lodge ceremonies, burned in smudges, branches boiled to purify the air or to help relieve lung conditions.
- Repels insects, mold, bacteria, and fungi.

COLD INFUSION: Steep 1 tbsp. fresh or dried leaves per cup in cold water for several hours or overnight. Take ¼–½ cup twice a day.

TINCTURE: Fresh herb 1:2 in 50% alcohol, 2–5 drops a day. Do not exceed recommended dose.

COMBINATIONS: Often used with Witch Hazel to treat eczema. Add Burdock root or Oregon Grape root to cool hot skin conditions. With Devil's Club or Figwort for chronic fatigue. With Peppermint or Rosemary for steam decongesting.

CAUTION: Avoid if pregnant as it can induce menstruation, although steam from simmering Red Cedar may be inhaled to stimulate labour if it is delayed. Contains thujone, a neurotoxin, so prolonged use is not recommended, although short-term use is considered safe. Avoid use of essential oils with infants. External use may cause allergic sensitivities.

RED CLOVER

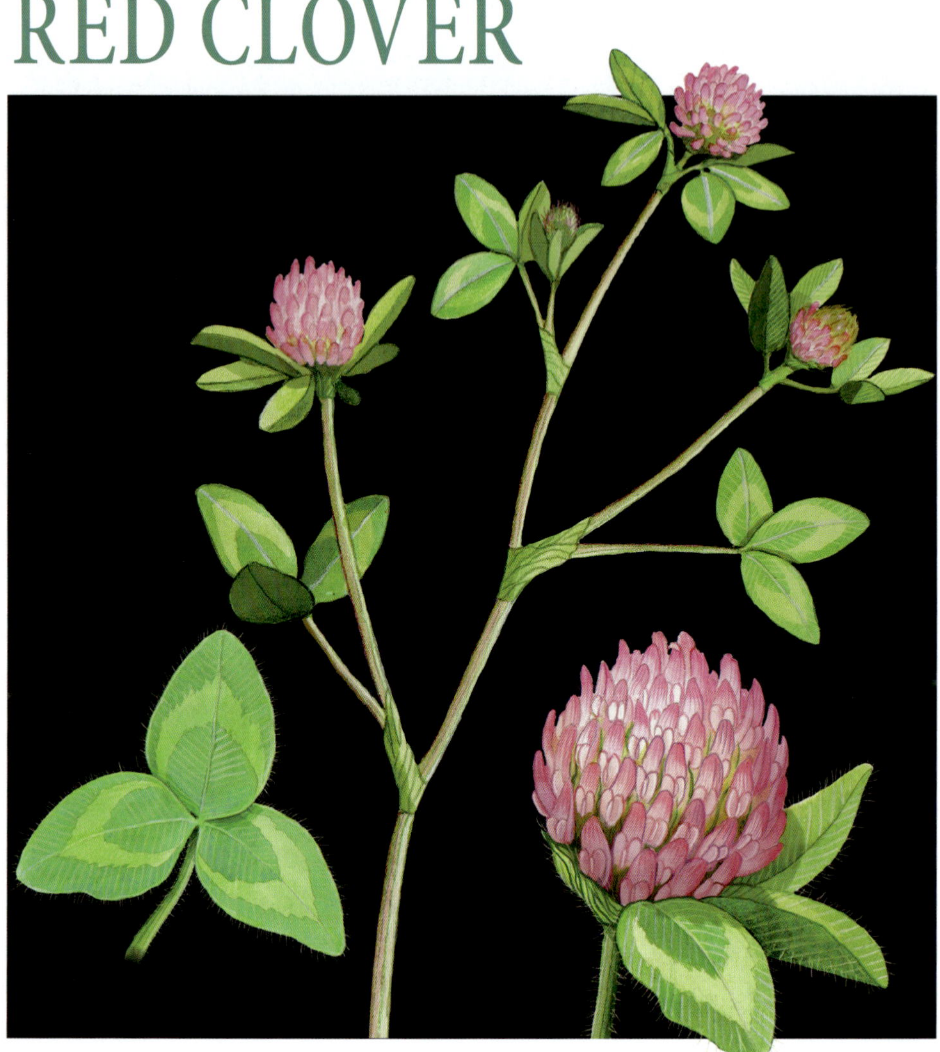

Trifolium pratense

FAMILY: Fabaceae (Leguminosae)

OTHER NAMES: Sweet Clover, Bee-bread, Meadow Clover, *Fr.* Trèfle rouge

PARTS USED: Flowerheads

CHARACTERISTICS: Sweet, salty, cool

ACTIONS: Alterative, antispasmodic, anti-inflammatory, expectorant, anti-tumour, antioxidant, nervine, sedative, tonic

RANGE: Introduced across Canada except Nunavut

Fields of Red Clover may be seen across Canada throughout the summer, its sweet scent permeating the air. Originating from Europe, it is often planted by farmers as a cover crop to improve the nitrogen levels in the soil, protect from erosion, and provide feed for animals, but it also grows wild almost everywhere. It is a short-lived perennial, with several stems 30 to 60 cm. high, arising from the one root and three oval leaflets with a V marked in a lighter green. The flowers are pink or red in a round dense terminal and bloom from June to September. It has been used as a medicinal remedy for centuries, and the young flowerheads, leaves, and sprouts can be eaten. Pick the flowerheads in early summer and dry for later use.

MEDICINAL USES:

PMS, skin diseases, coughs, congestion, fevers, menopause

- Known for its phyto-estrogenic properties, it has been used to treat many conditions caused by hormone imbalances during adolescence, menopause, and throughout the menstrual cycle, particularly skin conditions like acne. A rich source of isoflavones, it can mimic estrogen, relieving hot flashes and other discomforts of menopause as well as PMS and helps balance these hormones. Although research is limited, it may prevent bone loss, improve bone density, and help fight osteoporosis.
- Blood purifier and blood thinner, it helps reduce cholesterol and increases flexibility in the arteries. Reduces the risk of cardiovascular disease, especially after menopause.
- Cleansing, alterative and antispasmodic, it clears congestion in the respiratory tract, relieving coughs, asthma, whooping cough, and bronchitis, stimulating the immune system to fight infection. Flowers were once dried and smoked for asthma.
- Used in salves and liniments for skin complaints, soothes skin ulcers, psoriasis, eczema, bee stings, burns, and even skin cancer.
- Regulates digestion, improves appetite, increases detoxification ability of the liver.
- Contains several compounds that have anticancer properties, and although little clinical research has been done to prove its effectiveness, it appears to limit the growth of cancer by preventing the growth of new blood vessels that feed the tumour.

INFUSION: Pour 1 cup of boiling water onto 1–3 tsp. dried flowers. Infuse 10–15 minutes. Take 3 times a day.

TINCTURE: Dried flower tops, 1:5, 30% alcohol, take 60–100 drops 3 times a day.

COMBINATIONS: As an alterative, may be combined with Burdock root, Mullein, Yellow Dock, and Dandelion root.

CAUTION: Women with hormone-related conditions such as endometriosis, uterine fibroids, breast, ovarian, or uterine cancers, or those using hormonal treatments such as birth control pills or hormone replacement therapy, should consult with a professional before taking Red Clover due to the presence of phytoestrogens. Avoid if using blood thinners, or if pregnant or breastfeeding.

RED ROOT

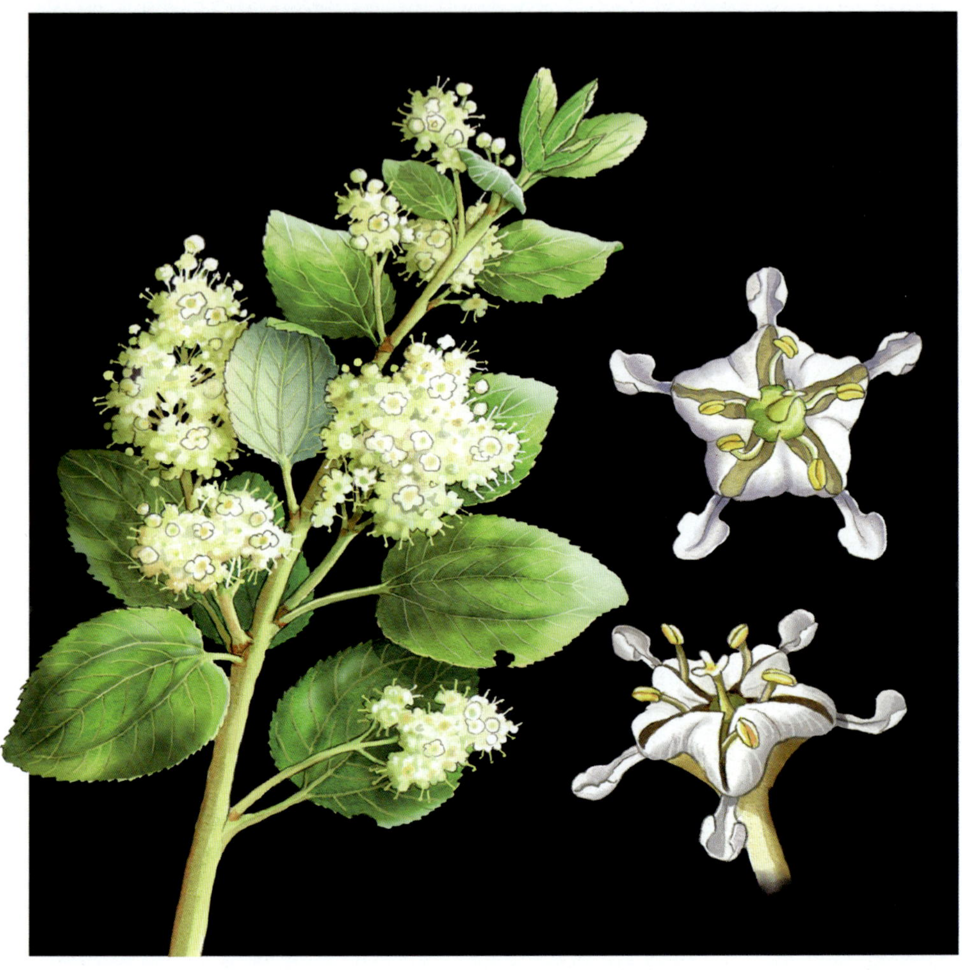

Ceanothus americanus

FAMILY: Rhamnaceae

OTHER NAMES: New Jersey Tea, *Fr.* Céanothe d'Amérique

PARTS USED: Root bark, leaves

CHARACTERISTICS: Astringent, bitter, cooling

ACTIONS: Astringent, anti-inflammatory, expectorant, antimicrobial, antioxidant, stimulant, antispasmodic

RANGE: Native to Ontario and Quebec

Many species of Ceanothus, some of which have similar medicinal uses, grow throughout North America, but Red Root is one of the most well-known mainly for its action on the lymph nodes. Native to Central Canada, this resilient deciduous shrub grows to about 1 m. tall and has been used by Indigenous Peoples for centuries. It is often one of the few survivors on land cleared by forest fires, its seeds and roots surviving the devastation. Its leaves are alternate and oval-shaped, finely serrated with a blunt tip, with three prominent veins and fine hairs, particularly on the underside. The small white aromatic flowers grow in clusters from June to August, each one having 5 spreading spoon-shaped sepals and 5 triangular sepals that fold into the centre. The red roots may be harvested in spring or fall, being careful to remove from only one side of the plant and filling in the hole so as not to kill it. Chop up when still fresh and dry for later use.

MEDICINAL USES:

Swollen lymph glands, congested liver, coughs, high blood pressure

- Noted for its action on the lymph nodes, it helps process waste quickly and reduces the time of recovery. Good for swollen glands, as well as chest congestion, and any catarrhal conditions with lots of mucus in the lungs or digestive tract. It loosens stuck fluids, drains and reduces swelling and inflammation, slowly increasing movement and blood flow. Best for cold, chronic conditions rather than hot, acute infections.
- Clears chronic bronchial and sinus congestion, sore throat, asthma, whooping cough, tonsillitis, mumps, colds.
- In Traditional Chinese Medicine, it relieves chronic indigestion due to a congested liver, removes dampness in the spleen, melancholy, sluggishness, poor digestion, and headache after eating. It opens and restores flow while the tannins in the root bark tighten and tone tissues. Tannins stimulate blood flow and dilate the blood vessels, reducing blood pressure. Stimulates blood flow to the brain, removing brain fog and that "stuck" feeling, when creativity seems to be blocked.
- Decoction of the root may be used topically to treat sores, eczema, cancerous lesions, rashes, hemorrhoids, and venereal disease.

OTHER USES:

- Contain saponins, which will produce a lather when mixed with water.
- Flowers and leaves make a nice shampoo.
- Ground leaves can be used as baby powder.

TINCTURE: Dried root bark 1:5, fresh 1:2 in 50% alcohol, 1–2 ml. up to 3 times a day.
DECOCTION: 1 tsp. dried herb in 1 cup water. Take 4–8 tbsp. up to 3 times a day.

COMBINATIONS: Used mostly with Echinacea for lymph congestion; promotes drainage and fights infection. For liver stagnation with constipation and distention, add Mahonia and Dandelion root. Other supporting herbs are Calendula, Lobelia, Yarrow, and Mullein.

CAUTION: Avoid use if spleen is inflamed. Do not use while taking blood thinners.

RED TRILLIUM

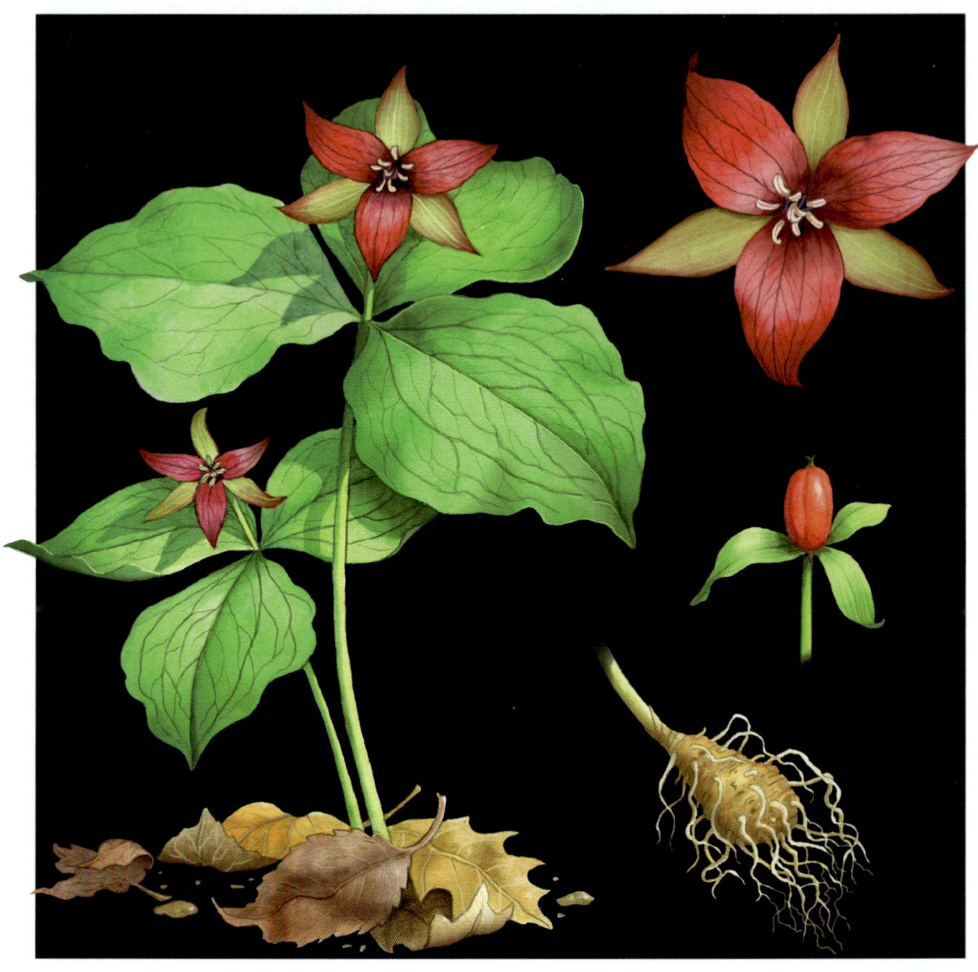

Trillium erectum

FAMILY: Liliaceae

OTHER NAMES: Beth Root, Birth Root, Wake Robin, Stinking Benjamin, *Fr.* Trille rouge

PARTS USED: Root, leaves

CHARACTERISTICS: Acrid, sweet, warming

ACTIONS: Antibacterial, astringent, aphrodisiac, alterative, expectorant, tonic, antiseptic

RANGE: Native from Ontario to the Maritimes

Red Trillium or Beth Root has been considered a sacred women's herb by many North American Indigenous Peoples for hundreds of years. Although typically a woodland flower, it is now cultivated in gardens for its showy, solitary nodding red or white flowers that bloom in early spring, often emitting a scent resembling rotting meat to attract flies and beetles, which pollinate them. The 3 petals, 3 sepals, and 3 diamond-shaped leaves give it its name, Trillium, which derives from the Latin word *trilix* meaning "triple." It prefers the shade or semi-shade and moist, humus-rich, slightly acidic soil of the woods, growing to a height of around 40 cm. It usually only flowers after five years, and the seeds can take three years to germinate, so it is not easily spread and has become endangered in some provinces. Only pick roots from places where it grows in abundance, or better still, from cultivated plants, after the leaves have died back in the fall. Leaves have similar uses, and can be picked in late summer after seed capsules have ripened.

MEDICINAL USES:

Childbirth, heavy menstruation, bleeding, chronic coughs, stomach upset, skin inflammation

- The root of this plant was traditionally used to aid in childbirth, induce labour, prevent excess bleeding, and help the uterus return to normal after parturition. Aids with pelvic weakness, endometriosis, menorrhagia, uterine prolapse, and menopausal bleeding. The root is rich in steroidal saponins, which have a hormonal effect and may help the body reduce inflammation, however there has been little research done on this plant.
- Stops hemorrhaging in the uterus, urinary tract, bowels, kidneys, lungs, stomach, and bladder.
- Astringent action eases stomach upset, diarrhea, dysentery, and leukorrhea.
- Decoction or powdered root used externally for tumours, inflammation, ulcers, snake and insect bites, and to prevent gangrene. Poultice of the plant soothes sore nipples. Raw root grated or boiled and mashed to a paste can be used as a poultice on aching joints.

OTHER USES:

- Young leaves edible in salads or cooked as a pot vegetable.
- Some claim it works as an aphrodisiac.

TINCTURE: Fresh plant 1:2 in 50% alcohol, 15–25 drops, up to 3 times a day.

CAUTION: Do not use during pregnancy, as it is stimulates labour. Use with caution if using steroids or heart medications. Large doses may cause nausea. External application may cause irritation in some people.

RHODIOLA

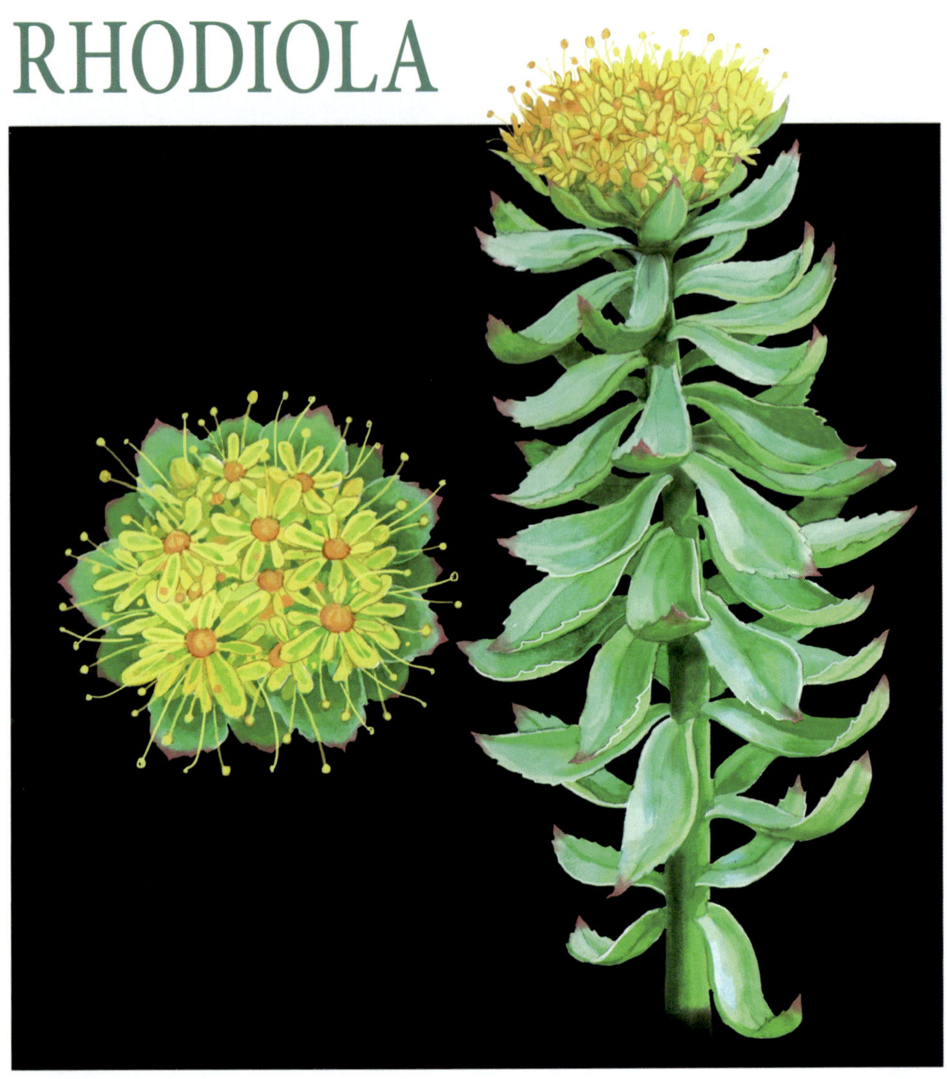

Rhodiola Rosea

FAMILY: Crassulaceae

OTHER NAMES: Arctic Root, Golden Root, Rose Root, King's Crown, *Fr.* Orpin rose

PARTS USED: Root and rhizome

CHARACTERISTICS: Slightly bitter, astringent

ACTIONS: Anti-inflammatory, antioxidant, antibacterial, antiviral, adaptogen, antidepressant, cardioprotective, tonic

RANGE: Native to Nunavut, Quebec, New Brunswick, Nova Scotia, Newfoundland and Labrador; cultivated in Alberta

Noted for its longtime traditional use in Northern Europe, Russia, and China, this perennial is mainly found on sea cliffs in high altitudes and coastal regions in cool, temperate, and subarctic areas of the Northern hemisphere. Used as a ground cover, it grows up to 40 cm. high. Several stems originate from one rootstock, with alternate, succulent leaves. Flowers have 4 petals and 4 sepals, female flowers are yellow and turn reddish when fertilized, male flowers remain yellow. The scaly roots smell like rose petals and should be at least 5 years old before harvesting. Remove only a portion of the rhizome if wild harvesting as it is endangered and is very slow-growing. Slice up the chunkier rhizome and dry for later use.

MEDICINAL USES:

Anxiety, depression, fatigue, burnout, altitude sickness

- Classified as an adaptogen, it is known for increasing resistance to physical and psychological stressors, combatting fatigue, anxiety, and burnout.
- Helps prevent high-altitude sickness, increases pulmonary efficiency.
- Aids recovery from long-term illness, chronic fatigue. Increases energy.
- Improves physical performance and endurance, reduces soreness after workouts.
- Helps to balance neurotransmitters in the brain, acts as an antidepressant but milder with fewer side effects than pharmaceuticals.
- May improve learning and memory, help with impotence, and slow down age-related diseases by reducing the negative effects of stress on the body.
- Has a protective effect on the liver, as well as the cardiovascular system, lowering blood pressure.

CAPSULES: Verify label to ensure they contain 3% rosavins and 1% salidrosides, the active ingredients, which are the natural proportions in the Rhodiola root. Take on an empty stomach but not before bedtime. Take 400–600 mg. per day or as directed on the product.

TINCTURE: Dried root, rhizome 1:4, 50% alcohol, take 1–5 ml. 1 time daily in the morning before eating. Start with smaller dose, increase gradually, and cut back if you start to have problems sleeping.

RESEARCH: A large number of clinical trials have supported the traditional uses of Rhodiola, although most studies are small and the results occasionally contradictory, often due to inconsistencies in dosage, presence of impurities, and location and timing of harvest.

One study administered 170 g. per day of *R. rosea* extract to fifty-six healthy male and female 24–35-year-old physicians working the night shift for a period of 14 days. There was a significant improvement in mental clarity, reaction speed, and short-term memory. Patients with chronic fatigue and burnout noticed a significant improvement after receiving the herb over an 8–12-week period, with increasing mental performance and decreasing cortisol effects. In small and medium doses, there was a significant effect on the central nervous system, stimulating the neurotransmitters noradrenaline, serotonin, dopamine, and acetylcholine receptors; however, in larger doses it tends to have more of a toning effect. Protects the heart and brain from damage due to stress and anxiety.

CAUTION: Generally considered safe if taken 6–12 weeks. May cause dizziness, exacerbate autoimmune diseases, or lower blood pressure. Avoid if pregnant or breastfeeding. May interact with some medications, consult with your healthcare professional before using.

SAGEBRUSH

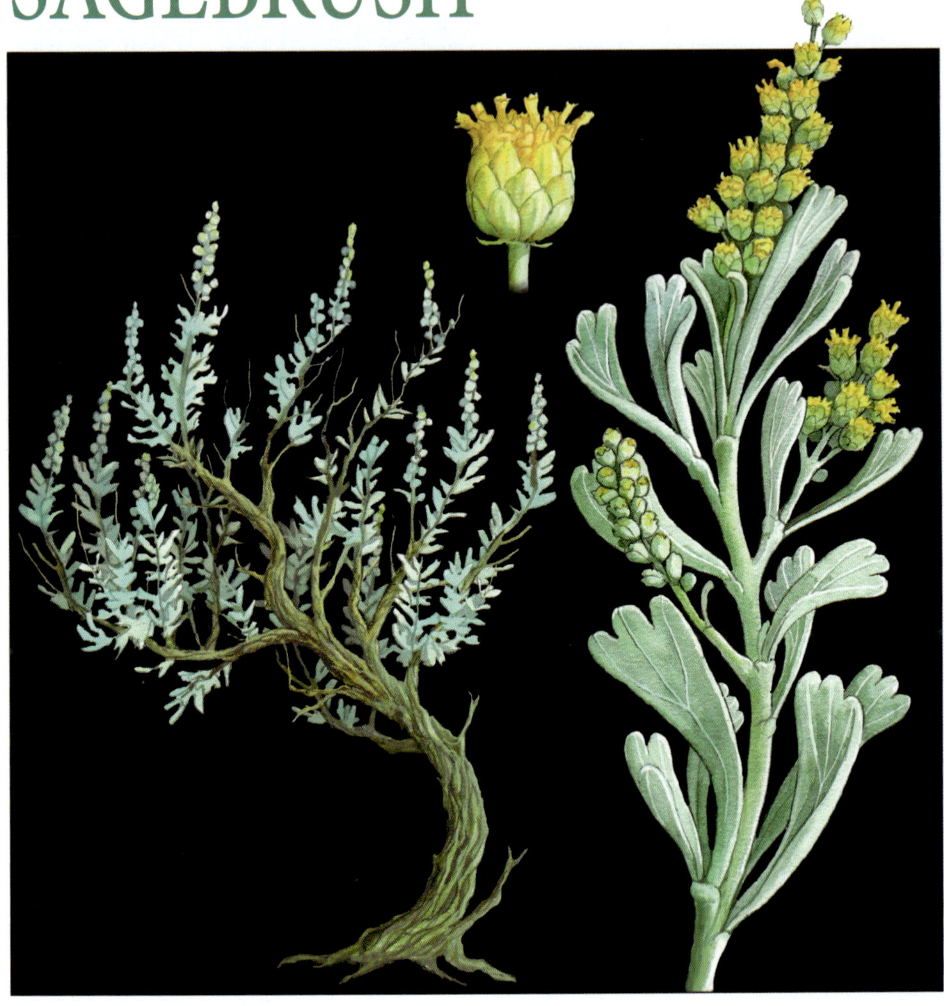

Artemisia tridentata

FAMILY: Asteraceae

OTHER NAMES: Big Sage, Big Sagebrush, *Fr.* Armoise tridentée

PARTS USED: Leaves, flowers

CHARACTERISTICS: Bitter

ACTIONS: Antirheumatic, antifungal, antiseptic, diaphoretic, digestive, emetic, febrifuge, sedative, antimicrobial

RANGE: Native to southern British Columbia and Alberta

This woody, aromatic, evergreen shrub is one of around 150 species of *Artemisia* in North America, many of which are widely used by Indigenous populations for medicinal and other purposes. Named after the Greek goddess Artemis, it is unrelated to the garden herb Sage, which belongs to the genus Salvia, though its scent is somewhat similar. Usually growing up to around 2 m. high, Sagebrush is mostly found on dry, sunny ranges, deserts, and hillsides, and doesn't tolerate cold temperatures or wet conditions. Its deep taproot has adapted to reach several metres into the soil in search of water. The silvery-grey, wedge-shaped leaves are covered in fine, soft hairs that help it to conserve moisture, and have three teeth at the tip, hence the name *tridentata.* At the tips of the branches there are clusters of yellow flowers that appear in late summer or early fall. As the bush ages, the bark starts to peel away in fibrous strips that can be used to make ropes or baskets. Harvesting is best done while the plant is in flower. Strip away small stems and leaves from mature plants, wash to remove dust, and hang upside down to dry. They will keep for about 2 years.

MEDICINAL USES:

Fungal infections, arthritis, parasites, colds, coughs, congestion, fevers, digestive problems, diarrhea

- Contains thujone, making it antimicrobial and antiparasitic; however, it needs to be used with caution as it can be toxic if taken internally in large doses. Used to treat worms and food- and water-borne illnesses such as salmonella and amoebic infections (traveller's diarrhea).
- Applied topically for wounds and ulcers as well as fungal infections such as ringworm or athlete's foot. Relieves pain from sprains or chronic diseases like arthritis. May be used in compresses or by applying wet leaves as a poultice.
- A tea or decoction is bitter-tasting but can be sipped slowly to help digestive upsets, clear mucous in coughs, bronchitis, and colds, and promote sweating to relieve fever. Used as a mouthwash it can help mouth sores and relieve toothache. When mixed with salt and used as a gargle it can help sore throats.
- Steam from boiling the herb can relieve headaches and clear sinus congestion. Infused oil is used for chest congestion and sprains.
- Settles nerves and anxiety, eases cramping and helps regulate menstruation.

OTHER USES:

- Leaves and buds produce a yellow dye.
- Bark fibre used to make mats, baskets, rope, and to stuff pillows.
- Leaves and branches used as a ceremonial smudge for purification.
- Seeds can be eaten raw or dried or ground into meal.
- Bug repellent.

COLD INFUSION: 1 tbsp. in 1 cup water, infuse 4–8 hours, take 2–4 tbsp. up to 3 times a day.

CAUTION: Do not use if pregnant or nursing. Discontinue use if dizziness, nausea, or headache occur. Toxic if taken in large doses or over a long period of time. Do not use for more than 1 week consecutively.

SEA BUCKTHORN

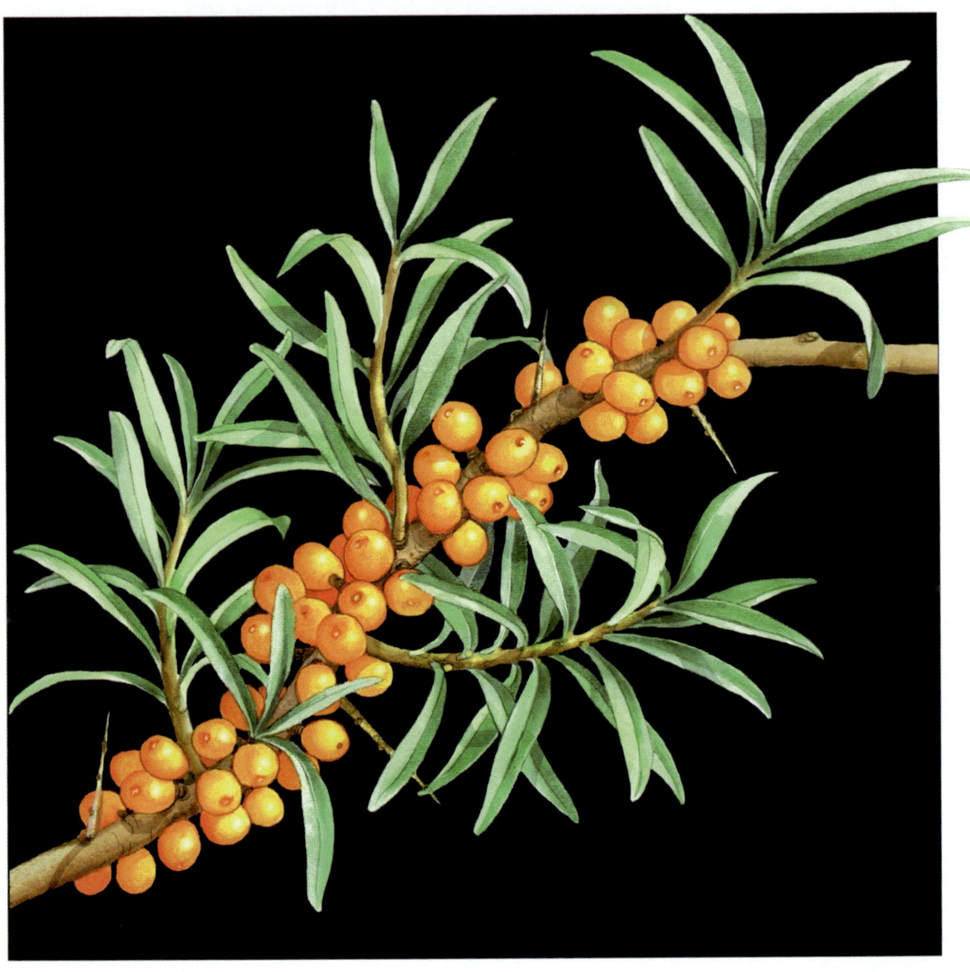

Hippophae rhamnoides

FAMILY: Elaeagnaceae

OTHER NAMES: Siberian Pineapple, Sandthorn, Seaberry, Sallowthorn, *Fr.* Argousier

PARTS USED: Whole plant, mainly berries, leaves, seeds

CHARACTERISTICS: Acidic, astringent

ACTIONS: Anti-inflammatory, antimicrobial, antiviral, antihypertensive, hepatoprotective, neuroprotective, tonic, antioxidant, antifungal

RANGE: Introduced in the Yukon, Alberta, Saskatchewan, Ontario, Quebec, New Brunswick

Originating in China, Tibet, and the Himalayas, this attractive deciduous shrub was introduced into Europe and North America for its abundant nutritive and medicinal properties. Usually found growing in coastal areas, it is often used to help erosion, and it improves soil quality by fixing nitrogen through its root nodules. It prefers moist but not boggy conditions and can tolerate salt spray, but it's a hardy plant that will grow in poor soil as long as there is full sun. Its bright orange berries are used around the world for their oil, mostly in skin products, but recent studies have shown that it may have potential for its ability to help with other conditions, from ulcers to heart disease and even cancer, although more research is needed. Growing to around 8 m. or even taller in some countries, it has silvery-green, lance-shaped leaves and thorny branches. Male and female plants are separate, and both are needed to produce berries, which grow in dense clumps along the branches. Each berry produces one shiny brown seed, usually in September or October. Fruit is usually harvested before the first frost, but must be done with care due to the thorns and the fact that they don't let go easily. Use a pair of pruning shears to remove one by one or simply snip off a branch and freeze, as the berries come away easier when frozen. Be careful not to overharvest, as you can kill the plant, and only prune every second year to give it time to recover.

MEDICINAL USES:

Ulcers, digestive problems, liver injury, high cholesterol, skin diseases, cancer, obesity, joint inflammation

- Very nutrient-rich, the berries contain vitamins A, B12, C, E, riboflavin, niacin, phosphorus, potassium, calcium, magnesium, iron, amino acids, lutein, and omega fatty acids. Used in the food industry to boost nutrients in food or juices.
- Balances oil levels on the skin and scalp, reducing acne and inflammation. Moisturizes and softens skin, improves elasticity, repairs free-radical injury from sunburn, helps eczema, psoriasis, dermatitis, dryness in the vagina. May be taken orally and/or topically.
- Lubricates and repairs the mucous membrane of the intestinal tract, improves slow digestion, gastric ulcers.
- Protects cardiovascular system, lowers LDL (bad) cholesterol, thins the blood. Has been shown to prevent atherosclerosis by reducing triglyceride levels, blood pressure, inflammation and oxidative stress.
- Shows promise in treatment of some cancers, particularly colon and stomach cancer and in prevention of prostate cancer, but more research is needed.
- May have an effect on obesity by reducing the appetite and improving the gut microbiome.
- Helps repair liver injuries and inflammation.
- Its neuroprotective properties may prove promising in treatment of Alzheimer's disease.
- Taking an oil supplement may reduce symptoms of dry eyes and reddening.
- Branches and leaves also produce an oil used for burn ointments.

CAUTION: No known toxicity, may slightly lower blood pressure. Thins the blood; avoid using within 2 weeks of surgery or if taking blood-thinning medication. Avoid during pregnancy. May cause yellowing of the skin if used over a long period of time.

SENECA SNAKEROOT

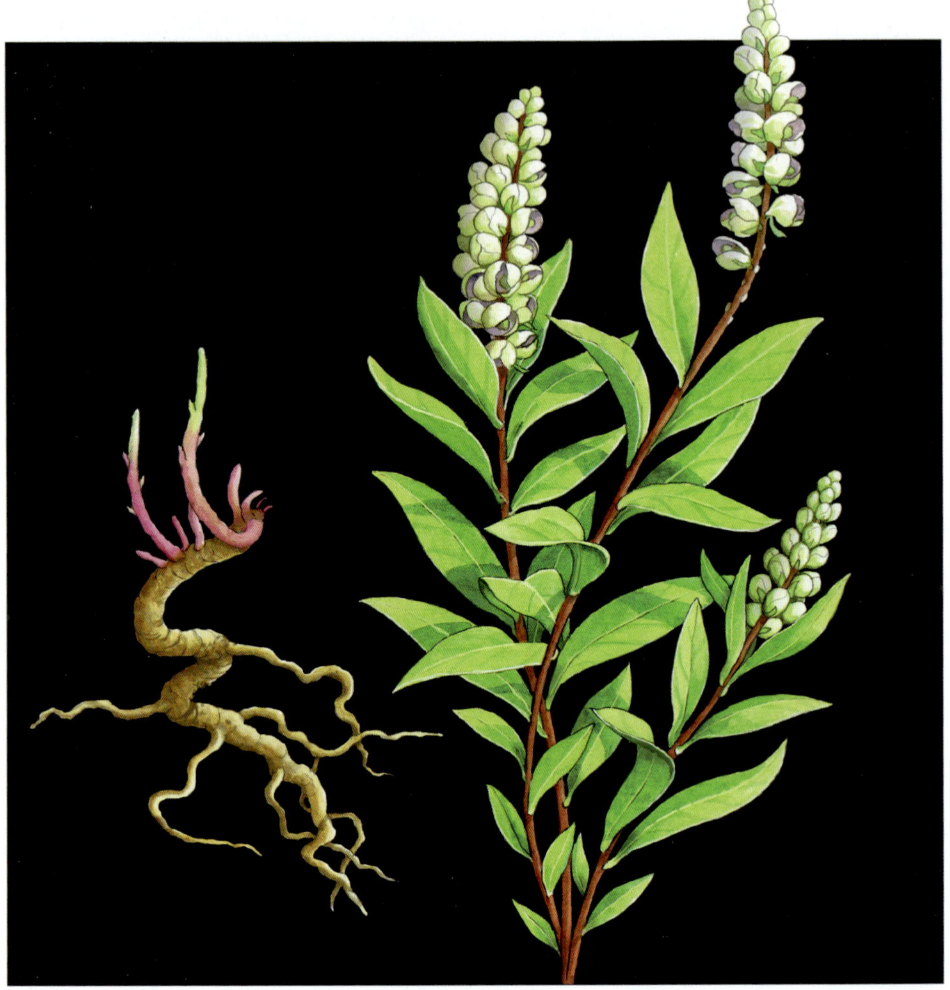

Polygala senega **or** ***Senega officinalis***

FAMILY: Polygalaceae

OTHER NAMES: Seneca Milkwort, Senega Root, *Fr.* Polygale sénéca, Polygale de Virginie

PARTS USED: Dried root

CHARACTERISTICS: Bitter, acrid, warm

ACTIONS: Anti-inflammatory, cathartic, diuretic, diaphoretic, emetic, emmenagogue, expectorant, stimulant, sialagogue, analgesic, antispasmodic

RANGE: Native to southern British Columbia, Alberta, Saskatchewan, Manitoba, Ontario, Quebec, New Brunswick

As its name suggests, this plant was originally used as a remedy for snakebites by Indigenous Peoples, specifically the Seneca Nation living just south of Lake Ontario. Up until the 1950s, Indigenous Peoples in Manitoba grew and harvested three quarters of the world's supply, exporting to Europe, Japan, and the US as an effective cough remedy. Since the discovery of synthetic replacements, the market has somewhat decreased, although it is still popular with herbalists. This small perennial from the Milkwort family grows from 15 to 40 cm. tall, thriving on rocky soils, woodlands, prairies, and abandoned fields across Canada, although mostly absent from NS, PEI, and NL. Leaves are lance-shaped and alternate along the vertical stems sprouting from the rootstock, becoming small and scale-like toward the bottom of the stem. The white, pinkish, or greenish flowers bloom in late June or July, looking very much like the rattle of a rattlesnake atop the unbranched stem, each flower having a bud-like appearance, even in full bloom. The root is twisted and snake-like, taking at least four years to grow large enough to use as medicine. There is a distinctive ridge on one side, and the odour and taste are pretty disagreeable, although they diminish as it dries. The best time to harvest is in the fall, although it's best to mark the plants while still in bloom so they can be identified later.

MEDICINAL USES:

Snakebites, respiratory problems, earaches, rheumatism, amenorrhea

- Known for its value as an expectorant for respiratory issues, this herb is still widely used by herbalists and Indigenous Peoples. Contains triterpenoid saponins which produce a soap-like foam when mixed with water. This irritates the gastric mucosa and causes secretion of mucous in the bronchioles, breaking up phlegm and reducing its viscosity. Used for deep, rattling coughs with excessive excretions such as chronic bronchitis, bronchopneumonia, bronchial asthma, laryngitis, whooping cough, and pleurisy. Reduces inflammation and improves breathing.
- Traditionally used by Indigenous Peoples for snakebites by chewing the root and placing the pulp over the wound after sucking out the venom. Root used by the Cree as a toothache remedy, and the juice swallowed for colds and sore throats.
- Brings on menstruation; uterine stimulant.
- Emetic and cathartic (laxative) when taken in large doses.
- Some research has shown it to be effective in reducing cancer cell growth, specifically in lung cancer.

TINCTURE: Fresh 1:2, dry 1:5, 65% alcohol. Take 10–45 drops up to 4 times a day, depending on how much is tolerated. Small, frequent doses work best to avoid nausea.

DECOCTION: Boil 2 tbsp. dried root in 3 cups water, reduce to 2 cups. Take 1 tbsp. at a time at 1-hour intervals.

CAUTION: Do not exceed recommended dose; may cause violent vomiting and diarrhea. Do not use if pregnant or lactating or if you have peptic ulcers or inflammatory bowel disease.

SHEPHERD'S PURSE

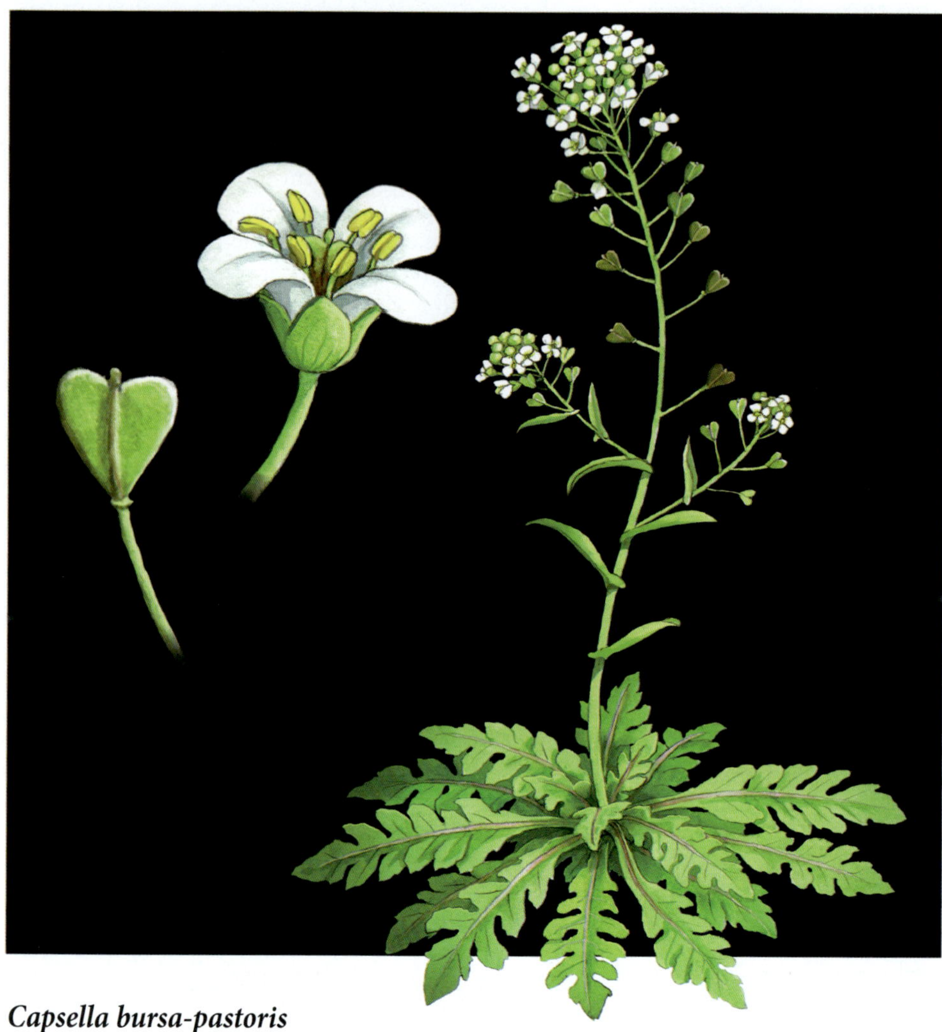

Capsella bursa-pastoris

FAMILY: Brassicaceae

OTHER NAMES: Lady's Purse, Pickpocket, Witches' Pouches, *Fr.* Bourse à pasteur, Capselle bourse-à-pasteur, Tabouret

PARTS USED: Whole plant

CHARACTERISTICS: Slightly bitter, warm, drying, pungent, salty

ACTIONS: Anti-inflammatory, antibacterial, antiscorbutic, astringent, diuretic, emmenogogue, haemostatic, hypotensive, oxytocic, stimulant, vulnerary, antimicrobial, tonic, antioxidant

RANGE: Introduced across Canada

This common annual or biennial weed originated in Europe but is now found in most corners of the world. It usually grows to a height of 30–60 cm., preferring cultivated soil, gardens, and waste places that get sun most of the day. A member of the Cabbage, Mustard, and Broccoli family, it is distinguished by its flat, green, heart-shaped fruits growing along the flower stalk that emerges from a rosette of lobed basal leaves about 23 cm. across and resembles that of a Dandelion without the milky sap. The tiny white 4-petalled flowers grow in terminal clusters on the erect stem and are replaced by the heart-shaped seedpods. Below the flowers and seedpods are small arrow-shaped leaves clasping the stem. Harvest the plants in the summer and use fresh, or dry for later use. Should be used within 1 year as it quickly loses its potency.

MEDICINAL USES:

Bleeding, menorrhagia, postpartum bleeding, cystitis, stones, hemorrhoids, prolapse

- Used for centuries throughout Europe, Asia, and North America as a remedy for all types of internal and external bleeding, this herb is also highly nutritious and contains vitamins A, C, and K, iron, calcium, and omega-3 fatty acids. Leaves can be mashed and applied to the skin as a poultice to staunch wounds, reduce bruising, cool inflammation, and reduce infection. A cotton ball may be soaked in infusion and inserted into the nostril for nosebleeds.
- One of the best herbs for heavy uterine bleeding, it is effective for menorrhagia, dysmenorrhea, uterine weakness, fibroids, or endometriosis. Reduces pain and congestion. Some herbalists advise waiting until the second day of menstruation before starting to take it. Has proven uterine-contracting properties. Used during childbirth to aid labour, tone the uterus after childbirth, and reduce bleeding. Not for use during pregnancy as it may provoke miscarriage. Helps prevent prolapse of the uterus. Constricts smooth muscles surrounding the blood vessels, especially in the uterus; improves clotting. Best if used under supervision of a professional. Stop use shortly after delivery if breastfeeding as glucosinolate constituents may transfer into breast milk.
- Valuable herb for the urinary system, it is a mild diuretic, astringent and antimicrobial, useful in treating urinary tract infections and blood in the urine. Helps to remove stones and gravel, reduces bedwetting.
- Its astringent action also helps with diarrhea and dysentery, and relieves hemorrhoids when used internally or topically.

OTHER USES:

- Seeds placed in water attract mosquitoes and stick to their mouths.
- Is toxic to mosquito larvae.
- Often planted on marshy land to absorb the salt and improve soil quality for gardening.

TINCTURE: Fresh herb 1:2, recently dried 1:5 in 50% alcohol, take 1–2 ml. every 1–2 hours until bleeding has stopped. For postpartum bleeding, take ½–1 tsp. every ½ hour.

INFUSION: 3–4 tsp. fresh herb in 2 cups boiling water. Steep 15 minutes, strain, and cool. Take until it starts working. It tastes unpleasant but is effective if you continue until it takes effect.

COMBINATIONS: With Lady's Mantle, Raspberry leaf, Stinging Nettle, and Yarrow for heavy periods. With Licorice root in a mouthwash as an antibacterial.

CAUTION: May cause uterine contractions, do not take during pregnancy or breastfeeding. May interfere with medications for blood pressure or thyroid. Contains oxalic acid and should be avoided if you have kidney stones.

SILVERWEED

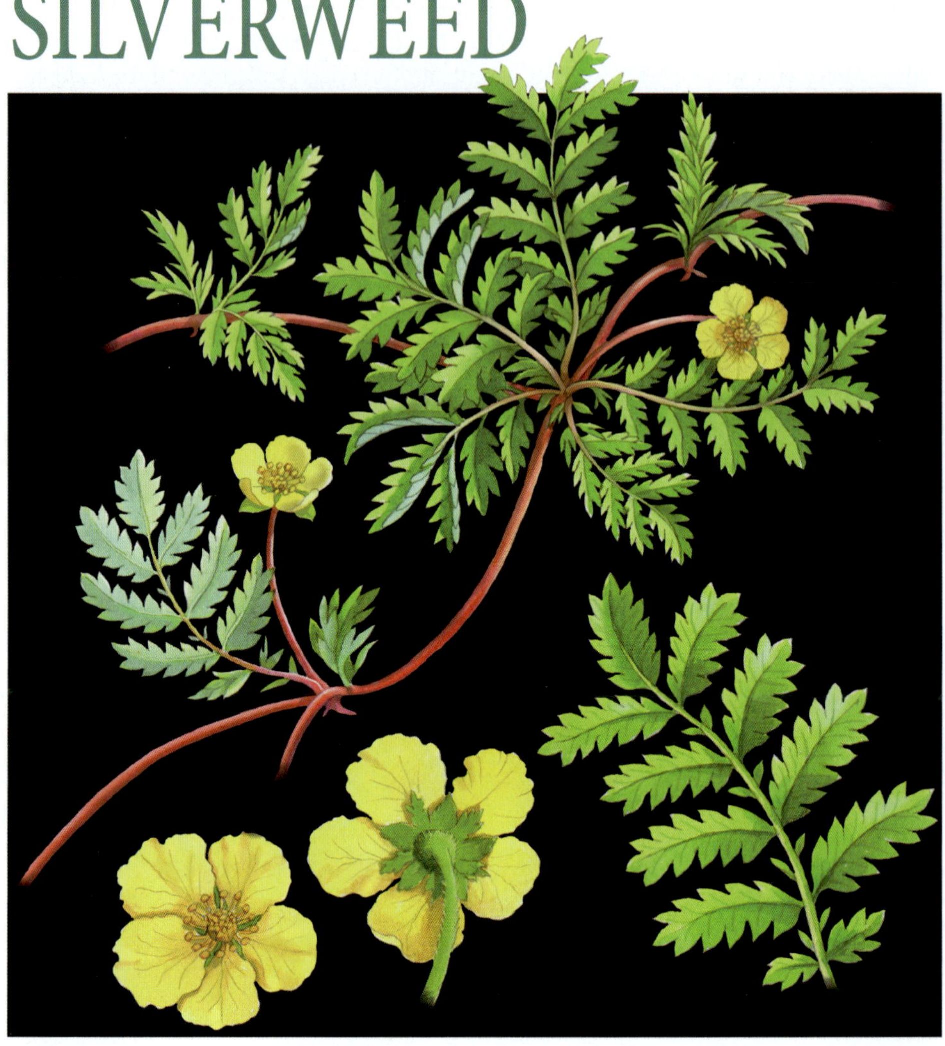

Argentina (Potentilla) anserina

FAMILY: Rosaceae

OTHER NAMES: Argentine, Crampweed, Goosewort, Moon Grass, Trailing Tansy, Silvery Cinquefoil, *Fr.* Potentille des oies, Argentine

PARTS USED: Root, herb, dried

CHARACTERISTICS: Bitter, sweet, cooling

ACTIONS: Astringent, anti-catarrhal, diuretic, anti-inflammatory, antispasmodic, hemostatic, tonic, analgesic

RANGE: Native across Canada

This ground-hugging native perennial usually grows to a height of only 20–40 cm. in the wild, but has red-coloured runners that can reach up to 1.8 m. long. Each tuft of leaves arising from the runners produces 1 yellow 5-petalled flower on a leafless stalk. They bloom between June and August and close at night and on cloudy days. The compound leaves are pinnately divided into up to 20 toothed leaflets, some smaller ones mixed in with the larger ones. They are hairy and either green or silver on the top, and woolly and silver underneath. Silverweed grows in ditches and roadsides as well as fields and is a favourite snack of geese, hence the name "Goosewort." The roots can be harvested late in the summer or fall and dried; the leaves should be picked in early summer and dried in the shade.

MEDICINAL USES:

Coughs, hemorrhoids, diarrhea, gingivitis

- The roots exert a gentle action on the gastrointestinal tract. Antispasmodic, it eases cramps in the stomach and abdomen, its astringent and tonic action helps diarrhea and bleeding hemorrhoids, and its antibacterial properties heal the lining of the intestines. May be taken internally in infusion, or applied to the affected areas with compresses.
- Diuretic, it can be useful for blood in the urine or in removing gravel or fine urinary stones.
- A decoction contains tannins, which are useful as a mouthwash or gargle for gingivitis, loose teeth, or sore throat.
- Eases menstrual cramps and excessive menstrual bleeding.
- Rootstock may be dried and ground to a powder for use in salves, compresses, or bath preparations. Used as a local analgesic and anti-inflammatory to treat hemorrhoids, swelling, burns, and skin ailments. Bruised leaves may be applied directly on the skin for the same purpose.

OTHER USES:

- Very rich in vitamin C and minerals, the young shoots can be added to salads or the leaves may be used as a pot herb. The root was used for centuries by some Indigenous Peoples as a nutritious food when no other food was available. It can be eaten raw, boiled, or roasted, and has a nutty and somewhat starchy flavour. The leaves may also be eaten raw or cooked.
- A leaf placed in the shoe can prevent blisters and sweaty feet.
- An infusion was said to remove freckles.

INFUSION: 1–2 tsp. dried herb in 1 cup boiling water, steep 10 minutes. Drink 2–3 times a day.

TINCTURE: Dried herb 1:5 in 50% alcohol, up to 2 ml. 3 times a day.

CAUTION: May cause stomach irritation if taken in large doses. Not recommended during pregnancy but otherwise safe.

SKULLCAP

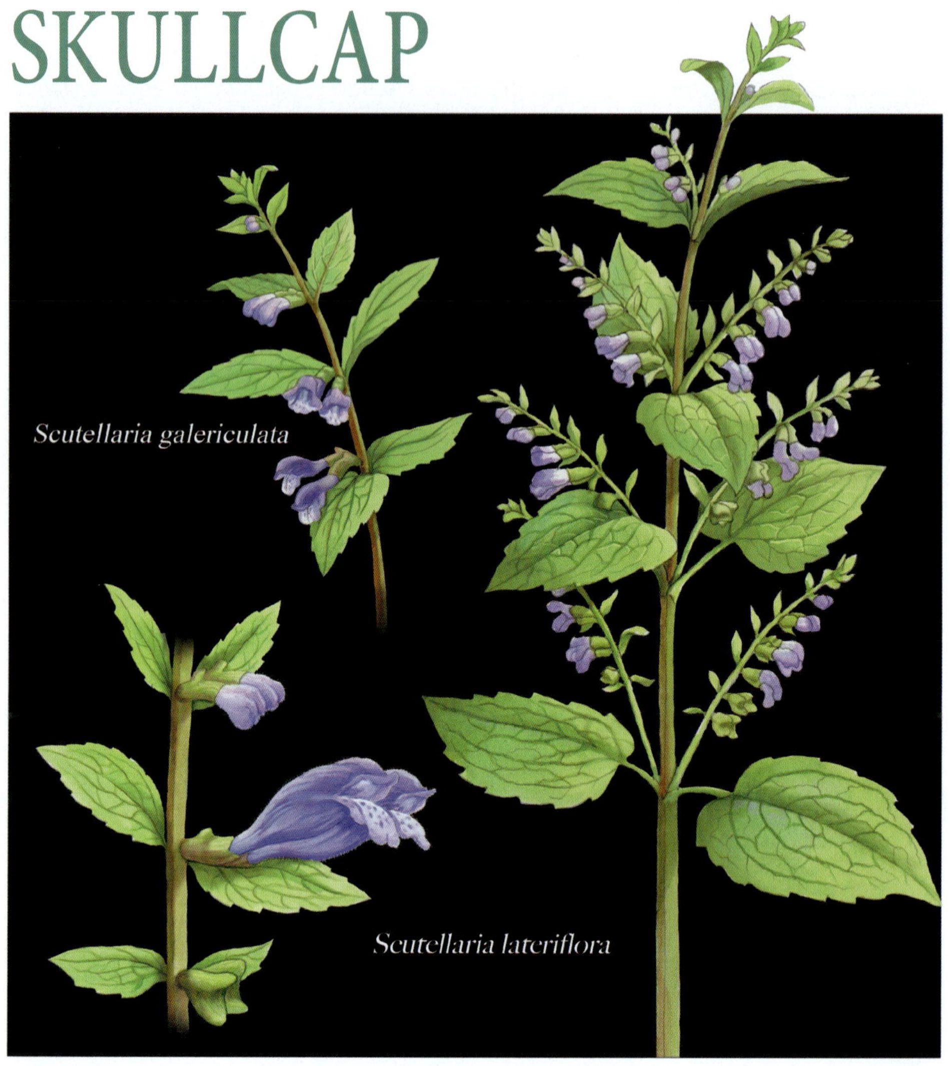

Scutellaria lateriflora (Blue); *Scutellaria galericulata* (Marsh)

FAMILY: Lamiaceae

OTHER NAMES: *S. lateriflora*: Mad-dog Skullcap, Virginia Skullcap, Madweed, *Fr.* Scutellaire latériflore; *S. galericulata*: Hooded Skullcap, *Fr.* Grande toque, Scutellaire à casque

PARTS USED: Aerial

CHARACTERISTICS: Bitter, cold, drying, sweet

ACTIONS: Sedative, anti-inflammatory, antioxidant, nervine, tonic, antispasmodic, emmenagogue, febrifuge, antibacterial, antiviral

RANGE: *S. lateriflora* native to British Columbia, Saskatchewan to Newfoundland and Labrador; *S. galericulata* native across Canada except Nunavut

A perennial plant native to North America, Skullcap has been used for centuries by Indigenous Peoples due to its effectiveness in treating nervous disorders and menstrual problems. It prefers partially shaded wetland areas and its erect square stem grows to a height of 45–60 cm. with occasional branches. It has broad, lance-shaped, toothed leaves in opposite pairs, and from July to September bears blue-lavender, two-lipped, tube-shaped flowers, the upper lip forming a hood, the lower having two lobes, somewhat resembling a helmet or cap. *S. lateriflora* is easily identified by a protuberance on the upper calyx. It should not be confused with the Chinese variety (*Scutellaria baicalensis* or *Huang qin*), which has different medicinal properties. Skullcap should be harvested while the flowers are in full bloom and dried for future use, although better used fresh in making tinctures if possible.

MEDICINAL USES:

Nervous disorders, insomnia, epilepsy, suppressed menstruation

- Excellent remedy for relaxing nervous tension and anxiety, this herb is widely used in cases of palpitations, panic attacks, muscle tension, phobias, tremors, and epilepsy. It acts as an antispasmodic and nervous system tonic, relaxing the mind and easing muscle tension. Not a true sedative, however it works well combined with other herbs for insomnia, particularly for people who are "tired and wired," calming a busy mind without causing lethargy or brain fog. May be used over a long period of time for a cumulative effect.
- Eases PMS symptoms, promotes menstruation. Relieves breast pain and encourages the expulsion of the placenta after childbirth.
- Contains scutellarin, a flavonoid with antispasmodic properties, used for epilepsy, convulsions, and spasms. Eases symptoms of neuralgia and fibromyalgia.
- Helps with alcohol and drug withdrawal, lessens the severity of symptoms and detoxifies.
- May relieve digestive upsets caused by anxiety and nervous tension.

FOLKLORE: In the eighteenth century it was claimed to be a cure for rabies, hence the names Mad Dog and Madweed, but this was soon discredited, although it does relieve some of the symptoms.

TINCTURE: Fresh herb 1:2 in 50% alcohol, take 1–4 ml. up to 3 times a day.

INFUSION: ¾–1½ tsp. freshly dried herb in 1 cup boiling water. Infuse 15 minutes. Take up to 3 times a day.

COMBINATIONS: With Valerian for sleep, with Cramp Bark for menstrual pain and cramping, with Feverfew for headaches, and with Blue Vervain for muscle spasms and tremors caused by stress. A tea can be made combining Skullcap with Lemon Balm, Chamomile, Passionflower, and Lavender to calm the mind and promote sleep.

CAUTION: Generally safe, although care should be taken to use herbs that are pure and unadulterated as they may be mixed with other herbs. Do not exceed recommended dosages.

SLIPPERY ELM

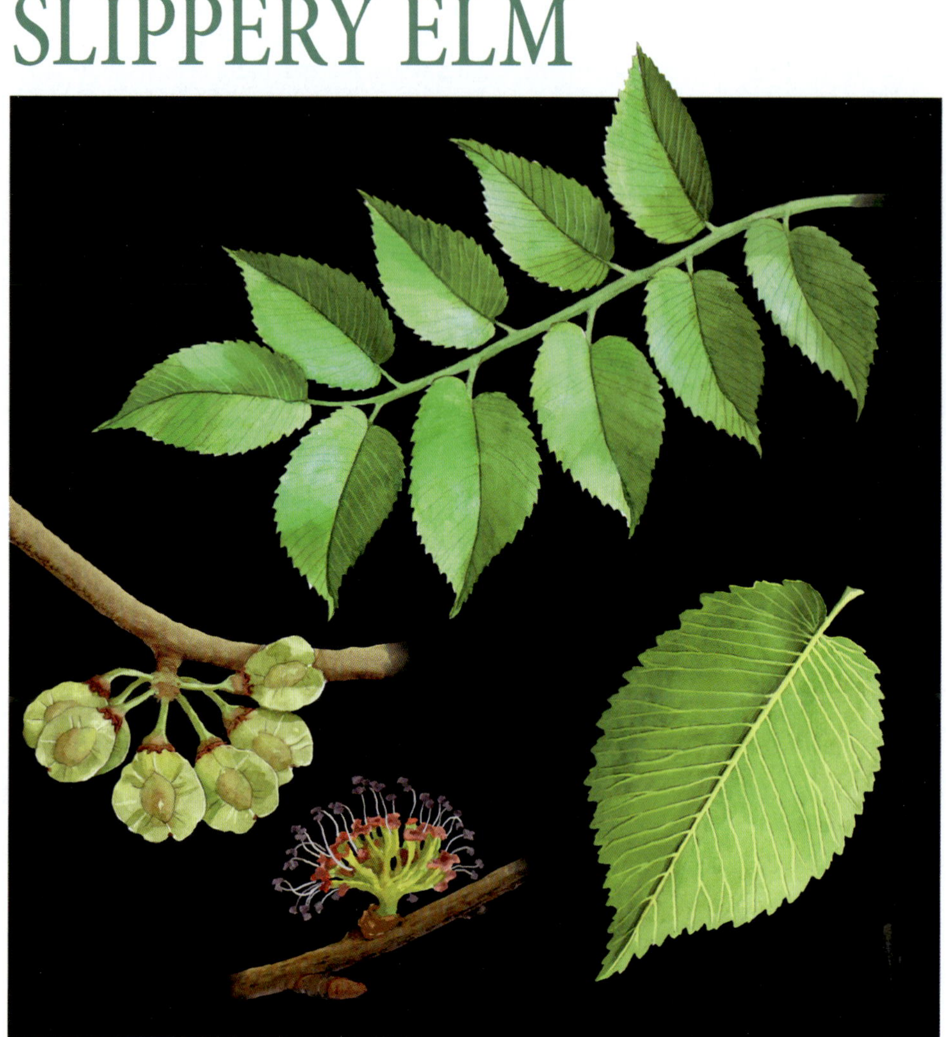

Ulmus rubra (U. fulva)

FAMILY: Ulmaceae

OTHER NAMES: Red Elm, Sweet Elm, *Fr.* Orme rouge, Orme gras

PARTS USED: Inner Bark

CHARACTERISTICS: Sweet, cooling

ACTIONS: Anti-inflammatory, demulcent, emollient, nutritive, astringent, laxative, vulnerary, expectorant

RANGE: Native to Ontario, Quebec, New Brunswick; introduced in British Columbia

Known for its mucilaginous qualities, this deciduous tree's inner bark was commonly used for centuries in North America by Indigenous Peoples and later on by European settlers as a medicine and food. Living for around 125 years, it grows 15–25 m. high and is found along streams and on adjacent slopes and rocky hillsides. Its alternate leaves are doubly toothed, 10–17 cm. long with a distinctly rough surface, an asymmetrical base, and an elongated pointed tip. Flowers appear before the leaves and are reddish-green in tassel-like clusters. Bark should be harvested in the spring from a tree that's at least 10 years old, preferably from low-hanging branches or recently fallen trees so as not to damage the tree. If you must use the trunk, cut a narrow vertical strip; it will not kill the tree and will grow back in a few years. It pulls away easily in strips; remove the outer bark and dry. May be ground into powder or chopped for later use.

MEDICINAL USES:

Digestive problems, arthritis, skin conditions, gum irritations, coughs, sore throat, urinary tract infections

- Very mucilaginous; when water is added, its mixture of polysaccharides creates a gelatinous fibre that lubricates, relieves dryness and irritation, coats mucous membranes, and soothes inflammation.
- Creates a protective barrier that lines the digestive tract, soothing indigestion, irritable bowel, dysentery, heartburn, GERD, and bloating, and easing constipation or diarrhea.
- Soothes and coats irritated membranes in the throat and lungs, eases coughs and helps expel stuck mucus, helpful for bronchitis, laryngitis, and tonsillitis.
- Eases the pain and discomfort of urinary tract infections.
- Anti-inflammatory action helps with arthritic pain.
- Used topically as a paste, poultice, or salve, it reduces inflammation in skin conditions like eczema, psoriasis, minor burns, and hemorrhoids. Hydrates, protects, promotes healing, and reduces irritation and itching, providing immediate relief. Draws out splinters or insect stings.
- Used as a mouthwash, it helps heal gum irritations and injuries.
- Nutritionally similar to oatmeal, it is easily tolerated by those who are recovering from stomach flu and debilitating illness when made into a gruel.

GRUEL: Mix 1½ tbsp. powdered bark and 1 tsp. sugar or honey with a little cold water, heat up 250 ml. milk, or almond or rice milk if you are avoiding dairy, and when it is close to boiling, slowly stir in Elm mixture. Keep stirring for 10 seconds and pour into a cup, drink warm. Add Cinnamon or Nutmeg if desired.

INFUSION: 1 tbsp. dried bark steeped in hot water for 10 minutes.

COMBINATIONS: With Marshmallow root, Licorice root, Ginger, Aloe Vera for digestive problems, gastritis, inflammation. With Turmeric and Licorice root for GERD, acid reflux.

RESEARCH: It has been found that Slippery Elm can act as a prebiotic to protect the mucosal barrier in gastrointestinal illnesses and keep the microbiome healthy by repopulating gut flora. May prove effective in healing leaky gut and reducing inflammation.

Recently studied for its use as a supplement for Irritable Bowel Syndrome and some promising research has confirmed the antioxidant effects, although more studies are needed.

CAUTION: Generally safe, some may experience allergic reactions. May interfere with absorption of certain medications. Avoid in pregnancy and breastfeeding.

SOLOMON'S SEAL

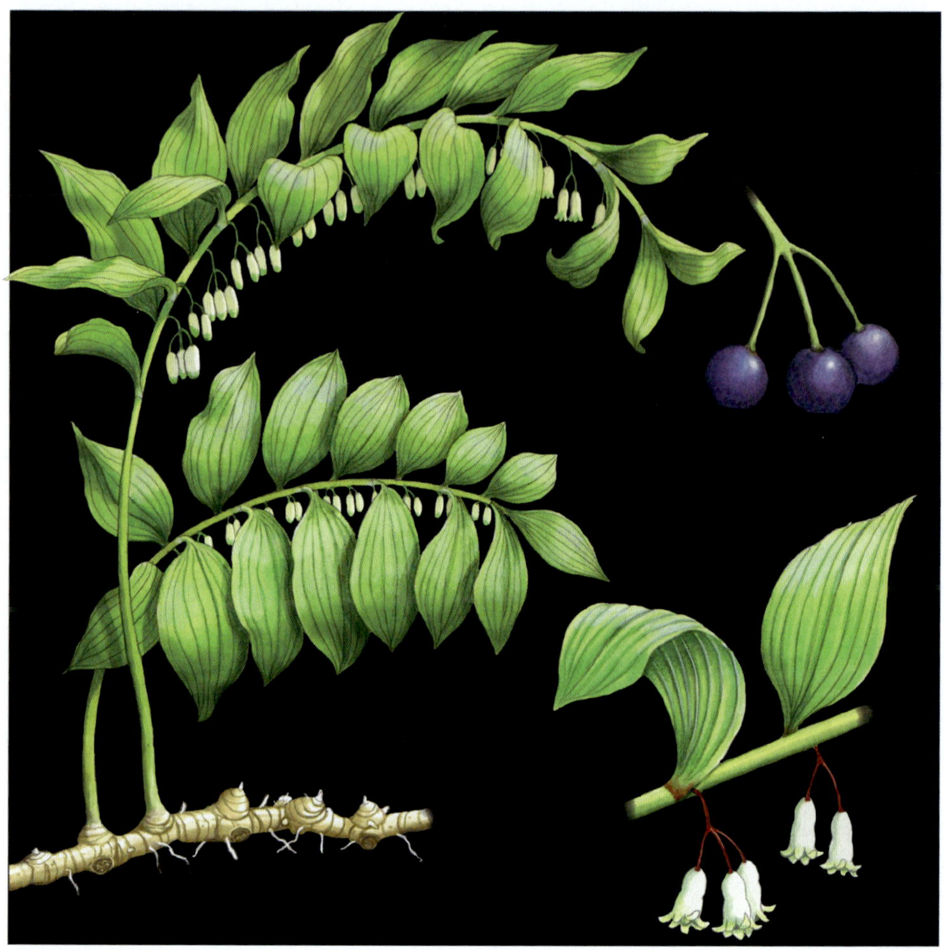

Polygonatum pubescens
Polygonatum biflorum

FAMILY: Asparagaceae

OTHER NAMES: *P. pubescens:* Hairy Solomon's Seal, *Fr.* Sceau de Solomon poilu; *P. biflorum:* Smooth Solomon's Seal, *Fr.* Seau de Solomon à deux fleurs

PARTS USED: Root

CHARACTERISTICS: Sweet, slightly acrid, cool, moist

ACTIONS: Mild sedative, antimicrobial, astringent, anti-inflammatory, antibiotic, antioxidant, demulcent, tonic, hemostatic, expectorant

RANGE: *P. pubescens* native to Ontario, Quebec, New Brunswick, Nova Scotia; *P. biflorum* native to Saskatchewan, Manitoba, Ontario

The use of Solomon's Seal as a wound-healer dates back several thousand years, and is still popular among herbalists. It is a native perennial herb found in woodlands and often grown in shade gardens throughout Canada. Its graceful, arching stems are 30–90 cm. tall with elliptical leaves. Unlike *P. biflorum,* the leaves of Hairy Solomon's Seal are slightly hairy on the underside along the veins, and both are arranged alternately along the stem. Its white to greenish, dangling, bell-shaped flowers hang from the leaf axis in groups of 1 to 3. The berries are dark blue and considered poisonous. The roots are fleshy with knobby circular scars from the previous year's growth. When harvesting the root in the fall, to avoid killing the plant, dig down gently with your fingers or a trowel until you find the rear portion, which will be away from the next year's bud. Run your fingers under it and cut a few cm. away from the stem, leaving the plant intact. This plant is endangered so it is important to collect it in a sustainable manner.

MEDICINAL USES:

Pulled ligaments and tendons, wounds, bleeding, sore joints, broken bones

- One of nature's best anti-inflammatory herbs for repairing sprains and broken bones and for chronic problems like arthritis and tendonitis. It tightens or loosens joints as needed, moistening and promoting production of joint fluid. May also be used externally for sprains, joint pain, and bruising when used in an oil infusion or poultice.
- Excellent demulcent for moistening and lubricating, it can be used in a decoction to loosen mucus when there is a dry cough, bronchitis, throat irritation, or other dry upper respiratory condition.
- Soothes irritated mucous membranes in the digestive tract, particularly in cases of diarrhea, tones and relieves inflammation.
- A mild sedative, it helps with PMS and stress. Strengthens abdominal muscles in cases of prolapse, and benefits vaginal dryness and infertility.
- Provides kidney and liver support, reduces blood pressure, tones the tissues.
- Heals wounds and stops bleeding, softens the skin.

TINCTURE: Dried root 1:5, 60% alcohol, 5–20 drops up to 3 times a day.

INFUSION: Steep ½ tsp. of herb in 1 cup hot water for 5 minutes. Take 2–3 times a day. Do not take for more than 7–10 days consecutively, and stop for 3 or 4 days before repeating treatment (if further treatment is necessary).

COMBINATIONS: With Vervain and Agrimony to strengthen and protect the liver and kidneys. With Horsetail, Stinging Nettle, Mullein root, Goldenseal, and Boneset for bone, tendon, and cartilage repair.

CAUTION: Do not consume berries; they are toxic. Avoid if pregnant or breastfeeding. Do not consume if taking heart medications. Avoid if you are diabetic, as it may decrease blood sugar levels. Do not exceed recommended dose as it may cause diarrhea or nausea.

SPRUCE

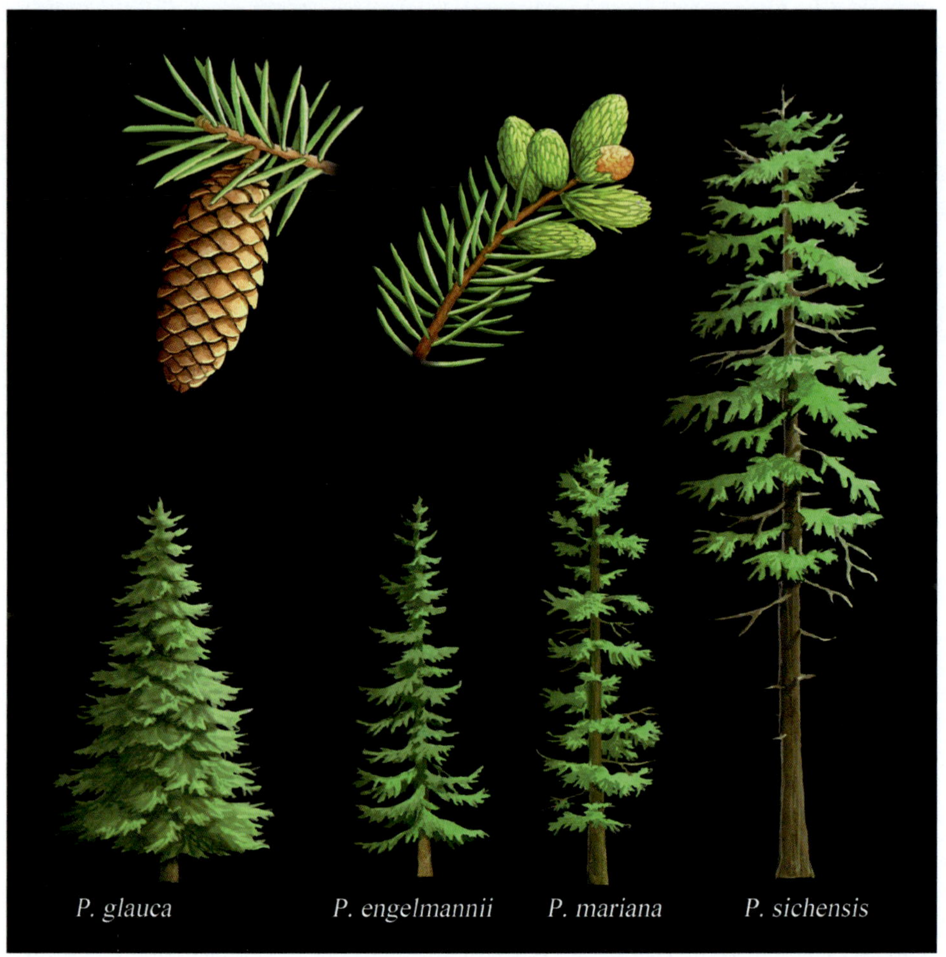

Picea engelmannii (Mountain Spruce); _Picea sitchensis_ (Sitka Spruce); _Picea glauca_ (White Spruce); _Picea mariana_ (Black Spruce)

FAMILY: Pinaceae

OTHER NAMES: *P. engelmannii:* Silver Spruce, Engelmann Spruce, *Fr.* Épinette d'Engelmann; *P. sitchensis:* Coast Spruce, Tideland Spruce, *Fr.* Épinette de Sitka; *P. glauca:* Canadian Spruce, Skunk Spruce, *Fr.* Épinette blanche; *P. mariana*: *Fr.* Épinette noir

PARTS USED: Pitch (resin), young tips, needles, cones

ACTIONS: Antiseptic, analgesic, antifungal, carminative, diaphoretic, diuretic, expectorant, laxative, antimicrobial, antioxidant, antibacterial

RANGE: *P. engelmannii* native to British Columbia and Alberta; *P. sitchensis* native to British Columbia coast; *P. glauca* native across Canada; *P. mariana* native across Canada

Spruce trees are one of the most common trees in Canada, found everywhere except for the northernmost regions. They are identified by their 4-sided, short, pointed needles arranged in spirals around the stem. Unlike Pine needles, which grow in clusters, Spruce needles grow singularly on small peg-like projections that remain when the needles fall, usually every four to ten years. The bark is scaly and cones hang downward after pollination. Indigenous Peoples rely heavily on this tree, not only as medicine, but for building materials, food, basket-making, and many other uses. The slow-growing Mountain Spruce is slender and conical, found in the high altitudes of BC and Alberta and averaging about 30 m. in height. The Sitka Spruce, on the other hand, grows more slowly but is the largest Spruce, sometimes reaching heights of up to 90 m., with few branches lower than 30 m. White and Black Spruce grow across Canada and are usually under 30 m. tall. The former smells a bit skunky and has shallow roots that make them prone to blowing over in a bad windstorm. Harvest Spruce tips in the spring as soon as the papery sheath falls off.

MEDICINAL USES:

Wounds, coughs, sore throat, colds, rheumatism, muscle pain

- Small bright green tips are rich in vitamins A and C and potassium, have a pleasant aroma, and make a nice tea for coughs, colds, or flu, or it can be made into jellies, glazes for meat, mixed into stuffings, or added as a pot herb. Used as a spring tonic.
- Decoction of needles and cones can be used as a wash for rashes, hives, burns, or as tea for colds, sore throat, or gargled for gum problems and toothache. The Nlaka'pamux use a decoction of needles and resin taken directly from the bark blisters to treat cancer, coughs.
- Resin or pitch is antiseptic and analgesic, can be applied to wounds or warmed and smeared on a piece of cloth, which is then warmed in the oven and applied to chest for coughs or back for backache. Boil resin in water for urinary or digestive problems.
- Ointment or infused oil made from resin can be applied to sore joints and muscles to relieve pain, or to insect bites, chapped hands, eczema, burns, or rashes.
- Inner bark made into an infusion is used for stomachaches, ulcers, mouth sores, and sore throats.

OTHER USES:

- Roots peeled and split for making ropes, baskets, and hats.
- Inner bark used as emergency food, or ground into meal and added to flour.
- Softened pitch used to waterproof boats; wood used for building, making canoes, snowshoes, and utensils, and it has acoustic properties for making pianos and guitars.
- Fresh shoots used to make spruce beer.

DECOCTION: Break several branches into small pieces and add with cones to 17 cups of water. Bring to a boil and simmer 20 minutes. Breathe in vapours for congestion or drink for colds and flu. Sip 2–3 tsp. 3 or 4 times a day.

SPRUCE TIP SYRUP: Place tips in a saucepan with just enough water to cover. Bring to a boil and simmer for 15 minutes. Allow to cool and refrigerate overnight. Strain out the tips, measure the liquid, and for every ½ litre of liquid add 3 cups white sugar. Bring to a boil and simmer for 15 minutes or until you get the desired consistency. Pour into sterilized, warm mason jars. Seal and store in a cool place. Can be taken by the spoonful or added to teas or juice, keep in fridge after opening.

CAUTION: Best when used in acute conditions over a short term and in small doses. Avoid during pregnancy.

ST. JOHN'S WORT

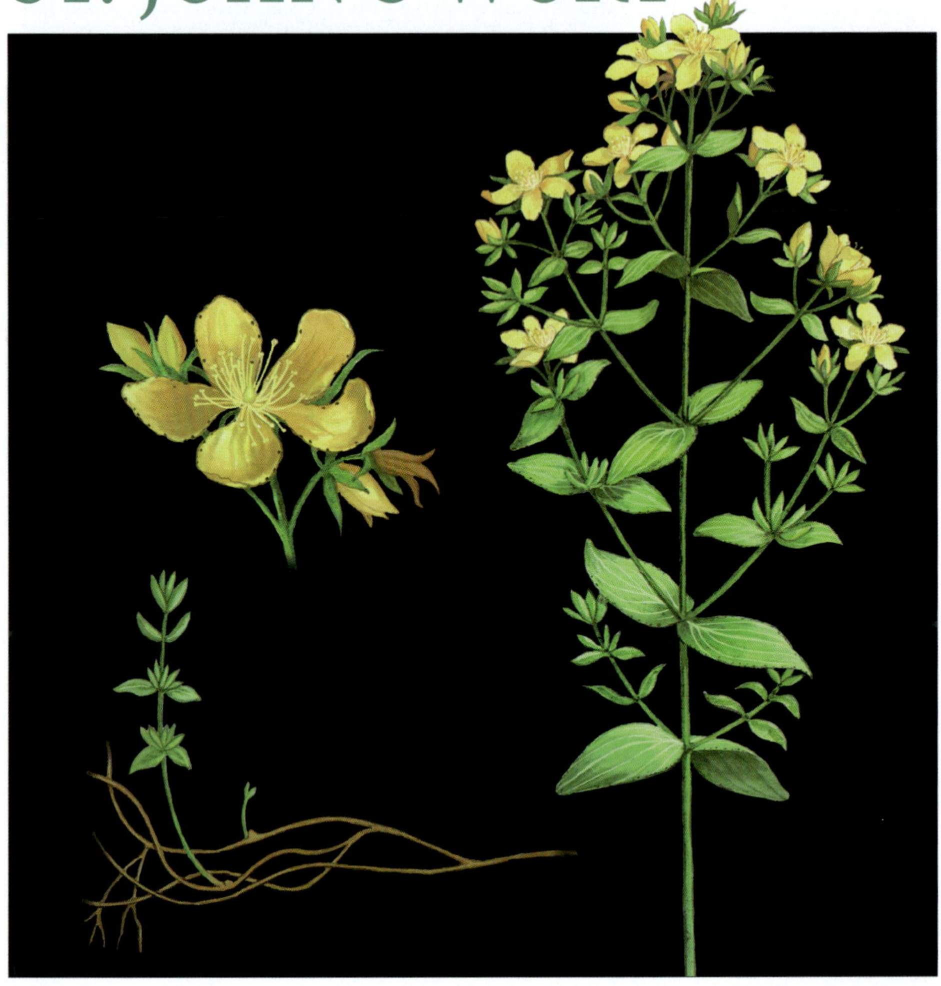

Hypericum perforatum

FAMILY: Hypericaceae

OTHER NAMES: Goatweed, Klamath Weed, *Fr.* Millepertuis commun

PARTS USED: Herb tops and flowers

CHARACTERISTICS: Cool, bittersweet, astringent, aromatic

ACTIONS: Sedative, anti-inflammatory, antidepressant, astringent, expectorant, nervine, external analgesic, antiviral, alterative

RANGE: Introduced in all provinces except Saskatchewan

St. John's Wort has been used as a medicinal herb for over two thousand years, with many stories and myths attached to it. A herbaceous perennial native to Europe, it has spread throughout North America, growing up to 1 m. high with a central stem branching out into several at the top. Leaves are opposite and have tiny translucent spots which are oil glands. The star-shaped flowers appear June to August and are yellow with 5 petals, with tiny black dots on the calyx and corolla. The root is a creeping rhizome, and the woody stem has 2 longitudinal ridges. Found in dry fields and along roadsides. Harvest leaves and flowers as plants bloom. Dry and store in airtight jar.

MEDICINAL USES:

Nervous system disorders, depression, anxiety, viral infections, arthritic pain

- Used internally and externally for centuries for pain relief and symptoms of anxiety and mild to moderate depression. Two ingredients—hypericin, which acts as an anti-depressant and an antiviral, and hyperforin, which influences neurotransmitters to modulate serotonin, dopamine, and norepinephrine—help manage seasonal depressive disorders, anxiety, menstrual and menopausal symptoms, and sleep problems. Anti-inflammatory actions reduce arthritic discomfort and have a calming effect on nervous system.
- Effective at easing nerve pain, lower back pain, rheumatism, arthritis, and chronic inflammation. Heals nerve trauma from injury or disease, assists recovery from illness, exhaustion, and fatigue. May be applied to skin as an infused oil or taken internally in a tincture.
- May be helpful for PMS and menopause with low energy, hot flashes, and insomnia.
- Oil made from flowers used since the Middle Ages for its astringent properties. Warming and soothing action penetrates skin and helps to heal wounds, bruises, insect bites, eczema, and hemorrhoids, and treats inflammation, joint pain, and arthritis.
- Once used by Indigenous Peoples in a tea to protect against tuberculosis and other respiratory ailments and fever.

FOLKLORE: Named after St. John the Baptist, as it usually flowers around June 24, St. John's Day. In Ancient Greece its fragrance was believed to chase away evil spirits. Used for centuries as a charm against witchcraft and in exorcisms. Medieval women would pick the herb on St. John's Eve with the dew still on the leaves; it was believed this would help her find a husband.

INFUSION: Add 1–2 tsp. herb to 1 cup boiling water, steep 10–15 minutes, drink up to 3 times a day.

TINCTURE: Fresh plant 1:2, 50% alcohol, 1–4 ml. 3 times a day.

OIL: Place flowers in a glass jar and add enough olive oil just to cover. Place jar in a sunny window for 2–3 weeks, shaking daily. Filter and place in dark glass container.

COMBINATIONS: With Cramp Bark for nerve pain or PMS symptoms, with Skullcap for restlessness, with Black Cohosh for menopause, and with Hawthorn for pain or loss.

RESEARCH: Studies have shown that St. John's Wort is as effective as pharmaceutical antidepressants at relieving mild to moderate depression, especially when there is anxiety, with fewer side effects. However, it may take a bit more time to build up and become effective.

CAUTION: Excessive use may cause photosensitivity or allergies in some people. Do not take in combination with other drugs, narcotics, alcohol, cold or hay fever medications, birth control pills, tryptophan, or tyrosine. Do not use during pregnancy.

STINGING NETTLE

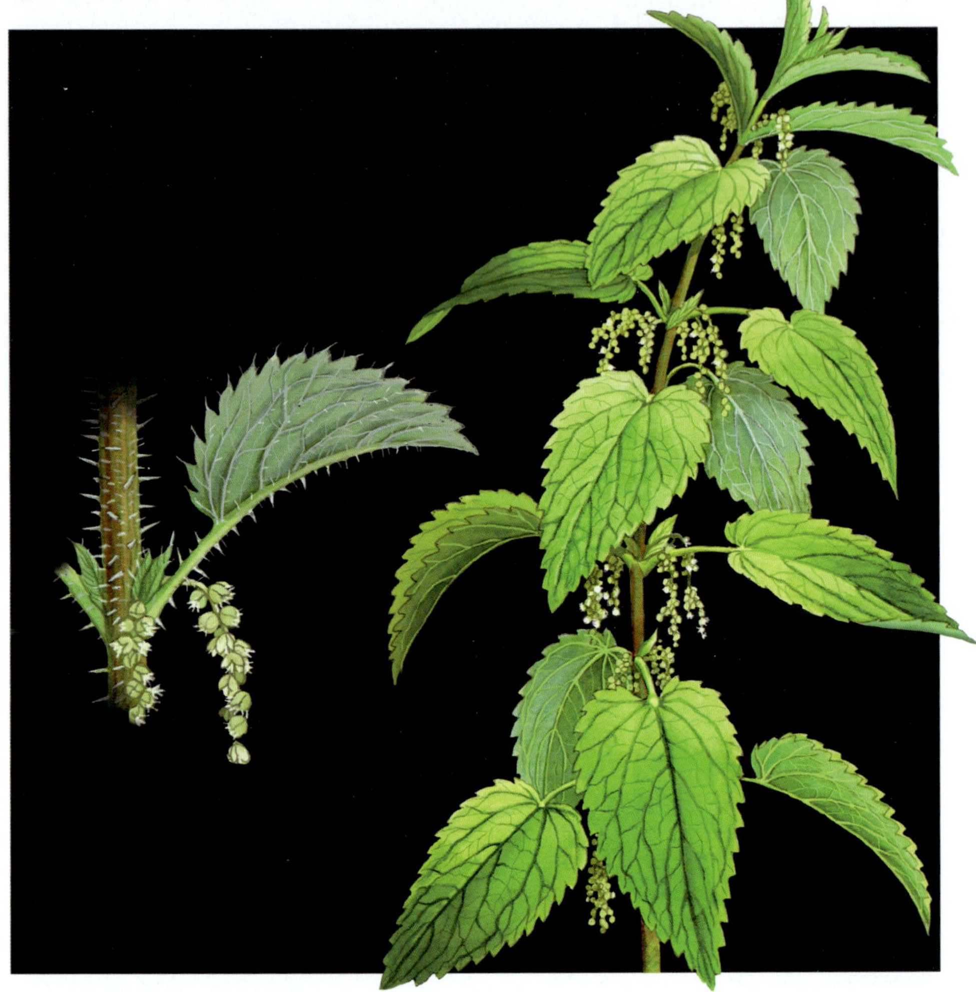

Urtica dioica (ssp.gracilis)

FAMILY: Urticaceae

OTHER NAMES: American Stinging Nettle, *Fr.* Grande ortie

PARTS USED: Leaves, root

CHARACTERISTICS: Bitter, cool, sweet, salty, dry

ACTIONS: Diuretic, astringent, tonic, hemostatic, galactagogue, expectorant, nutritive, antiseptic, anti-inflammatory, antioxidant, analgesic, antimicrobial

RANGE: Native across Canada except Nunavut

Although these plants have a bad reputation for their stinging hairs, if properly handled they are one of the best medicinal herbs, with a wide variety of applications. A perennial which grows 30–90 cm. high, it has oval leaves that are opposite, tapered to a point, and finely toothed. The roots are creeping rhizomes, so it multiplies easily. The flowers are greenish and hang in branched clusters. The stiff hairs covering the entire plant contain a small amount of formic acid, which give its sting, but it can be neutralized by rubbing Dock leaf or Plantain onto affected areas. It loses its sting after it's been dried or cooked, or even stored in the refrigerator for a day or so. It is usually found in waste places and ditches where the soil is moist; gather with rubber gloves in the spring or early summer when the leaves are free of dew, and hang to dry in a shaded area for later use.

MEDICINAL USES:

Arthritis, asthma, bronchitis, eczema, cystitis, stagnant mucous, enlarged prostate, stones, diarrhea, hemorrhoids, hay fever

- Stinging Nettle makes a wonderful spring tonic, cleansing herb, and blood purifier, as it is very nutritious and rich in vitamin C, A, iron, magnesium, calcium, potassium, and silicon. This makes it ideal for those with anemia or convalescing after illness, as it replenishes nutrients and restores energy. The young leaves when cooked taste like spinach, and if steamed for 30 minutes the juice may be squeezed out and 1 spoonful taken every hour to relieve PMS, menorrhagia, or excessive bleeding. Applied to skin, it stops bleeding and soothes itchiness, burns, bites, and stings.
- After childbirth, Stinging Nettle tea may be used to promote milk production and build up the blood. Combines well with Raspberry leaf for this purpose.
- Contains a high amount of sterols, especially in the root, and may be effective in treating enlarged prostate or benign prostatic hypertrophy, stimulating white blood cells to counteract inflammation.
- Removes stagnant mucous in the lungs and sinuses; useful for asthma, pneumonia, pleurisy, bronchitis, and allergies. Traditionally it was burned and the smoke inhaled for lung infections.
- An effective diuretic, it is useful for lowering uric acids through urine, which can prevent or treat gout, arthritis, and kidney or bladder stones. Seeds especially good for urinary tract infections.
- Antihistaminic effect calms allergic responses on skin, as in eczema or dermatitis, and also seasonal respiratory allergies such as hay fever and asthma. Restores balance, calms an overactive immune system, removing stagnant mucus in the lungs and sinuses.
- Relieves diarrhea, dysentery, hemorrhoids, mucous in the stool, or any cold, damp conditions.
- Compresses reduce pain of arthritis, rheumatism. Purposefully stinging oneself causes increased blood flow to the skin, relieving inflammation of the joints.

OTHER USES: Fibres used to make fabrics and clothing, rope, netting.

COLD INFUSION: 2 tbsp. dried herb in 2–3 cups cold water. Steep for a couple of hours or overnight, strain, and drink throughout the day.

HOT INFUSION: Mix 1–3 tsp. dried herb in 1 cup boiling water; infuse 10–15 min. Drink 1 cup up to 3 times a day.

TINCTURE: Dried herb 1:5 in 40% alcohol, 1 dropper 2–3 times a day.

COMBINATIONS: With Elder flower, Sage leaf, Eyebright, and Peppermint for allergies and hives. With Saw Palmetto for prostate.

RESEARCH: Studies have found that Stinging Nettle leaf extract given to patients with osteoarthritis or rheumatoid arthritis over a 3-week period dramatically improved symptoms. Most participants said it relieved symptoms, 26% said they would go off anti-inflammatory drugs, and 32% said they would reduce the amount of their medication.

CAUTION: Handle with gloves. Not recommended for pregnant women. Could interfere with blood thinning drugs or diuretic drugs. May lower blood pressure. Do not apply to open wounds.

STONEROOT

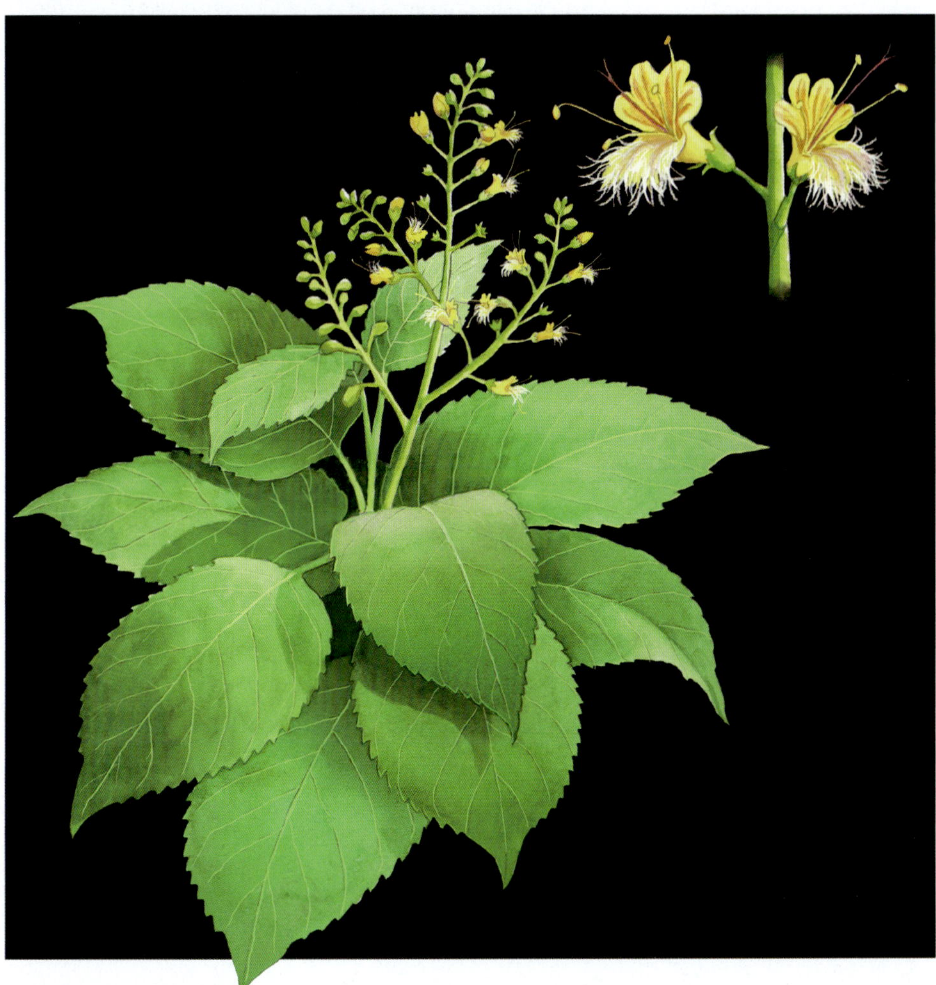

Collinsonia canadensis

FAMILY: Lamiaceae

OTHER NAMES: Horse Balm, Broadleaf Collinsonia, Richweed, Hardrock, Knob Root, *Fr.* Racine de Pierre, Collinsonie du Canada

PARTS USED: Root (fresh), leaves

CHARACTERISTICS: Pungent, bitter, spicy, drying, warm

ACTIONS: Anti-inflammatory, antioxidant, antispasmodic, alterative, astringent, diaphoretic, diuretic, emmenagogue, sedative, stimulant, stomachic, tonic, vasodilator, vulnerary

RANGE: Native to Ontario

Stoneroot is a perennial widely used by Indigenous Peoples and early settlers and is common to damp wooded areas or floodplains of southern Ontario. Growing up to about 1.2 m. tall, it has a square, slightly hairy stem and large, lemony-scented heart-shaped leaves that are sharply toothed. The tubular yellow-green flowers grow in loose clusters at the top of the stem, with a fringed lower lip and protruding stamen. Like its name suggests, the root is hard, knotty, and rock-like and smells rather disagreeable. It may be harvested in the fall, broken up and dried for later use; however, it is more potent if used fresh. Keep in a paper bag or box to keep from spoiling.

MEDICINAL USES:

Kidney stones, urinary tract infections, diarrhea, indigestion, dysmenorrhea, varicose veins, hemorrhoids, memory problems, sore throat

- The root is used to relieve mild urinary tract infections and kidney stones. Diuretic action enhances urine flow and helps to flush out stones, relax the urethra, and relieve pain.
- Tannins and saponins in the root help lower inflammation in the digestive tract and reduce symptoms of diarrhea, or alternating diarrhea/constipation, toning the mucosa and easing stomach pain. Good remedy for indigestion, tones the gastrointestinal tract and improves appetite.
- Tightens, tones, and strengthens vein walls, reducing venous pressure, helping with varicose veins and hemorrhoids and improving blood circulation.
- Mucilage contained in the root also protects and lubricates the throat, easing pain and inflammation of laryngitis, pharyngitis, sinus infections, bronchitis, and hoarseness.
- Fresh leaves are only used topically, as they cause vomiting when ingested. Used as a poultice they are good for bruises, cuts, sores, poison ivy, and sprains.

INFUSION: 1 tsp. fresh root in 1 cup hot water (do not boil). Infuse 10–15 min. Drink 2–3 cups a day.

TINCTURE: Fresh root 1:2, in 60% alcohol, 20–40 drops, 3 times a day; dried root 1:5 in 60% alcohol, 45–60 drops up to 4 times a day.

COMBINATIONS: With Witch Hazel or Calendula for hemorrhoids, with Gravel Root or Parsley for urinary stones.

RESEARCH: Several compounds in Stoneroot have been found to be beneficial to improving memory and in the treatment of Alzheimer's Disease, including rosmarinic acid, thymol, carvacrol and saponins, which are anti-inflammatory and have antioxidant properties which can improve cognitive function and shield neurons from oxidative stress. However, more research is needed to fully understand its effects on the brain.

CAUTION: Fresh leaves are strongly emetic; even a small amount may cause vomiting. Not recommended for prolonged use or in large doses. Avoid if using blood thinners or on blood pressure medications. May interact with some pharmaceuticals. Not recommended if pregnant or breastfeeding, or with severe kidney or liver disease.

SUMAC

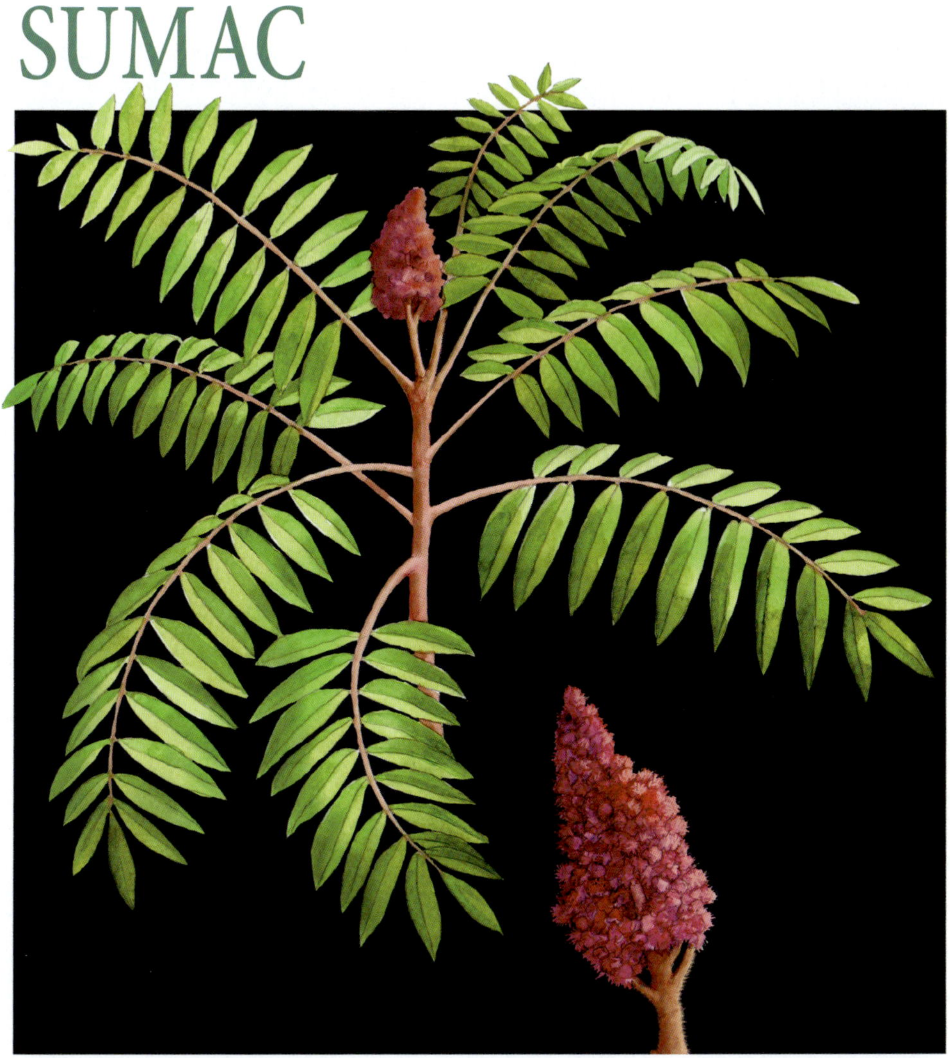

Rhus glabra; Rhus typhina

FAMILY: Anacardiaceae

OTHER NAMES: *R. glabra:* Smooth Sumac, *Fr.* Sumac glabre; *R. typhina:* Staghorn Sumac, Velvet Sumac, *Fr.* Sumac vinaigrier

PARTS USED: Bark, root bark, berries, leaves

CHARACTERISTICS: Cool, dry, sour, astringent, slightly bitter

ACTIONS: Antimicrobial, antibiotic, antioxidant, antifungal, anti-inflammatory, antiviral, astringent, alterative, diuretic, galactagogue, haemostatic, rubefacient, emmenagogue

RANGE: *R. glabra* native to British Columbia, Manitoba, Saskatchewan, Ontario; *R. typhina* native to Ontario, Quebec, New Brunswick, Nova Scotia, Prince Edward Island, introduced in British Columbia and Newfoundland and Labrador

These large shrubs are just 2 out of 4 species of Sumac found in North America; the others have similar medicinal properties but are not as potent. Their cousin, *R. coriaria,* has been used as a cooking spice in Eastern Europe for hundreds of years, particularly in a mixture of spices called za'atar. Dense colonies of *R. glabra* and *R. typhina* are common in full sun along roadsides and forest edges across Canada, growing 3–6 m. tall. The compound leaves are lance-shaped and serrated, with 11–31 leaflets that turn bright red or orange in the fall. Clusters of small green flowers appear from July to August, growing in a distinct upright cone that turns to bright red berries in the fall. The Staghorn Sumac, as its name suggests, has branches resembling the fuzzy antlers of a stag, and its berries also are covered with fine hairs. The Smooth Sumac is very similar but without the hairs on the stems and less obvious on the berries. Root and stem bark can be harvested in spring or fall and dried for later use. The tart berries are more flavourful if harvested when young and not after a rainstorm, although they often stay on the tree all winter. Dry and grind to a fine powder for herbal remedies and cooking. Do not confuse with Poison Sumac (*Toxicodendron vernix*), which has white berries.

MEDICINAL USES:

Diarrhea, sore throat, skin sores, painful menstruation, bacterial and fungal infections

- Bark is astringent, useful for toning soft tissues, tightening up mucous membranes and soothing inflammations. Bark, leaves, and berries are antimicrobial.
- Infusion of bark used for colds, sore throat, painful urination, and urinary tract infections. Its astringency also treats edema, diarrhea, hemorrhoids, fevers, and mouth sores.
- Decoction of branches, bark, and seed heads used topically for itchy scalp, blisters.
- Infusion of leaves used for asthma, mouth sores, post-nasal drip. Its diuretic and astringent properties reduce water retention and damp conditions such as post-nasal drip or wet cough.
- Poultice of leaves used for rashes, acne, sore gums, lips, fungal infections; leaves smoked for asthma.
- Berries are diuretic and high in vitamin A and C, as well as emmenagogue, antioxidant, and antimicrobial. They help regulate blood sugar, lower LDL cholesterol, ease sore throat and urinary tract infections. They are a remedy for bedwetting, and help diarrhea.
- Roots boiled and used as an antiseptic for wounds and skin ulcers. Juice used to remove warts. Emetic if ingested.
- Once used in treatment of bacterial diseases like dysentery, gangrene, and sexually transmitted diseases.

OTHER USES:

- Berries, particularly of the European variety, are dried and ground, filtering out the seeds, for use as a spice in Mediterranean cooking.
- Plant contains tannic acid used for tanning leather.
- Young shoots eaten peeled and raw in the spring.
- Red dye extracted from berries, yellow from the inner bark.

WARM BERRY INFUSION: Put 1 part berries and 2 parts hot water in a bowl, infuse for about 30 minutes. Strain through a filter to remove tiny hairs. Add honey and Cinnamon if desired.

COLD BERRY INFUSION: Soak berries in cold water for up to 24 hours, crushing periodically to extract juice. Strain to make a refreshing drink, add sugar, maple syrup, lemon, or Mint if desired.

RESEARCH: Research on phenolic compounds in Sumac, specifically *R. coriaria,* which is very similar to our Canadian species, has shown it has powerful antioxidant, antifungal, anti-inflammatory, and antimicrobial activity, which could be useful for treating cardiovascular disease, skin disorders, cancer, and diabetes, as well as possible use in the food industry as a natural preservative.

CAUTION: May cause skin irritation. Avoid if allergic to cashews or mangoes, as it is in the same family. Do not confuse with Poison Sumac, which is toxic if handled or ingested.

SUNDEW

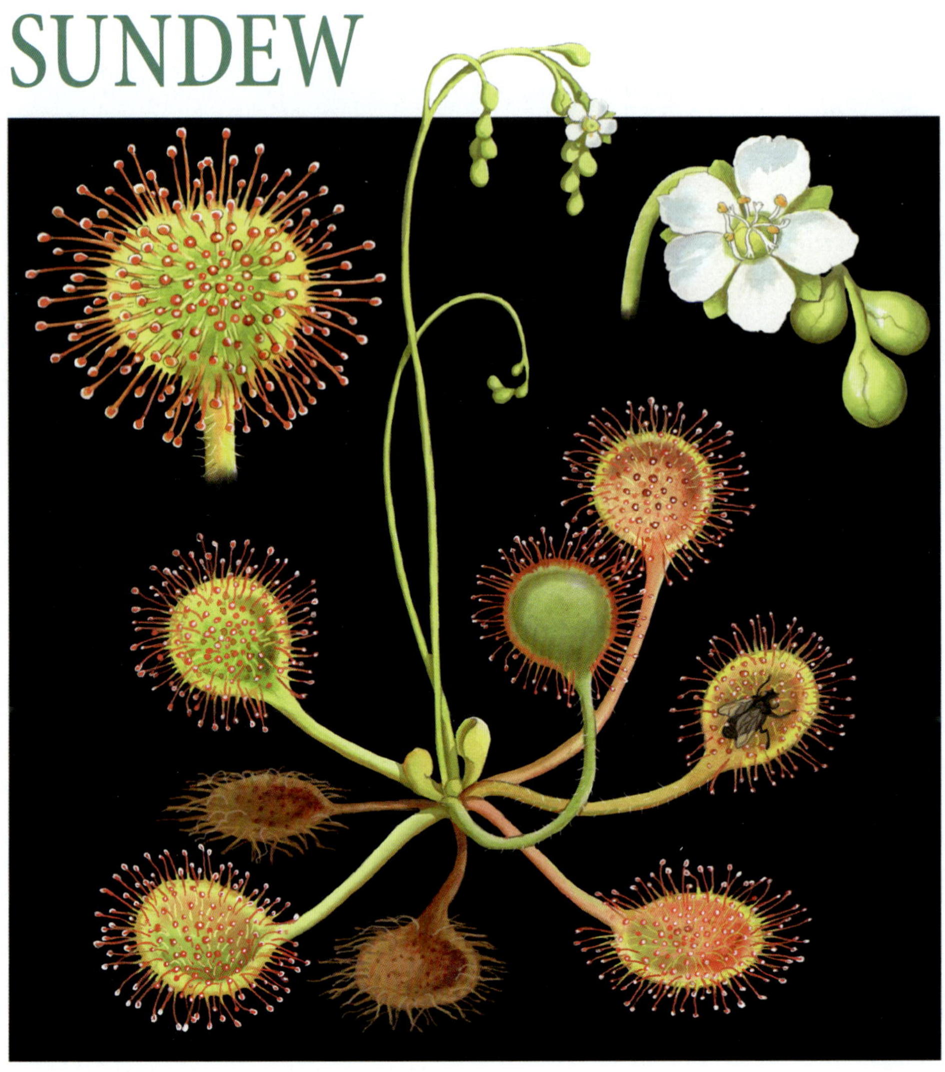

Drosera rotundifolia

FAMILY: Droseraceae

OTHER NAMES: Dew Plant, Red Root, Herba Rosellae, Round-leaf Sundew, Lustwort, *Fr.* Droséra à feuilles rondes, Rosée du soleil

PARTS USED: Whole plant

CHARACTERISTICS: Bitter, acrid, cool

ACTIONS: Anti-spasmodic, antibiotic, demulcent, expectorant, antimicrobial, anti-inflammatory, antifungal, antioxidant, astringent, antiviral

RANGE: Native across Canada

This tiny native aquatic plant can be found in acidic peaty soil alongside ponds, rivers, or in damp woods. An insectivore (or insect-eating) perennial, its leaves grow close to the ground in basal rosettes, and are covered with red glandular hairs, which exude sticky mucilaginous drops that resemble morning dew. They lure and catch insects, holding on to them as their leaves fold over and digest them. The tiny 5-petalled white or pink flowers emerge from the middle of the rosette on erect leafless stems 5–15 cm. high, and appear in summer or early fall. This plant is endangered, so it should be left where it is unless it's cultivated or growing in abundance in the area. Gather in mid-summer and air-dry for later use.

MEDICINAL USES:

Tuberculosis, coughs, asthma, whooping cough, bronchitis, warts, stomach ulcers

- Its antispasmodic and antibiotic properties make it effective in treating lung infections with dry coughs and inflamed respiratory tract issues. It has a relaxing effect on the involuntary muscles and thins the mucus, making it easier to cough up, reducing coughing spasms and soothing tissues. Specifically recommended by herbalists in Europe for dry cough, whooping cough, asthma, and bronchial spasms.
- The juice of the plant contains enzymes that will dissolve warts, bunions, and corns.
- Has been reported to have aphrodisiac effects.

FOLKLORE AND OTHER USES: Was once employed in Sweden to sour milk in the making of cheese. The "dew" on the leaves was once believed to endow long life or restore youth to anyone who drank it.

INFUSION: Add 1 tsp. dried herb to 1 cup steaming water; infuse 10–15 minutes. Strain and drink 3 times a day.

TINCTURE: Fresh plant 1:2 in 50% alcohol, 5–15 drops up to 3 times a day.

CAUTION: May cause gastrointestinal irritation if taken in large doses. Contains substances that may cause dermatitis in some people. Do not exceed recommended doses. Do not take if pregnant or breastfeeding.

SWEET FERN

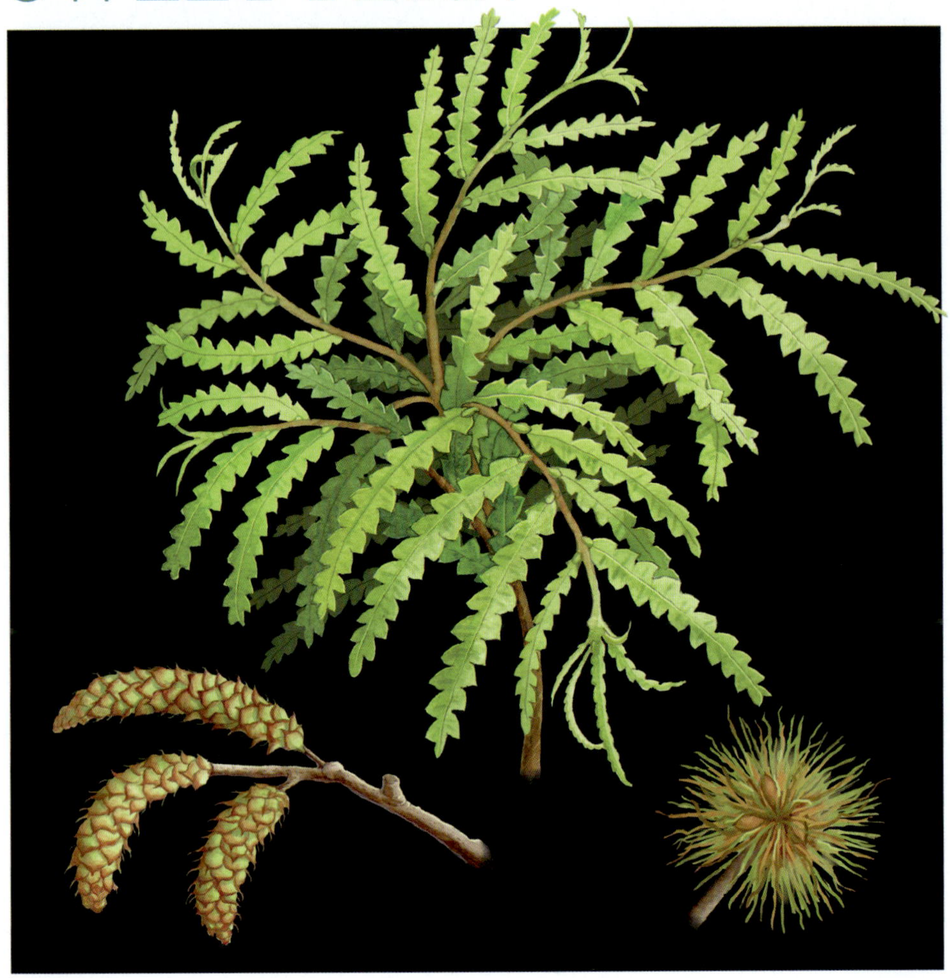

Comptonia peregrina

FAMILY: Myricaceae

OTHER NAMES: Meadow Fern, Sweet Bush, Fern Gale, Fern Bush, *Fr.* Comptonie voyageuse

PARTS USED: Leaves, flowers, nutlets

CHARACTERISTICS: Warm, spicy, bitter

ACTIONS: Astringent, anti-inflammatory, antibacterial, antifungal, analgesic, expectorant, digestive, immune and lymphatic tonic, emollient, sedative

RANGE: Native to Ontario, Quebec, Maritimes

Despite its name, this plant is not really a fern but a low-growing shrub from the Bayberry family that spreads by rhizomes, forming dense colonies 0.9–1.5 m. tall. It thrives in poor, acidic areas that have been opened up by fires or logging, with brown, woody, loosely branched stalks. Its roots are equipped with nodules that fix nitrogen in the soil, adding nutrients and helping to stabilize embankments and reduce erosion. Leaves are alternate, narrow, and lance-shaped, with a soft, hairy down, rounded lobes or teeth, and dotted with yellow glands. When crushed they are extremely aromatic, and the scent can even be detected from a distance on a warm day. Male and female flowers grow on the same plant before leaves emerge. The male clusters of flowers or catkins are cylindrical and drooping, and the female catkins are soft and burr-like, developing nutlets in early fall that are edible. Leaves are best harvested in early summer and dried to be used later as a refreshing tea.

MEDICINAL USES:

Diarrhea, headache, fevers, poison ivy stings, rheumatism, swollen lymph nodes

- Well-known by Indigenous Peoples as an aromatic tea, it is used medicinally for diarrhea, coughs, rheumatism, and externally as an anti-itch treatment. It is also burned as incense in ceremonies. Contains tannins, terpenes, and flavonoids that are anti-inflammatory, antioxidant, and antimicrobial.
- Leaves can be crushed and used as a poultice for toothaches, sprains, poison ivy, and bleeding.
- Infusion of the leaves is astringent and useful for diarrhea, headache, fever, and coughs. Externally in cold infusion it eases itching and stings, poison ivy, ringworm, and dermatitis.
- Strong decoction applied externally relieves arthritic pain or bruises.
- With an affinity to the lymphatic system, it moves and clears swollen lymph nodes and clears brain fog.

OTHER USES:

- Natural insect repellent.
- Used when storing fresh fruit and berries to delay spoiling.
- Crushed and added to potpourri or used as a cooking herb.

INFUSION: Put 1 tsp. dried (2 tsp. fresh) herb in 1 cup boiling water, infuse 5–10 minutes. Will become bitter if infused for too long. Drink 1–2 cups a day.

COMBINATIONS: With Mallow root, Elder flowers in infusions as a blood purifier and to remove mucus from the lungs, for bladder inflammations and swollen lymph glands. With Yarrow as a liniment for swellings.

RESEARCH: Contains gallic acid, which has been shown to have potent antimicrobial activity against a wide range of bacteria. Also contains cytotoxins, which may prove to play a role in fighting colon and lung cancers.

SWEET FLAG

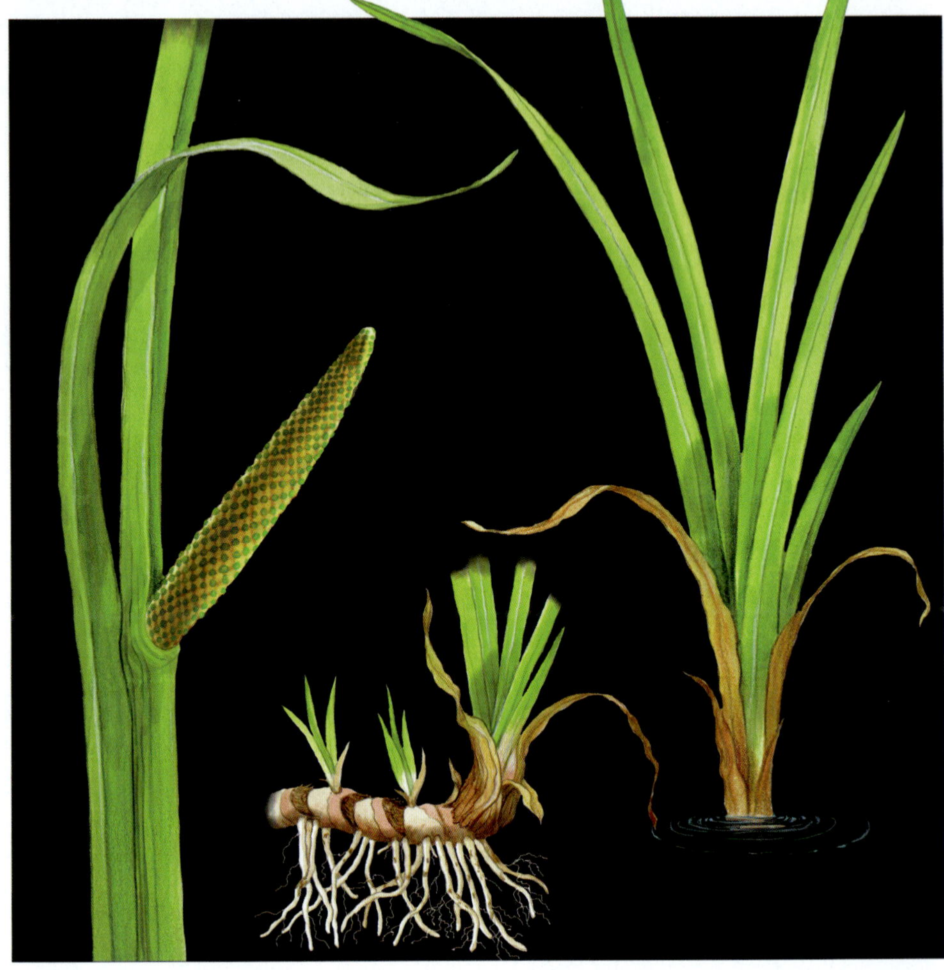

Acorus calamus
Acorus americanus

FAMILY: Acoraceae

OTHER NAMES: Calamus, Muskrat Root, Rat root, *Fr.* Acore, Belle-Angelique

PARTS USED: Rhizome, dried

CHARACTERISTICS: Acrid, slightly warm, aromatic, pungent, bitter

ACTIONS: Anodyne, antispasmodic, anti-inflammatory, antioxidant, antimicrobial, anticancer, aphrodisiac, aromatic, carminative, diaphoretic, emmenagogue, expectorant, febrifuge, hypotensive, nervine, sedative, stimulant, stomachic, mildly tonic, and vermifuge

RANGE: *A. calamus* introduced in Ontario, Quebec, and Nova Scotia; *A. americanus* native across all provinces and Northwest Territories.

There has been much confusion and disagreement concerning the native status of these species. Most botanists consider them to be separate, as there are a couple of differences: *A. calamus*, or the Asian variety, has only one raised vein on its basal leaves and wavy leaf margins, whereas *A. americanus,* the native species, has two or more raised veins and is generally flat. Although they are very similar medicinally, *A. americanus* seems to lack the carcinogen present in *A. calamus*; however, the presence of toxins is also debated, as it has been used in Asia for thousands of years without reports of cancer.

Both are semi-aquatic perennials that are found around marshes and lakes and look very similar to Cattails until their flowers emerge. Also, Sweet Flag is distinguished by its pleasant smell when the leaf is broken. It has erect, sword-shaped leaves growing to almost 1 m. tall, with a brown sheath at the base and the rhizome buried in the mud. The flower stem looks similar to the leaves, a spadix projects outward from the stem like a finger, with the actual yellow-green, inconspicuous flowers growing on it. The rhizome can be collected in late fall or early spring. Avoid plants older than 3 years as the root is often hollow. Dry before using.

MEDICINAL USES:

Stomach disorders, diarrhea, coughs, failing memory, anxiety, epilepsy

- With its combination of bitter and spicy properties, it has a long history of use in Traditional Chinese Medicine and Ayurveda, and is considered a sacred herb by Indigenous Peoples. The root is often carried around to prevent disease, or chewed on to relieve indigestion, clear the throat, or increase endurance or concentration.
- Used extensively for deficient, sluggish digestion, it relieves ulcers, hyperacidity, upset stomach, gastritis, gas, and headaches associated with weak digestion, as well as diarrhea, dysentery, colic, and cramps. Increases appetite, helps cases of anorexia.
- Rejuvenates the brain and nervous system, improves memory, focus, and intellect. Helps recovery from stroke, aids dementia, nervous disorders, epilepsy, and depression. Used in cases of numbness, debility, and vascular disorders.
- Good for colds, flu, bronchitis, chest congestion, and damp, wet coughs; clears congestion from the sinuses. Strong antibacterial action helps ease sore throats, laryngitis.
- Antispasmodic, analgesic, and sedative, it relieves stress and relaxes the body.
- Relieves pain of toothaches, rheumatism, and headaches.

OTHER USES:

- The highly aromatic volatile oil is used for perfumes.
- Can be used as a spice or flavouring for beer or gin.
- Burning dried leaves can be used as a smudge.
- As a strewing herb to keep away insects.

COLD INFUSION: Steep the root in a jar (2 cups) of cold water for 10–12 hours; drink throughout the day.

HOT INFUSION: ½ tsp. powdered root or dried leaves in 1 cup boiling water.

TINCTURE: Dried root 1:5 in 60% alcohol, 1–4 ml. up to 3 times per day.

CANDIES: Cut root into thin slices and parboil in water, changing once or twice to reduce the bitterness, then simmer in simple syrup (2 parts sugar, 1 part water), just to cover, until most of the syrup is absorbed. Drain, roll in sugar if desired. Preheat oven to 200°F and bake mixture on a cookie sheet until dry.

RESEARCH: Showed significant anti-inflammatory activity, up to 45%, in studies on rats. Found to reduce epilepsy attacks by up to 50% with no repeat attacks after 2 years of treatment. Calamus oil was tested in cases of diarrhea and colic pain and found to be an effective antispasmodic. Effective at reducing chest pain and lowering blood pressure, improving ECGs, decreasing LDL cholesterol and increasing HDL. In a clinical trial on patients with moderate to severe bronchial asthma, the fresh rhizome was chewed for 2–6 weeks, and was found to have anti-asthmatic potential without side effects. Caused suppression of blood glucose levels in mice. Leaf and rhizome have antimicrobial and high antifungal activity, and moderate activity against yeasts due to α- and ß-asarones, particularly effective against candida. Shows neuroprotective activity in vitro for Alzheimer's and Parkinson's disease.

CAUTION: *A. Calamus* has been banned in the US due to possible carcinogenic properties because of the presence of ß-asarone, although there have been no known cases in Asia, where it has been used for centuries. However, caution is advised, do not use in large doses. *A. americanum* does not contain this carcinogen. May cause vomiting in large doses. Avoid during pregnancy or breastfeeding.

TANSY

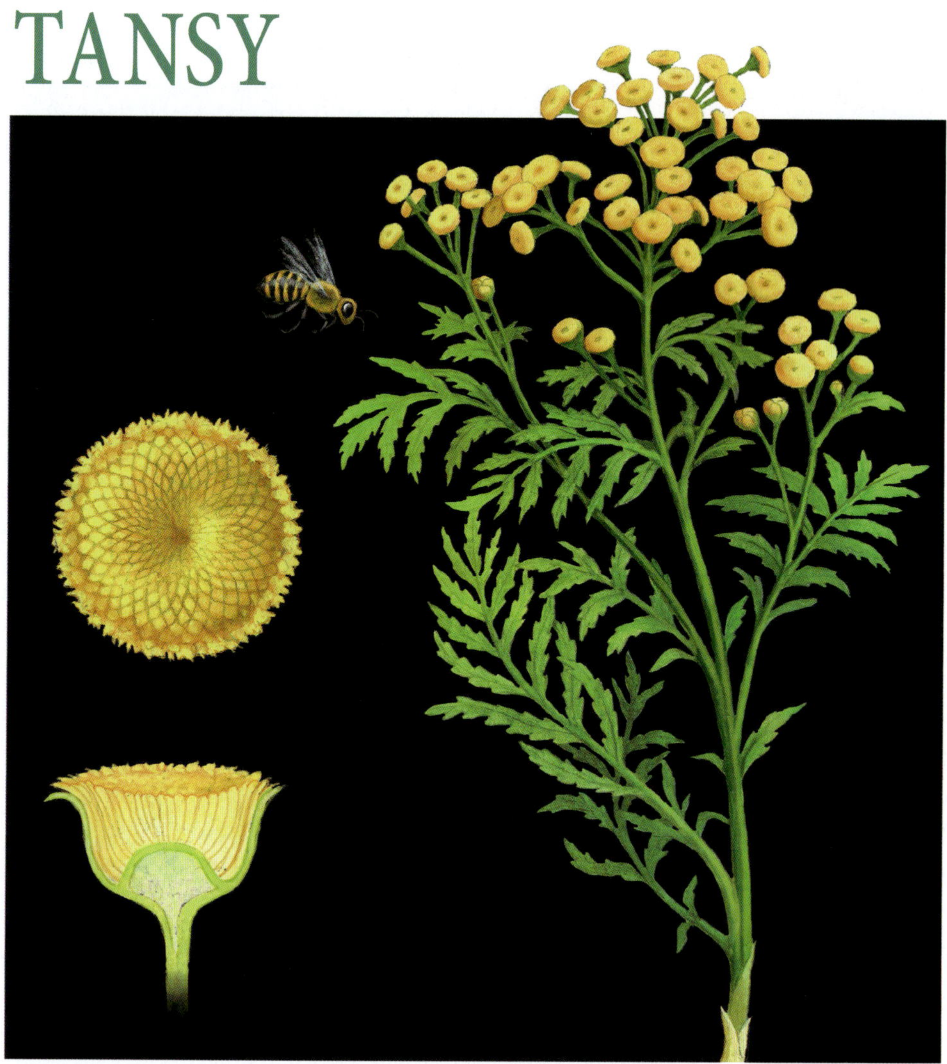

Tanacetum vulgare

FAMILY: Asteraceae

OTHER NAMES: Golden Buttons, Stinking Willie, *Fr.* Tanaisie commune, Tanacée

PARTS USED: Aerial

CHARACTERISTICS: Bitter, aromatic, cooling

ACTIONS: Anthelmintic, antispasmodic, antiseptic, anti-inflammatory, emmenagogue, insecticide, carminative, vermifuge, diuretic, antihypertensive, abortifacient, diaphoretic

RANGE: Introduced across Canada except Nunavut

Tansy is an aromatic perennial that is rarely used anymore as a medicinal herb due to its thujone content, which can be toxic in large doses—although in small amounts it can be quite effective to remove parasites. It has a hardy, erect stem about 75 cm. high, which is grooved and angular, with fern-like, feathery, alternate leaves. It is distinguished by its round, yellow, composite flowers that grow in clusters and look like small buttons, with an odour much like a mixture of camphor and Rosemary. It blooms from July to September, and is found in fields and along roadsides. Harvest as it is coming into flower and dry for later use.

MEDICINAL USES:

Parasites, rheumatism, indigestion

- This herb is no longer recommended for internal use, but it was historically used to expel worms in children, as an emmenagogue for suppressed menstruation, as an abortifacient, and to prevent gout and jaundice. It is high in thujone, which is insecticidal and toxic when ingested in large doses, and since the amount differs from plant to plant, it is difficult to predict a safe dose. It also has diaphoretic and antimicrobial actions. It is moderately safe to use externally.
- Fresh leaves crushed and applied to the skin can relieve swelling, bruises, varicose veins, scabies and lice. Essential oil when diluted and applied to clothing may repel ticks and mosquitoes.
- When heated in a fomentation, it will relieve rheumatism, gout, neuralgia, and muscle pain.
- A weak infusion stimulates digestion, aids in dyspepsia, and relieves flatulence.

OTHER USES:

- As a strewing herb it was scattered on floors as a disinfectant and to repel insects.
- Used as a companion herb in gardens to repel many destructive insects.
- When dried, the flowers last a long time in bouquets.
- Flowers were once used as a dye.

FOLKLORE: Leaves once used in Tansy cakes throughout England during Easter; its bitter taste helped cleanse the body after Lent and symbolized the suffering of the Jews at Passover. Irish folklore claimed bathing in Tansy and salt would cure joint pain.

ALTERNATIVE HERBS: For intestinal worms: raw Garlic, Wormwood, Mugwort; for indigestion: Dandelion root, Gentian, Fennel, and Angelica.

COMBINATIONS: With Lavender, Lemongrass, or Lemon Balm for an insect repellent spray.

CAUTION: Not recommended for internal use. Contains thujone, which can cause severe gastritis, vomiting, miscarriage, liver damage, and convulsions. May cause dermatitis in some people. Avoid use externally in high concentrations or over long periods of time.

THYME

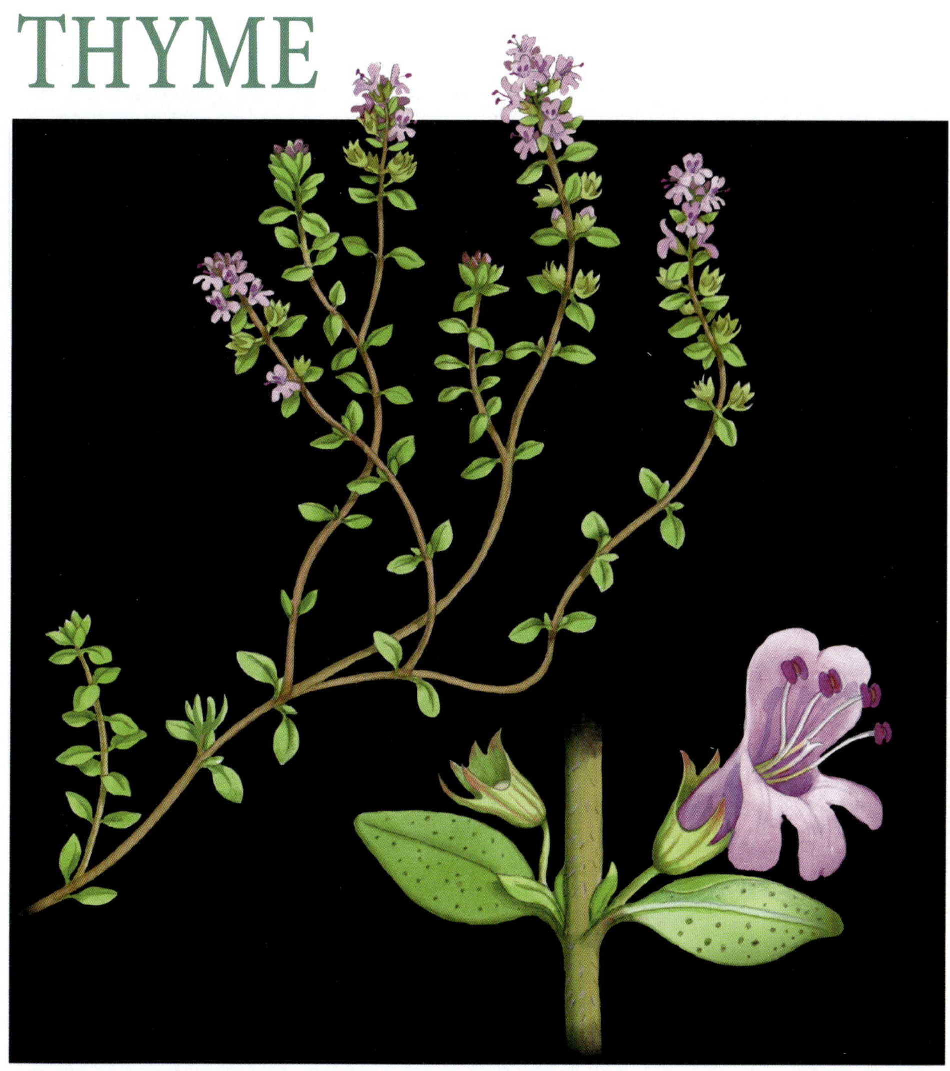

Thymus pulegioides

FAMILY: Lamiaceae

OTHER NAMES: Creeping Thyme, Garden Thyme, Wild Thyme, Lemon Thyme, *Fr.* Thym

PARTS USED: Aerial

CHARACTERISTICS: Spicy, warm, slightly bitter, drying, aromatic

ACTIONS: Carminative, antiseptic, expectorant, antitussive, sedative, anthelmintic, antispasmodic, diaphoretic, tonic, antimicrobial, antifungal, anti-inflammatory, astringent, antioxidant

RANGE: Introduced in British Columbia, Alberta, Ontario to Maritimes

Thyme is a common garden herb that originated in Europe but now also grows wild throughout much of Canada, with similar properties to the garden variety (*Thymus vulgaris*) although to a lesser degree. It is a perennial evergreen shrub, but rarely grows higher than about 10 cm. in the wild, creeping along roadsides and lawns in dense masses. The stems and roots are woody, reddish brown, with tiny green oval leaves set in opposite pairs. The pink or mauve flowers bloom from early summer to early fall, and the entire plant gives off a distinct fragrance that can be detected from several metres away. It should be gathered when in full flower and can be dried for later use.

MEDICINAL USES:

Powerful antiseptic, gastrointestinal problems, headaches, coughs and colds, mouth and throat infections, menstrual cramps

- The essential oil of Thyme contains thymol and carvacrol, and is a potent antibiotic, antifungal, and antiseptic, but should be used with caution as it is very concentrated and should be diluted with almond or other oils. Can be rubbed on the chest to relieve congestion. The herb taken in infusion or tinctures has an antispasmodic and relaxing effect on the respiratory tract, easing spasms and dry coughs. It also has a carminative effect on the digestive tract, soothing gas pains and indigestion.
- Traditionally used for upper respiratory infections, it treats dry, irritating, and unproductive coughs, loosens phlegm, and makes it easier to clear the airways. A specific for whooping cough but also helpful for colds, fever, bronchitis, asthma, and strep throat.
- Improves sluggish digestion, bloating, diarrhea, food poisoning, candida, and bowel disorders. Slightly bitter, it stimulates digestive secretions, relieves spasms, and improves gut microbiome. Soothes menstrual cramps.
- Useful as an antiseptic mouthwash or gargle for sore throats, gum disease, or laryngitis.
- When added to massage oils or liniments, it relieves aching joints and muscles or arthritis.
- Sprigs of Thyme can be added to a bottle of olive oil to improve LDL levels (high cholesterol).

FOLKLORE: Scottish highlanders made a tea from Thyme to give them strength and courage and to prevent nightmares. Pliny the Elder (23 AD–79 AD), a Roman naturalist and author, claimed it to be a cure for snakebites. In the Middle Ages it was included in a recipe that would enable a person to see fairies.

INFUSION: 1 heaped tsp. dried herb in 1 cup boiling water, steep covered for 15 minutes. Strain and drink in small doses.

TINCTURE: Dried herb 1:5 in 50% alcohol, take 2–4 ml. up to 3 times a day.

ESSENTIAL OIL: Diluted with 2 parts vegetable oil for topical use.

COMBINATIONS: Use with Lobelia for asthma, or with Mullein and Coltsfoot for coughs.

CAUTION: Herb is safe when used in recommended doses. Essential oil is very concentrated and irritant and for external use only. Dilute with a carrier oil before using.

TRUE UNICORN

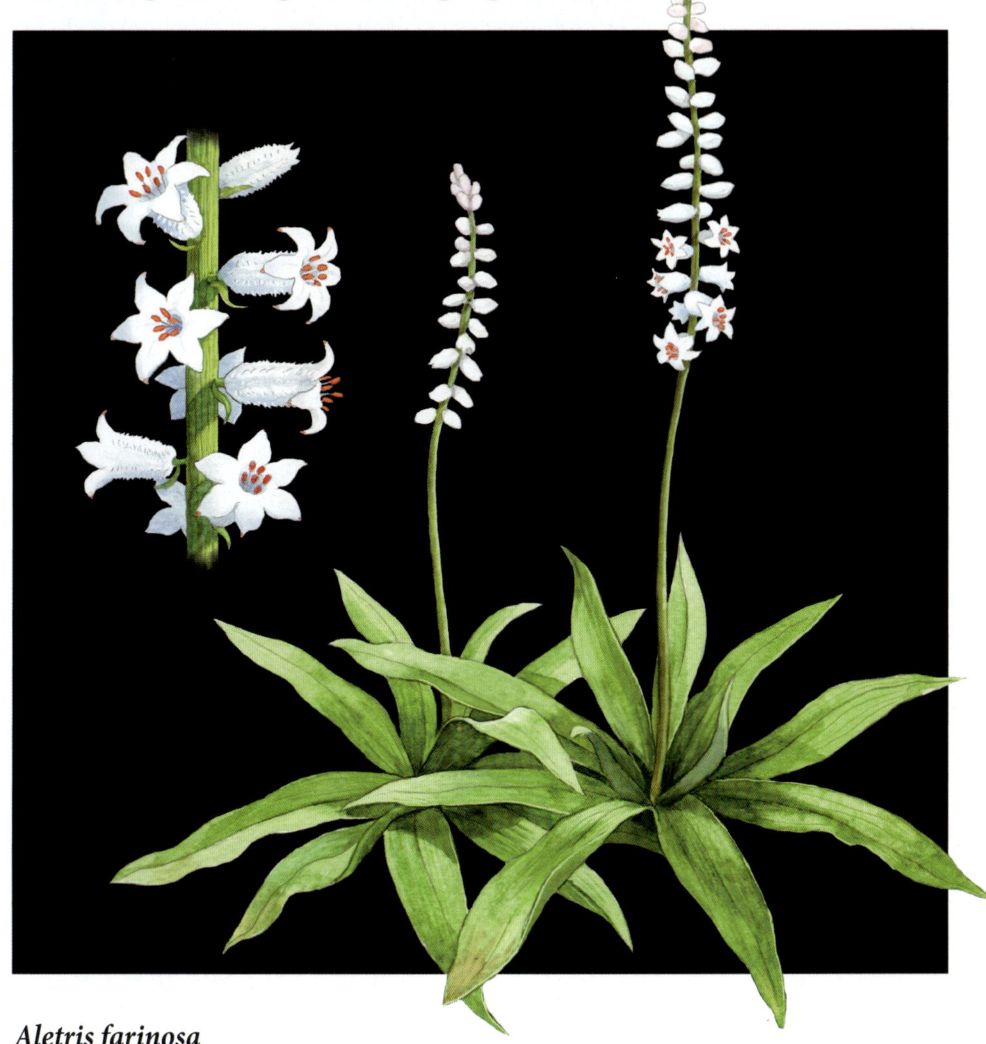

Aletris farinosa

FAMILY: Nartheciaceae

OTHER NAMES: Colic Root, Star Grass, Ague Root, Unicorn Root, *Fr.* Alétris farineux

PARTS USED: Dried root, rhizome, leaves

CHARACTERISTICS: Bitter

ACTIONS: Anti-inflammatory, antioxidant, antispasmodic, appetite stimulant, diuretic, relaxant, tonic

RANGE: Native to Ontario

True Unicorn is a herbaceous perennial that has become more and more rare in Canada and is now restricted to the southernmost portions of Ontario due to loss of habitat from urban and industrial development and invasive species. Its leaves are mainly basal, pale yellow-green and lance-shaped, with usually one upright flower stalk that arises from the leaf rosette in early summer, growing from 30 cm. to 1 m. tall. The flower spike has small, tubular white flowers with an unusual rough, grainy texture and 6 orange stamens. It blooms from June through to August, bearing similar capsules in the fall which split open to release 2 or more seeds. Avoid using wildcrafted plants as they are endangered.

MEDICINAL USES:

Diarrhea, reproductive and menstrual problems, rheumatism, indigestion, colic

- This plant's roots have a long history of traditional use as a women's herb, to improve women's reproductive health and help relieve menstrual difficulties. Contains diosgenin, a steroid sapogenin, which acts as an anti-inflammatory and has some estrogenic activity.
- Eases cramps and pain from dysmenorrhea, amenorrhea, stimulates the uterus improving blood circulation and balancing hormones. Tones the reproductive organs, helping prolapse and improving fertility. When taken before conception it has been used to prepare the uterus for pregnancy when there is risk of miscarriage. Not for use while pregnant.
- Improves appetite and digestion, eases stomachache, diarrhea, flatulence, colic, dysentery.
- Used traditionally to help coughs. Antioxidant properties boost immune system, maintain a balanced immune response.

TINCTURE: Dried root, 1:5 in 50% alcohol, 30–60 drops up to 3 times a day.

DECOCTION: 1 tsp. dried root in 1 cup water, boil 15 minutes. Take 1–2 tbsp. at a time, 3 times a day.

COMBINATIONS: With Red Trillium, Partridgeberry, Wild Yam for female complaints.

CAUTION: Fresh root is mildly poisonous; may cause dizziness, abdominal discomfort, diarrhea, vomiting. Should only be used dried in small doses. Avoid during pregnancy. Estrogen-like properties may interfere with hormonal drugs. Avoid if taking anticoagulants, non-steroidal anti-inflammatory drugs (NSAIDS), or if you have breast cancer.

VALERIAN

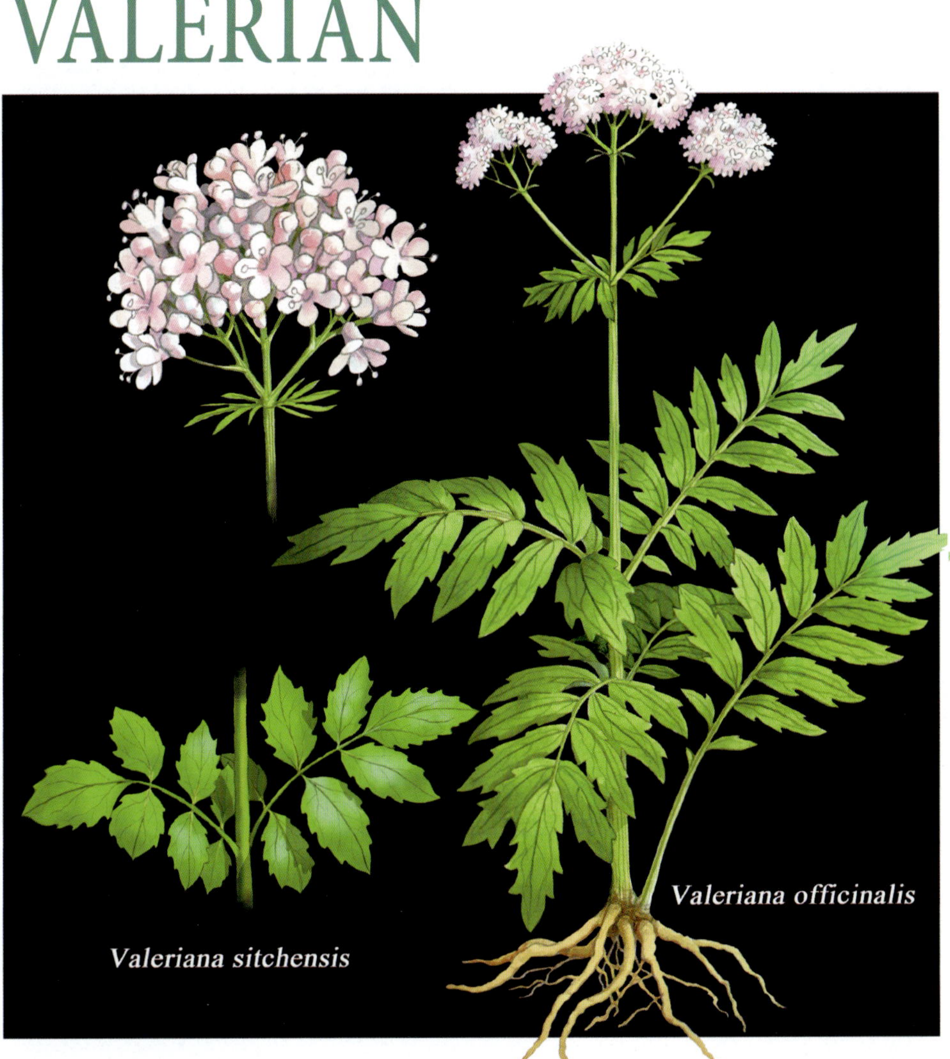

Valeriana officinalis
Valeriana sitchensis

FAMILY: Caprifoliaceae

OTHER NAMES: *V. officinalis*: Garden Valerian, European Valerian, *Fr.* Valériane; *V. sitchensis*: Sitka Valerian, Marsh Valerian, Pacific Valerian, *Fr.* Valériane de Sitka

PARTS USED: Root, rhizomes

CHARACTERISTICS: Spicy, bitter, warm, aromatic, astringent, sweet

ACTIONS: Sedative, hypnotic, nervine, antispasmodic, carminative, stimulant, anodyne, hypotensive, tonic, diuretic

RANGE: *V. officinalis* introduced in the Yukon and all provinces except Saskatchewan; *V. sitchensis* native to the Yukon, Northwest Territories, British Columbia, and Alberta

Valerian's genus comprises about 150 species, the most widely used in herbology Garden Valerian (*V. officinalis*), native to Europe and Asia but now present throughout most of Canada and escaped to the wild. *V. sitchensis* is a native to Western Canada and considered to have stronger medicinal activity than the European variety. Attaining a height of 0.7–1 m., it is smaller than Common Valerian, but often one of the most common wildflowers in the moist subalpine meadows of Western Canada. The pink or white fragrant flowers of both species grow atop a usually smooth stem in two or more clusters or cymes. There are 2–4 pairs of compound opposite leaves with 1–4 pairs of lobes below a terminal leaflet. The plant sends out runners, spreading quickly, and the roots give off a rather fetid odour, like smelly socks. The root is more potent if kept from flowering and should be at least 2 years old; dig them up after the leaves have died down in the fall. Tincture and infusions are best made from the fresh root, but it may also be dried for later use.

MEDICINAL USES:

Insomnia, hypertension, menstrual cramps, eczema, anxiety, hot flashes, headache, mild depression

- Known for centuries for its calming effect on the nervous system, Valerian is one of the most effective nervines available, soothing nerves, relieving anxiety, and making it easier to fall asleep. As effective as some medications for sleep, it does not make you groggy, has no after effects the next day, and is not addictive, although it doesn't work for everyone. It often takes several days of regular use to reach maximum effect.
- Promotes sleep, helps with restless leg syndrome, muscle pain, stress, anxiety, panic attacks, mild depression, tension headache, and migraine.
- Eases palpitations and reduces high blood pressure.
- Helps with menstrual pain, PMS, cramps, and hot flashes.
- Soothes nervous stomach, intestinal cramps, and IBS.
- Has a calming effect on people with obsessive-compulsive disorders, hypochondria, and epilepsy.
- Externally an infusion can be used as a wash or compress to treat eczema and minor injuries or relieve muscle spasms.

OTHER USES: May be used to speed up bacterial activity in compost heaps as well as being a good fertilizer in gardens, attracting earthworms and adding phosphorus to the soil.

TINCTURE: Fresh root 1:2 in 50% alcohol, 2–4 ml. up to 3 times a day. Start with a smaller dose, and find the dose that works for you.

COMBINATIONS: With St. John's Wort, Lemon Balm, Hops, Skullcap, Motherwort, or Passionflower for insomnia or anxiety. With Cramp Bark for muscle tension.

RESEARCH: Studies have shown that Valerian decreased the time it took to fall asleep, decreased waking episodes, increased REM sleep, and decreased sleepiness the next morning. Works to increase levels of GABA, a neurotransmitter that helps reduce stress and anxiety. Not all studies are conclusive, but one study lasting 28 days found that the differences in improvement between Valerian and the placebo increased between assessments done on days 14 and 28, suggesting effectiveness increases the longer it's taken.

CAUTION: Generally considered safe for short term use, avoid taking with other sedatives or driving while using.

VIOLET

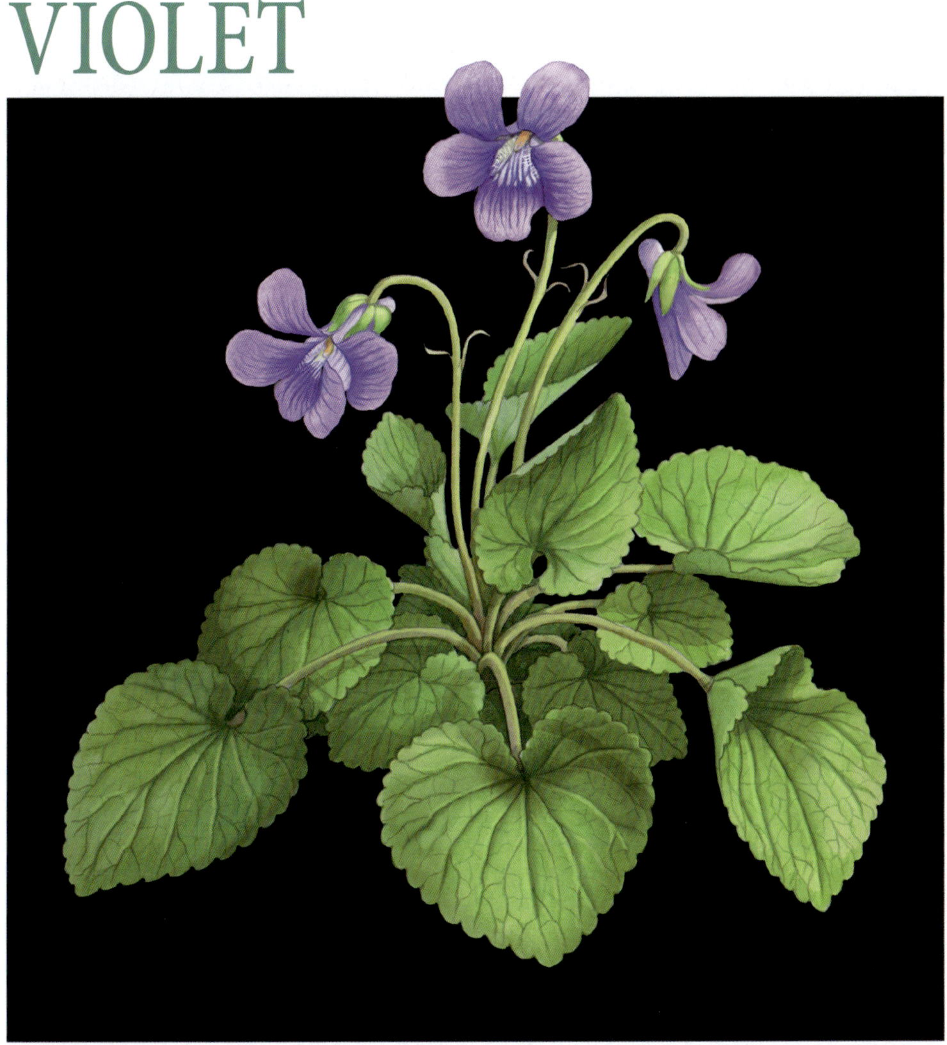

Viola odorata
Viola adunca

FAMILY: Violaceae

OTHER NAMES: *V. odorata:* Sweet Blue Violet, Garden Violet, *Fr.* Violette odorante; *V. adunca:* Dog Violet, Hooked Violet, *Fr.* Violette des chiens

PARTS USED: Aerial

CHARACTERISTICS: Sweet, mild but pleasantly bitter, cool, salty, moist

ACTIONS: Demulcent, expectorant, astringent, alterative, febrifuge, antiseptic, vulnerary, antispasmodic, anodyne, antiscrofulous, antibacterial, aromatic, anti-inflammatory, diuretic

RANGE: *V. odorata* introduced in British Columbia, Ontario, Quebec, Nova Scotia; *V. adunca* native across Canada, except Nunavut and Newfoundland and Labrador

Violets are pretty little creeping perennials, some of which are native to Europe and others to North America, and which belong to a genus of over nine hundred species, all with similar medicinal uses. Many foreign species have now naturalized throughout most of North America and are one of the first flowers to appear in the spring, traditionally symbolizing rebirth and bringing joy at the end of a long winter. Its leaves are heart-shaped, dark green, with scalloped edges, and grow in rosettes close to the ground. The fragrant flowers can be anywhere from deep purple to blue, pinkish, or even white. They are 5-petalled with a yellow beard in the centre and bloom from April to June. *V. adunca* is very similar to *V. odorata*, with a more elongated, hooked nectar spur on its flower. Oddly enough, the violet produces a second kind of flower later in the summer, growing colourless and hidden underground. Although they never see the light of day, they do produce viable seeds. If you pick only the leaves and flowers without disturbing the underground parts, they will continue to produce leaves all summer. Eat only the aerial parts, use fresh or dried, and store in glass away from heat and light.

MEDICINAL USES:

Dryness, inflammation, constipation, swollen glands, mastitis

- A gentle but nourishing medicine rich in vitamins A and C and minerals, it coats and soothes irritated tissues and eases inflammation due to its mucilage content, used both topically and internally. The leaves also contain salicylic acid, which reduces pain and swelling. Makes a nice addition to salads.
- Soothes sore throat and loosens mucus from the respiratory tract when there is a dry and unproductive cough. Useful for colds, bronchitis, whooping cough, and asthma, and makes an effective cough syrup.
- Mild laxative, the plant lubricates the intestines in cases of constipation.
- Used both internally and externally to treat a wide range of skin problems such as eczema, psoriasis, acne, bruising, and capillary fragility. Can be applied as a poultice for enflamed skin eruptions or bites. Infused oil massaged into the skin acts as a lymphatic stimulant for swollen glands, mastitis. A compress soothes dry, irritated skin or corns, hemorrhoids, abrasions.
- Has a relaxing effect on the nervous system, bringing comfort and reducing excessive thinking. Helps promote sleep. Contains methyl salicylate, a pain reliever, although in small quantity.

TINCTURE: Fresh plant 1:2 in 50% alcohol, 1–2 tsp. up to twice a day.

INFUSION: 1 tbsp. fresh plant in 1 cup boiling water, infuse covered for 15 minutes. Take up to 3 times a day.

COMBINATIONS: May be combined with equal parts Dandelion Leaf, Stinging Nettle, Red Clover, and Mint for a nutritious tea.

CAUTION: Generally considered safe, although may cause mild diarrhea or nausea if used in large doses. Underground parts should not be eaten as they can cause nausea and vomiting.

WHITE HOREHOUND

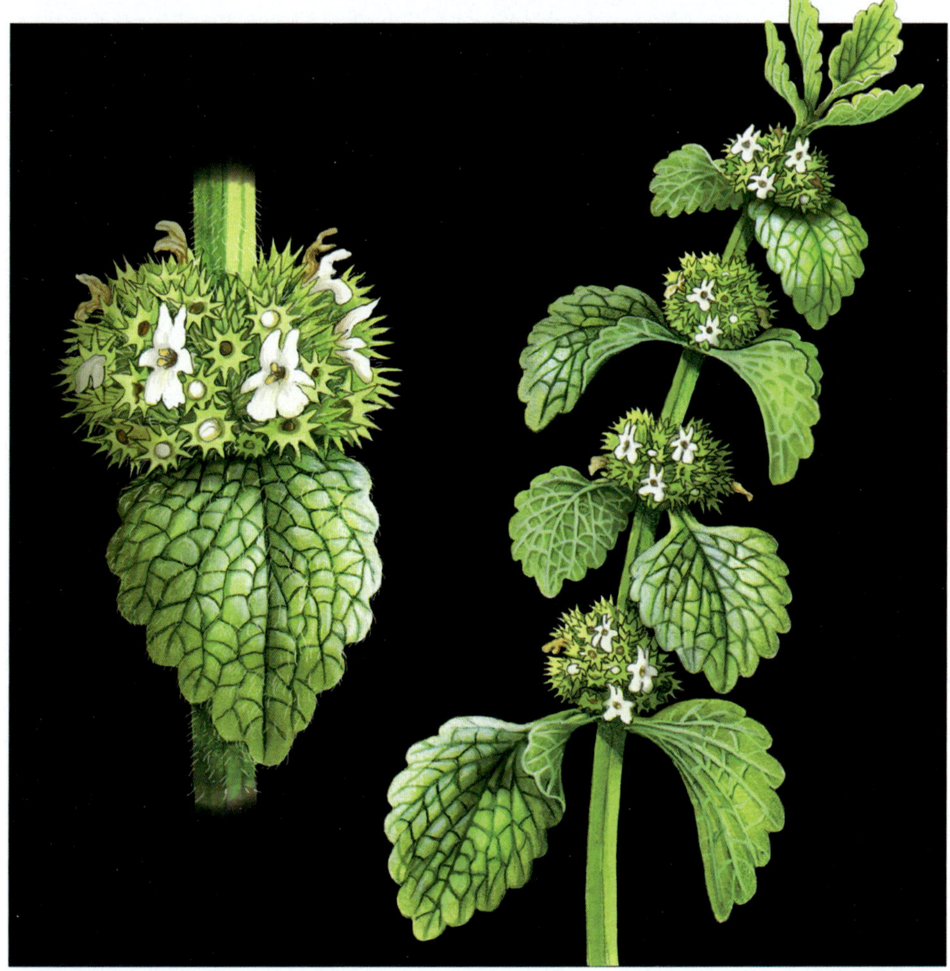

Marrubium vulgare

FAMILY: Lamiaceae or Labiatae

OTHER NAMES: Common Horehound, *Fr.* Marrube blanc

PARTS USED: Aerial

CHARACTERISTICS: Bitter, pungent, hot, dry

ACTIONS: Antibacterial, antispasmodic, antioxidant, anti-inflammatory, analgesic, cholagogue, diaphoretic, digestive, diuretic, emmenagogue, expectorant, hepatic, hypoglycemic, stimulant, tonic, hepatoprotective, antiviral, hemostatic, antimicrobial, antidiabetic

RANGE: Introduced in southern British Columbia, Saskatchewan, Ontario, Quebec, Nova Scotia

White Horehound, from the Mint family, is a native of Europe, northern Africa, and western Asia. Naturalized in North America, it's increasingly cultivated for medicinal use as a digestive herb and especially a cough remedy. Its branched stems, reaching 30–90 cm., are square and hairy; downy, wrinkled leaves round or ovate with rounded teeth, arranged in opposite pairs along the stems. Small, white, tubular flowers come out in spring, arranged in axillary whorls around the stem. As they mature, the calyces' spiny teeth once dried will cling to passersby to disperse their seeds. Found along roadsides and in fields, plants can be harvested in spring as they start flowering. Use fresh for tincturing or dried for later use in teas.

MEDICINAL USES:

Upper respiratory congestion, fever, indigestion, hypertension

- Highly recommended for millennia for coughs and respiratory problems, this herb is effective at loosening phlegm, breaking up congestion, and toning mucus membranes. Resolves difficult and chronic conditions with a dry, unproductive cough, facilitating mucus production, relaxing the bronchi and promoting expectoration. Add honey to teas or syrups to reduce bitterness.
- Used in infusions, lozenges, or cough syrups for bronchitis, asthma, whooping cough, pneumonia, hoarseness, sore throat, sinus congestion, colds and flus. A hot infusion will promote sweating when there is fever.
- In small doses it encourages bile flow, and its bitterness helps the liver, aids digestion, and stimulates appetite. Prepared in a cold infusion, it relieves dyspepsia, heartburn, and bloating, and protects the stomach from excess acid and ulcers. Avoid taking in large doses as it can become emetic and cathartic.
- May lower blood sugar and cholesterol levels, improving blood pressure and normalizing heart rhythm; however, care should be taken to not exceed recommended doses.
- Externally sometimes used to heal wounds, skin damage, and inflammatory conditions.

COUGH SYRUP: Bring 2 tbsp. of dried herb and 1 cup water to a boil, and simmer for 30 minutes covered. Strain, cool slightly, and add 1 cup unpasteurized honey. Add lime or lemon juice and ½ cup brandy if desired.

HOT INFUSION (DIAPHORETIC): ¼–½ tsp. dried herb in 1 cup boiling water, cover, and steep for 45 minutes. Strain and drink warm with molasses or honey.

COLD INFUSION (DIURETIC): Place 2 tbsp. dried herb into a cheesecloth bag and suspend in 4 cups of cold water. Leave overnight, then remove bag, squeezing out all the liquid. Take 4–8 tbsp. up to 4 times a day.

TINCTURE: Fresh 1:2, dried 1:5 in 50% alcohol. Take 30–90 drops, 4 times a day.

COMBINATIONS: With Elecampane and Wild Cherry bark for coughs, with Motherwort for amenorrhea.

RESEARCH: Ongoing studies show that oral administration resulted in significantly lowering blood glucose levels and suggest that it may be effective in treating diabetes mellitus. Studies on rats have shown it protects the liver from injury, and its high anti-inflammatory activity makes it a potential source for supportive treatment of cancer. An animal study where a water extract was given over 10 weeks showed a decrease in systolic blood pressure and had a significant antihypertrophic effect on the aorta and decreased LDL cholesterol. However, more clinical trials on humans are needed.

CAUTION: Avoid if pregnant or nursing. May cause diarrhea in large doses. Not recommended for children under twelve years old.

WILD BERGAMOT

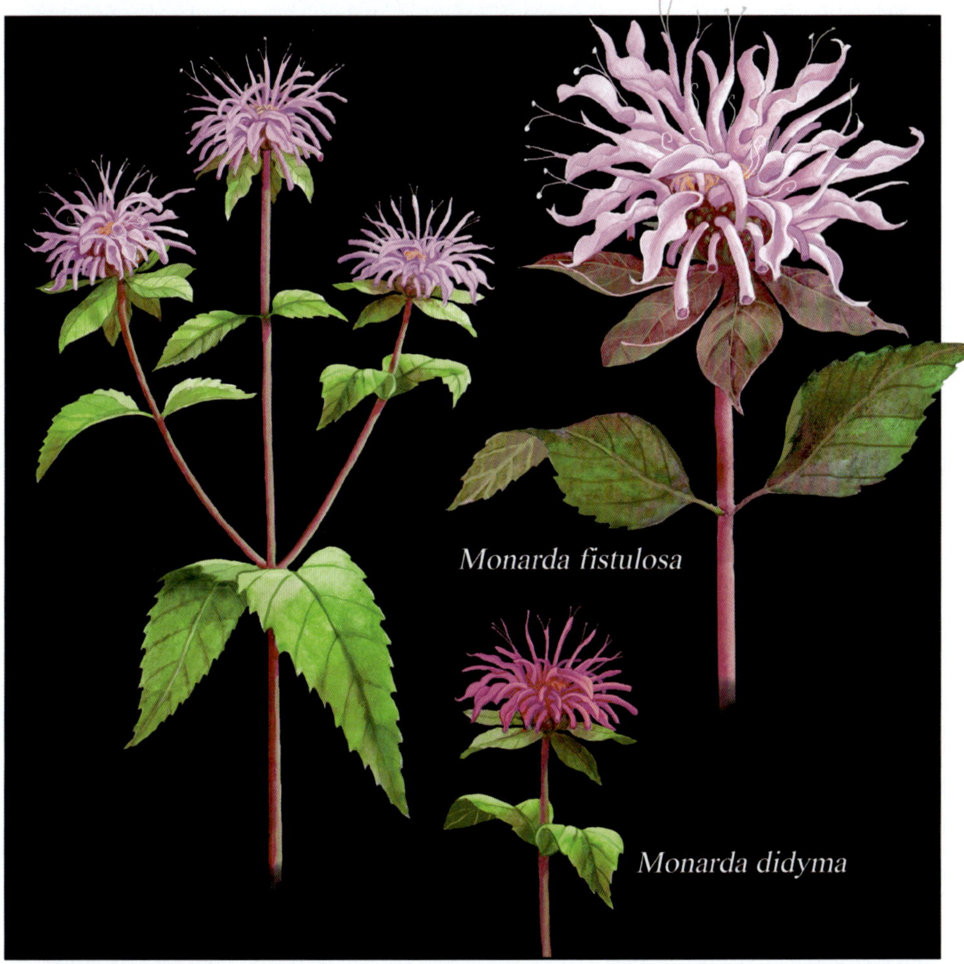

Monarda fistulosa
Monarda didyma

FAMILY: Lamiaceae

OTHER NAMES: *M. fistulosa:* Purple Beebalm, Sweet Leaf, *Fr.* Monarde fistuleuse; *M. didyma:* Scarlet Beebalm, Oswego Tea, *Fr.* Monarde écarlate

PARTS USED: Leaves and flowers

CHARACTERISTICS: Aromatic

ACTIONS: Antiseptic, antispasmodic, anti-inflammatory, antifungal, anthelmintic, antioxidant, carminative, diuretic, diaphoretic, sedative

RANGE: *M. fistulosa* native from British Columbia to Quebec, introduced in New Brunswick; *M. didyma* native to Ontario, introduced in Quebec, New Brunswick, and Nova Scotia

Wild Bergamot, still widely used by Indigenous healers, is one of their most important herbs, growing in dry fields, woods, and meadows throughout most of North America. The aerial parts are highly aromatic, making it a favourite for teas and as a cooking herb. *M. fistulosa* has purple, lavender, or white blooms, whereas *M. didyma* has bright red flowers; otherwise the two species are very similar, both in appearance and medicinal uses, the former being considered more potent. Growing 0.6–1.2 m. tall, it has a square stem that is slightly hairy and often branched with toothed, opposite, oblong leaves. The two-lipped, tubular flowers emerge in July and August, growing in dense, terminal heads that rest on a whorl of pinkish bracts. They are often grown in gardens to attract bees and butterflies; however, it is prone to powdery mildew, so care should be taken to avoid growing in dense clumps. Since the volatile oils are important to its healing properties, select plants with a buttery-sweet, pungent, hot taste and harvest at the beginning of flowering to maximize potency. Tie in bundles and hang to dry for later use.

MEDICINAL USES:

Digestive problems, colds, flu, fevers, upper respiratory infections, chronic bladder and yeast infections, Meniere's disease, fungal infections

- Strong antiseptic useful for flu, colds, fevers, upper respiratory infections.
- Eases bloating, nausea, diarrhea, soothes digestive tract, hyperacidity.
- Useful for chronic bladder and yeast infections.
- Used topically as a poultice for skin problems such as minor wounds, stings, and fungal infections. Flowers can be chewed up and placed on burns.
- A strong infusion is used as a mouthwash for sore throats, toothaches, and mouth sores.
- Leaves are steamed to clear sinuses, or added to bathwater for sore muscles.
- Calms the nervous system, warm poultice relieves sore eyes, headaches, muscle spasms.
- Infusion or tincture may ease the symptoms of Meniere's and tinnitus.

OTHER USES: Can be used as a cooking herb adjacent to thyme or oregano.

INFUSION: Standard, 1–2 tsp. dried leaves and petals in 1 cup boiling water, up to 3 times a day.

TINCTURE: 1:2 in 50% alcohol, 1–3 drops, up to 25 drops 3 times a day.

COMBINATIONS: Can be used with Yarrow, Elder flower, Mullein, or Spearmint to help clear the sinuses.

RESEARCH: Thymol, carvacrol, and cinnamyl carbanilate, three of the major components in Wild Bergamot, have been tested for their antifungal activity and were found to be a safe natural alternative to synthetic fungicides used on fruit and vegetables for preservation. Thymol and carvacol are also effective antimicrobial agents against gram-positive and gram-negative bacteria, and with thymoquinine are also antioxidant, anti-inflammatory, anticancer, and immunomodulatory. Thymol and carvacrol can alter the fluidity and permeability of cell membrane in a wide variety of bacteria and fungi, leading to cell death. Thymoquinone has also proven to be promising in treatment of several cancers including oral and prostate cancers by causing DNA damage and disrupting carcinogenic signalling pathways.

CAUTION: Generally safe, however, use with caution during pregnancy as there is very little data. May cause vomiting if combined with Valerian.

WILD GINGER

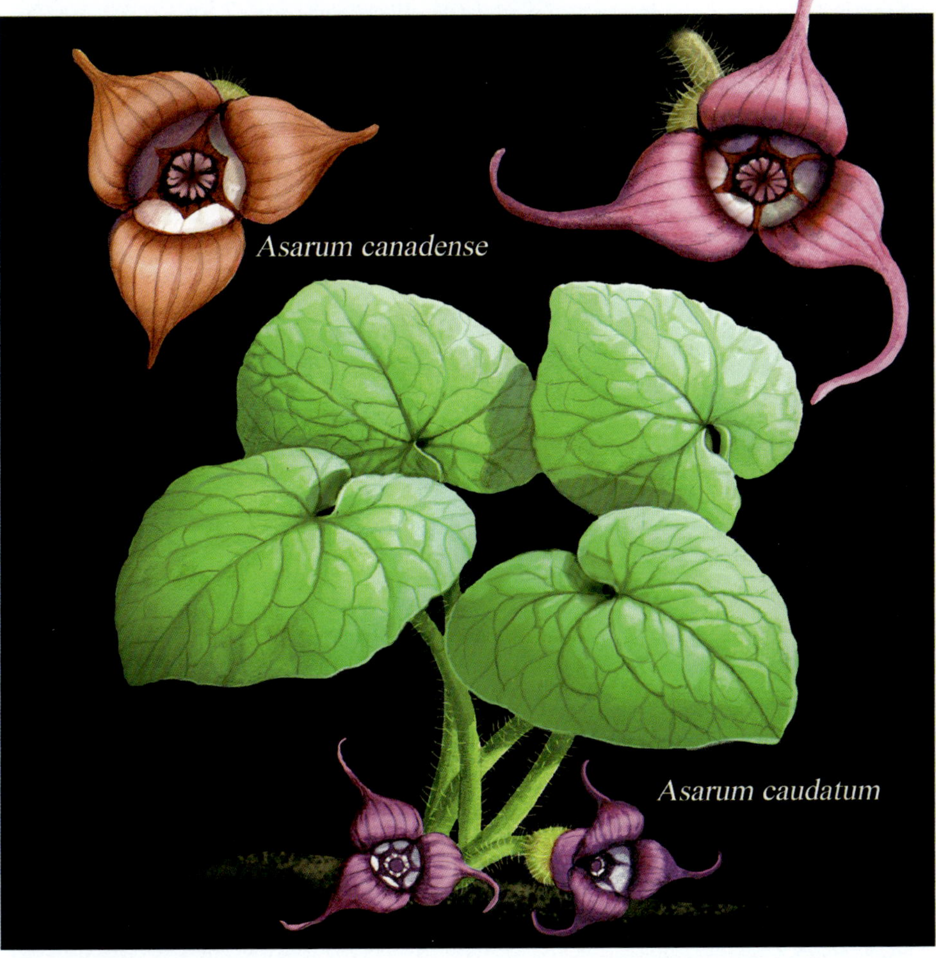

Asarum canadense*; *Asarum caudatum

FAMILY: Aristolochiaceae

OTHER NAMES: *A. canadense:* Canada Wild Ginger, Snakeroot, *Fr.* Asaret du Canada, Snicroûte; *A. caudatum:* Western Wild Ginger, Long-tailed Wild Ginger, *Fr.* Asaret caudé

PARTS USED: Rhizomes, leaves

CHARACTERISTICS: Pungent, aromatic, warming, bitter, stimulating

ACTIONS: Anthelmintic, analgesic, antirheumatic, carminative, diaphoretic, diuretic, laxative, stimulant, tonic, stomachic, antiviral, circulatory stimulant, anti-inflammatory, antibacterial, expectorant, antimicrobial, antispasmatic

RANGE: *A. canadense* native to Manitoba, Ontario, Quebec, New Brunswick; *A. caudatum* native to British Columbia

Wild Ginger, an evergreen perennial, is not related to culinary Ginger (*Zingiber officinale*), but its roots are occasionally used as a spice, exuding a mild ginger-like odour when crushed. A low-growing woodland plant about 15–25 cm. tall, it prefers shady, moist, acidic soils. The leaves grow in opposite pairs and are heart-shaped with a deep cleft at the base, the underside and stems covered in fine, white hairs. In the spring each plant produces a single, hairy, cup-shaped flower nestled beneath the carpet of leaves. They can be reddish, brownish-purple, or rust-coloured and have 3 triangular "petals" that are actually sepals; on the Western variety the tips are more elongated. Rhizomes grow close to the surface and are best harvested in the fall, although it is preferable to grow your own as it has become endangered in the wild. Be careful not to unearth more than is needed. Dry for later use.

MEDICINAL USES:

Viral infections, indigestion, dysmenorrhea, amenorrhea, poor circulation

- This plant, especially the leaves, stems, and flowers, contains aristolochic acid, which is a strong emetic and toxic to the kidneys, but has been used in herbal medicine for thousands of years with no toxic effects as long as it's used in the recommended doses. The root is used traditionally as an immune stimulant and expectorant to dispel viral infections, particularly colds and flu where there is pain, chills, and low fever with cough and clear nasal discharge.
- Rhizomes used in teas or tinctures in small amounts for viral infections, colds, coughs, fevers, nasal congestion, and bronchitis.
- A decoction of the rhizomes is used as a digestive aid to relieve bloating, gas, stomach pains, indigestion, nausea, cramps, and constipation. Stimulates the appetite and tonifies the digestive system.
- Effective at relieving menstrual cramps, absent or light periods, and menopausal symptoms.
- Increases peripheral blood circulation, improves heart function.
- Decoction used externally for headaches, joint pain. Fresh warmed leaves may be applied to wounds, boils, skin infections, and toothaches. Used in compounds for fractures.
- Strengthens the effect of other herbs when used in formulas.

OTHER USES:

- Dried root burned as incense.
- Repels insects.
- Decoction may be used as herbicide.
- Antibacterial, used for disinfecting hands.

DECOCTION: Standard decoction, sip 6–8 tbsp. up to 3 times a day.

INFUSION: ¼–⅓ tsp. dried rhizome in 1 cup boiling water, use once daily.

TINCTURE: Dried rhizome 1:5 in 50% alcohol, take 10–30 drops daily.

COMBINATIONS: Used by many Indigenous Peoples with Pine and Chaga during the COVID-19 pandemic to relieve viral infections.

CAUTION: Contains aristolochic acid, a toxin that is emetic and harmful to the kidneys. Do not exceed recommended doses and avoid using for more than 10 days. Do not use if pregnant or breastfeeding. Avoid in inflammatory conditions. Handling may cause dermatitis in some people.

WILD LICORICE

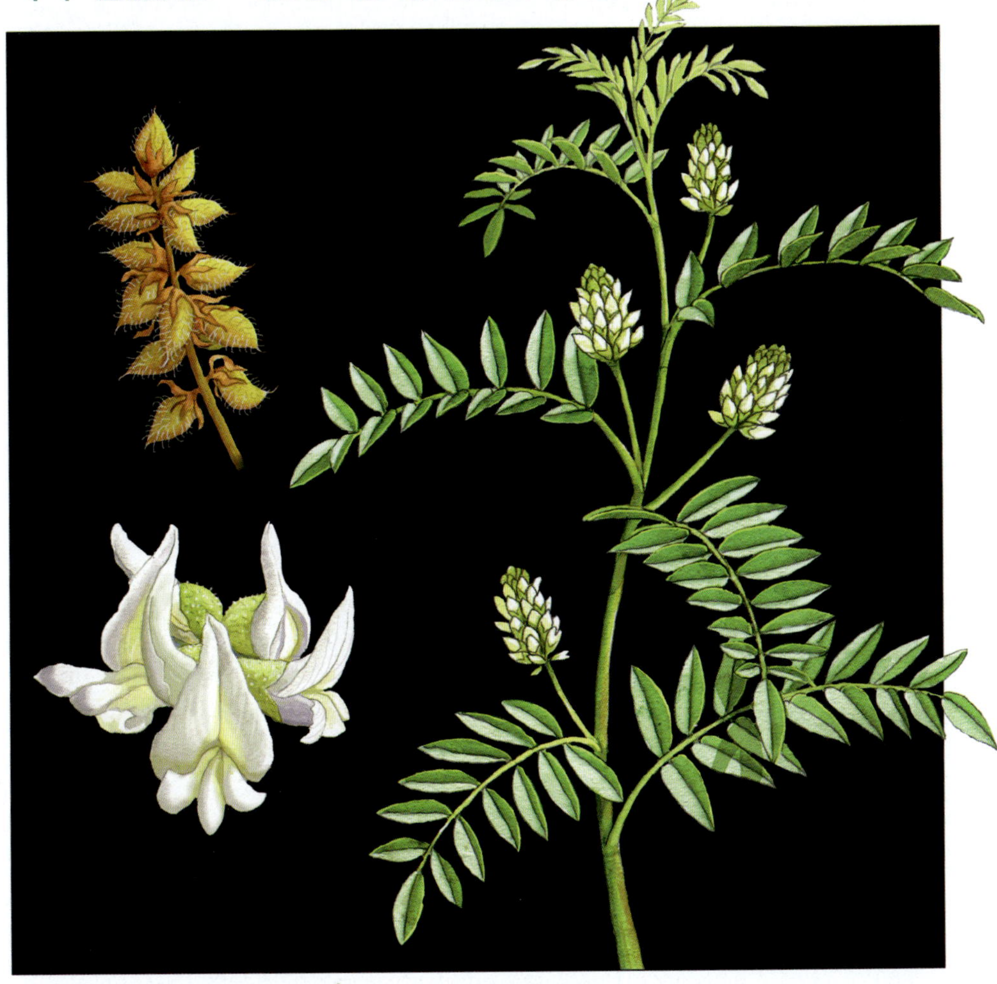

Glycyrrhiza lepidota

FAMILY: Fabaceae or Leguminosae

OTHER NAMES: American Licorice, *Fr.* Réglisse sauvage

PARTS USED: Root, leaves

CHARACTERISTICS: Sweet, moist, cooling, mucilaginous

ACTIONS: Antibacterial, antimicrobial, antioxidant, antifungal, anti-inflammatory, demulcent, expectorant, emollient, respiratory and kidney stimulant, tonic

RANGE: Native from British Columbia to Ontario

The European variety of Licorice (*G. glabra*) has a very long history of use around the world and has been cultivated both as a medicine and a flavouring for centuries. The American wild variety is perhaps less well-known, but is widely used by Indigenous Peoples across North America for much the same purposes. A perennial from the pea family, it grows up to around 1 m., its erect stem producing alternate compound leaves composed of up to 21 oblong toothless leaflets which often fold up when young. The flowers grow in mid to late summer from the leaf axils in spiky clusters and range from white to cream or pale yellow in colour. They are replaced by a green pod about 1.3 cm. long which is covered in hooked bristles and turns brown as it matures, often sticking to animal fur. Its woody roots or horizontal rhizomes, which are primarily used for medicines, taste like Licorice and are sweet due to the presence of glycyrrhizin, a substance fifty times sweeter than sugar. Plant should be at least 3 or 4 years old before harvesting. Dig up root in the fall, split lengthwise, and dry for later use.

MEDICINAL USES:

Coughs and upper respiratory problems, fever, stomachache, toothache, sores

- All parts of Wild Licorice, but particularly the peeled, dried roots, have been used by many Indigenous Peoples for a variety of ailments, but particularly in coughs, upset stomachs, and flus. It contains mucilage, which soothes inflamed mucous membranes of the respiratory tract, digestive and urinary systems. It strengthens and tonifies the adrenals and nervous system, and is often used in formulas to harmonize and strengthen the effects of other herbs.
- Root is used in decoction as an effective expectorant, commonly used for coughs and other inflammatory upper respiratory infections, bronchial asthma, sore throat, and fevers in children. Added to medicines and syrups to sweeten the taste.
- Sipping an infusion will speed up delivery of the placenta in childbirth.
- Good remedy for stomachaches, diarrhea, stomach flu, and peptic ulcers.
- Chewing the dried root is effective in easing toothache pain or sore throat. When saliva is swallowed after chewing, it helps strengthen the voice of singers.
- Externally, it can be used as a wash or poultice for swellings, and the mashed leaves may be applied to sores on both humans and animals.
- Taking 2 cups of infusion per day for 1 week lessens painful menstrual cramps.

OTHER USES:

- Roots may be eaten raw, cooked, or slow-roasted.
- Roots chewed by Indigenous Peoples as a tooth cleaner, or to cool the body in sweat lodges or Sun Dance ceremonies.
- Tender spring shoots can be eaten raw in the spring.
- Powdered roots are used as a sweetener.

DECOCTION: ½–1 tsp. chopped dried root in 1 cup water, simmer 15 minutes. Take 2–3 times a day.

COMBINATIONS: Works well with Mullein and Horehound for coughs, and with Echinacea, Ginseng, and Hawthorn for strengthening the immune and nervous systems, heart, and adrenals.

RESEARCH: Since Wild Licorice contains less of the active ingredient glycyrrhizic acid, most of the research has been done with *G. glabra*, *G. uralensis*, and *G. inflata*, which are grown in Europe and Asia. Research has found that these species exhibit a vast array of activities to enhance heath. They are highly antibacterial, inhibiting bacterial growth and biofilm formation, and may eventually serve as an alternative to some antibiotics. There is also potential to combat viruses, specifically HIV, atypical pneumonia, hepatitis, and some flu viruses. Glycyrrhizic acid is showing promise in inhibiting activity and inducing apoptosis in liver cancer stem cells, supports regeneration and repair, reduces inflammation, and has a protective effect on the liver. It also has cardioprotective, antidepressive, and neuroprotective activity. There is a great deal of potential for further research on the entire genus of these herbs.

CAUTION: Avoid if pregnant or nursing. May increase blood pressure; increased risk of edema, headaches, sluggishness if taken in large quantities. Generally safe if taken in recommended doses, use under supervision if you have kidney disease or are on heart or steroid medications.

WILD SARSAPARILLA

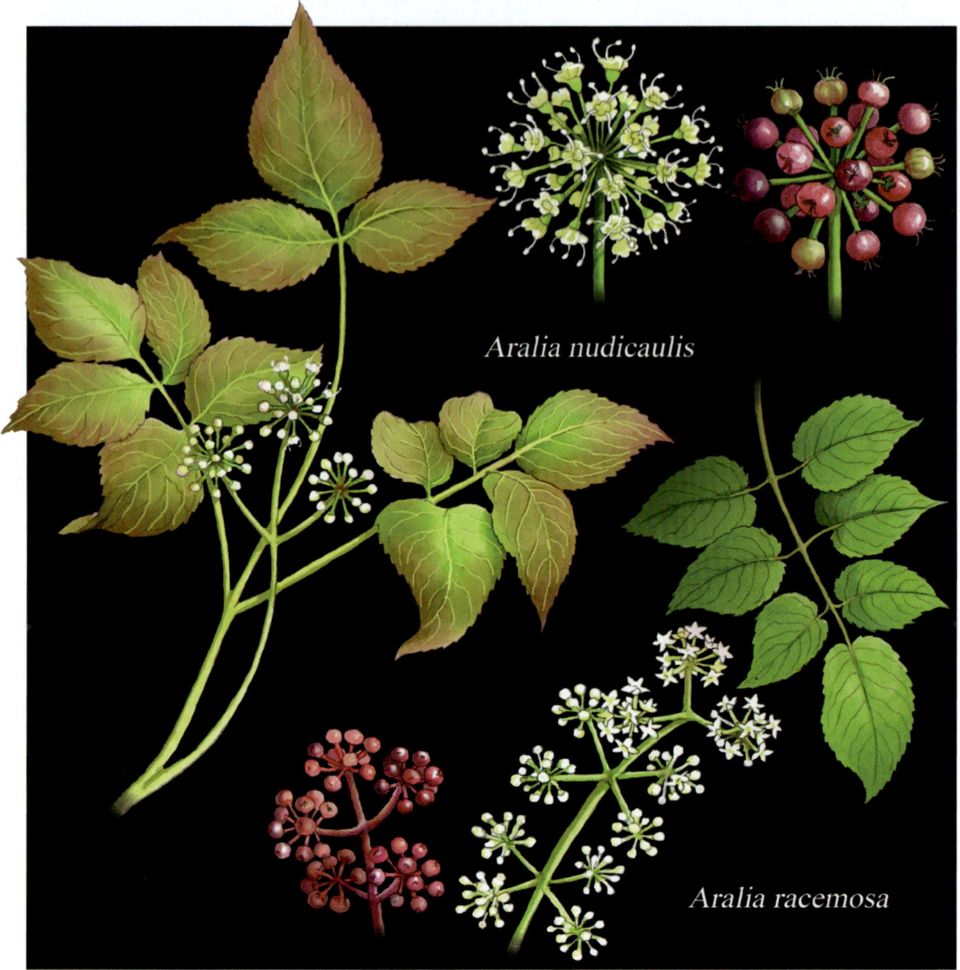

Aralia nudicaulis
Aralia racemosa

FAMILY: Araliaceae

OTHER NAMES: *A. nudicaulis:* Rabbit Root, False Spikenard, *Fr.* Salsepareille; *A. racemosa:* American Spikenard, *Fr.* Grande Salsepareille;

PARTS USED: Root, leaves, berries

CHARACTERISTICS: Sweet, pungent, aromatic, warm, moist

ACTIONS: Alterative, diaphoretic, diuretic, pectoral, stimulant, tonic, antioxidant, anti-inflammatory, antisyphilitic, nervine

RANGE: *A. nudicaulis* native across Canada except Nunavut; *A. racemosa* native from Manitoba to the Maritimes

Aralia nudicaulis, or Wild Sarsaparilla, has been widely used by Indigenous Peoples across North America for centuries, and as a substitute in formulas for the unrelated tropical variety, *Smilax ornata*. It is a perennial of the Ginseng family that grows to a height of 60 cm. with cord-like runners. The stems are smooth and grow out of the runners, dividing into 3 branches, each producing large, finely toothed compound leaves composed of usually 5 leaflets. The leaves are often reddish early in the spring and turn green as the plant matures. Usually, 3 globe-shaped clusters of tiny white flowers will appear on scapes the same height as the stems in June or July, and are followed by edible black berries that taste spicy and sweet. *Aralia racemosa*, or Spikenard, is quite a bit taller, often growing as high as 1.5 m. Its leaves are more heart-shaped and the flowers grow in many clusters along the stem. Both varieties prefer moist, shady woods, and are used for similar purposes. The rootstock, which has a sweet and spicy taste, is best collected in the fall and dried for later use.

MEDICINAL USES:

Pulmonary diseases, fevers, skin problems, rheumatism, sleep disorders

- Historically used for chronic respiratory problems, it works as a mild expectorant to break up thick mucus in cases of pneumonia, asthma, tuberculosis, and other chronic lung problems. Encourages sweating and helps with colds and flu. Boiling the root and adding honey makes a tasty cough syrup.
- Root is nourishing and rich in calcium, potassium, magnesium, iron, and zinc. Improves bone density and repairs connective tissue. Purifies the blood and removes stagnant waste from the joints, easing the discomfort of arthritis and rheumatism.
- Used as a nervine tonic to help with anxiety, stress, and sleep disorders. Mildly hypotensive and cardio-protective.
- Eases indigestion and stomachaches, tones the digestive tract, and increases appetite.
- Used externally as a poultice for rheumatism, burns, shingles, fungal infections, sores, eczema, and swellings.

OTHER USES:

- Rootstock has been used as a substitute for the tropical medicinal herb Sarsaparilla (*Smilax ornata*).
- Used as flavouring for root beer.
- Since the root is highly nutritious, it was often mixed with oil and used by Indigenous Peoples as an emergency food.
- Makes a pleasant herbal tea by boiling in water until it turns reddish-brown.
- Jelly or wine can be made from the fruit.

TINCTURE: Fresh or recently dried root 1:5 in 50% alcohol, 15–30 drops up to 3 times a day.

DECOCTION: 2 tbsp. chopped root infused in 2 cups boiling water, use within 24 hours.

CAUTION: Avoid if pregnant due to uterine-stimulating properties.

WILD YAM

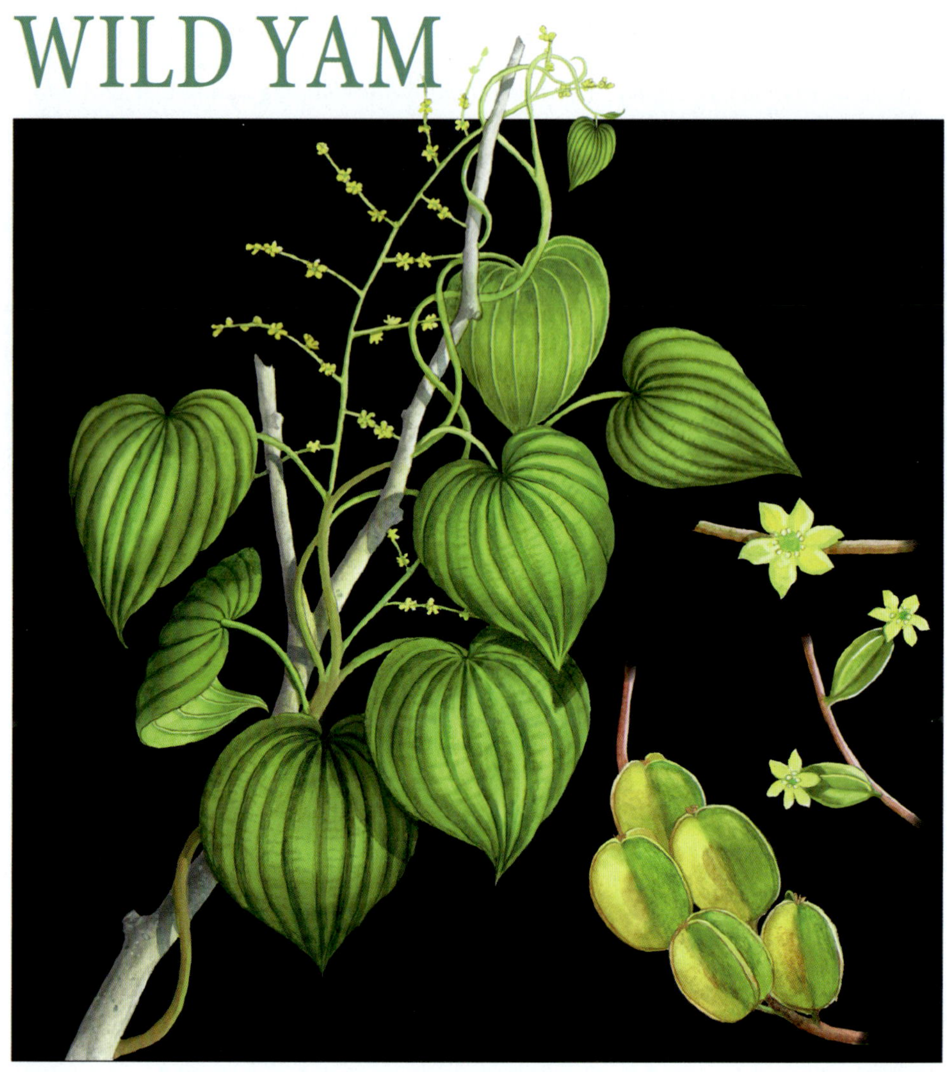

Dioscorea villosa

FAMILY: Dioscoreaceae

OTHER NAMES: Four-leaved Yam, Colic Root, Yam Root, Devil's Bones, *Fr.* Igname velue, Dioscorée velue

PARTS USED: Root

CHARACTERISTICS: Sweet, acrid, cool, bitter

ACTIONS: Anti-inflammatory, antioxidant, antispasmodic, cholagogue, diaphoretic, relaxant

RANGE: Native to Ontario

This twisting, perennial vine has been known for its tuberous medicinal roots since the eighteenth century. Its tiny, yellow-green to white flowers dangle in clusters from the leaf axils, the male and female flowers growing on separate plants. Several single female flowers grow along an unbranched raceme at the tip of an ovary, which develops 3 broad wings expanding to a 3-sectioned green capsule that turns brown as it ripens and is carried off by the wind. Its leaves are mostly alternate, heart-shaped and 2.5–12.5 cm. in length with a sharp pointed tip and veins that radiate from the base. The upper side is smooth, the underside may be downy. Its roots or tubers are woody, cylindrical, and pale brown and can be harvested in late summer or early fall.

MEDICINAL USES:

PMS, cramps, arthritis, digestive issues

- Most commonly used by herbalists to alleviate hormonal imbalances, menstrual cramps, dysmenorrhea, PMS, low sex drive, childbirth pain, and infertility. Some claim it relieves menopausal symptoms if taken internally, however there is little evidence for any of these claims.
- Antispasmodic action eases muscle spasms and cramps in the digestive tract, colic and gallstone pain, diarrhea, flatulence, and nausea, particularly when there are painful spasmodic contractions.
- Reduces inflammation in the joints, and in combinations can be effective at relieving pain from rheumatoid arthritis.
- Used alone or in formulas to release tension and as a relaxant for anxiety-related problems.

TINCTURE: Dried root 1:5, 2–4 ml. 2–3 times a day. For significant pain, take 1–2 ml. every 2 hours until pain subsides.

DECOCTION: ¼-½ tsp. dried root, cover with boiling water and simmer ½ hour. Take 1 cup 1–3 times a day.

COMBINATIONS: With Ginger or Angelica for intestinal problems. With Black Cohosh and Cramp Bark for rheumatoid arthritis and pain in the joints, taken in small, frequent doses throughout the day.

RESEARCH: Although the use of Wild Yam creams has gained popularity in the last few decades as a treatment for menopausal symptoms, researchers have refuted their claims, finding no proof that they have any effect. Wild Yam contains diosgenin, a steroidal saponin from which scientists can produce progesterone, estrogen, cortisone, and DHEA, but the human body cannot convert diosgenin into hormones by itself, so either the creams are ineffective or they have synthetic hormones added.

Wild Yam may be effective as an anti-inflammatory for arthritic pain, has been shown to lower blood sugar in diabetics, lower triglycerides in the blood, and may be promising in the treatment of breast cancer, but very little research has been done on humans to date.

CAUTION: Ingesting large doses may cause nausea and vomiting. Avoid if pregnant or breastfeeding, or if you have endometriosis, uterine fibroids, or are on birth control pills or hormone replacement therapy. Due to its estrogenic effect, it should be avoided by anyone with hormone-sensitive conditions like breast, ovarian, or uterine cancers. Creams may contain synthetic progesterone. Not effective as birth control. Long-term supplementation should be avoided, especially in people with kidney problems.

YARROW

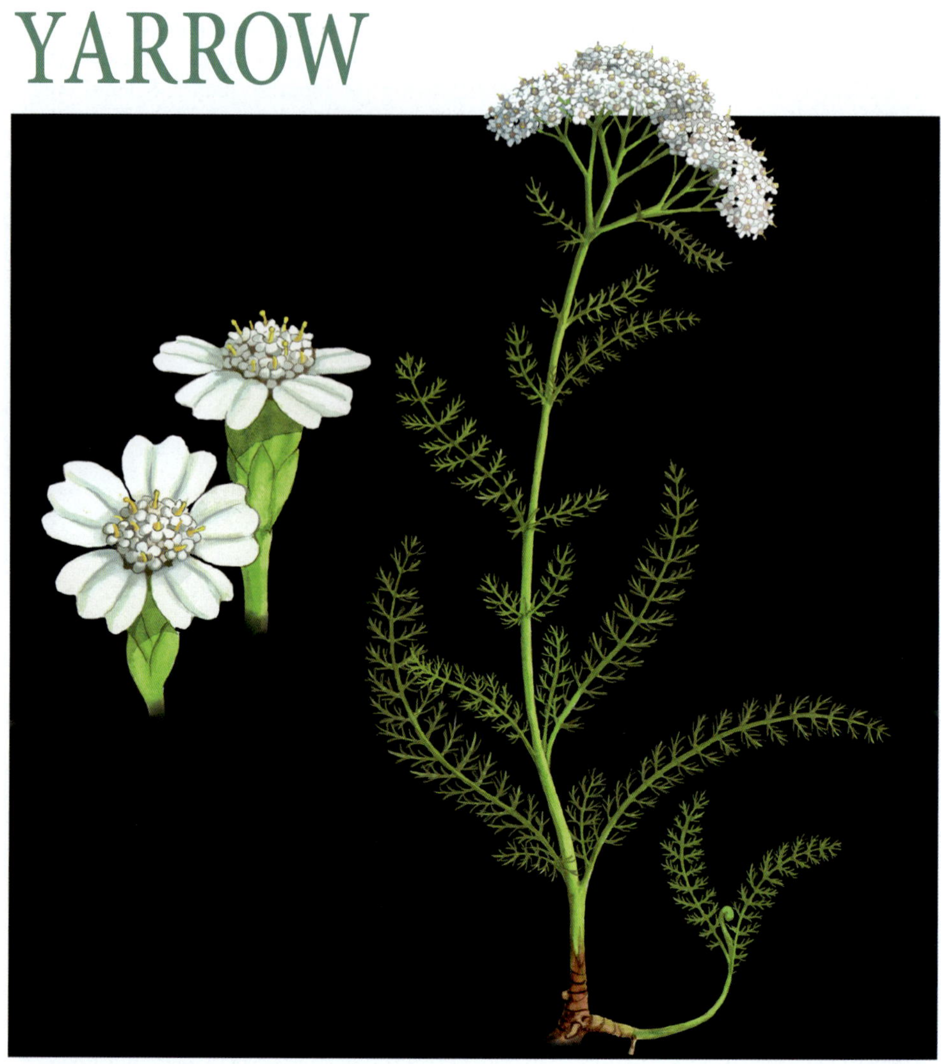

Achillea millefolium

FAMILY: Asteraceae

OTHER NAMES: Soldier's Woundwort, Nosebleed, *Fr.* Achillée millefeuille, Herbe à dindes

PARTS USED: Whole plant

CHARACTERISTICS: Bitter, pungent, cold, dry, sweet, salty, aromatic, astringent

ACTIONS: Diaphoretic, astringent, anti-inflammatory, antipyretic, carminative, hemostatic, antispasmodic, stomachic, tonic, alterative, stimulant

RANGE: Introduced across Canada, except Nunavut and the Yukon

This common perennial weed found throughout North America has been popular as a medicinal herb for centuries. It gets its name from the Greek myth of Achilles, who was invulnerable to arrows except on his heel, and it was traditionally used to stop the bleeding of soldier's wounds on battlefields. It grows 20–90 cm. tall, with stems branching near the top and alternate, highly segmented, feathery leaves. At the top of the stalk are clusters of tiny white or pink daisy-like flowers with 5 petals which bloom throughout the summer and fall. It grows in fields and on roadsides but is more potent if found in stony, sandy soils, and should be harvested early in the summer. Avoid using the woody stalks and mature leaves. Hang to dry.

MEDICINAL USES:

Wounds, fever, colds and flu, poor digestion, urinary tract infections, menstrual cramps, hemorrhoids

- Used as a wound remedy since Roman times, Yarrow is especially good for deep wounds that bleed profusely. It will stop hemorrhaging, but will also break up stagnant or congealed blood, bruises. May be taken internally or applied externally as a poultice or infused oil. Indigenous Peoples use it in teas or pound the plant into a pulp for sprains, bruises, or wounds. Has an antiseptic and anti-inflammatory action, particularly when used fresh.
- Relieves fever by causing sweating; good for colds, flu, and sinusitis, stimulates the immune system to fight infection. Especially good for children.
- Used for chronic urinary tract infections, incontinence, and leukorrhea. Tones urinary tract.
- Bitter, stimulates stomach acids to aid digestion of fats and proteins, helps heartburn. Soothes mild diarrhea and dysentery and stimulates appetite.
- Helps ease menstrual cramps and normalizes irregular periods. Stimulates and tones the uterus, brings on menstruation.
- Tones the blood vessels, relieves bleeding hemorrhoids and varicose veins as well as internal bleeding and ulcers. Also tones the mucous membranes of the digestive tract, particularly useful for dysentery, colitis, and leaky gut. Improves peripheral circulation.
- Can be used topically as a scalp and hair rinse, promotes growth of hair and helps prevent balding.
- May be used in a sitz bath to help with uterine fibroids, varicose veins, hemorrhoids, leukorrhea, rashes, or eczema.
- Anti-inflammatory action helps with osteoarthritis, rheumatism, and muscle pain. Many Indigenous Peoples pounded the roots to use as a poultice for sciatica and arthritis.

INFUSION: 1–2 tsp. dried herb in 1 cup boiling water, infuse 10–15 minutes. Drink hot 3 times a day. For fevers drink hourly.

TINCTURE: Dried plant 1:5 in 50% alcohol, take 1–4 ml. per day.

SITZ BATH: ½ cup whole cut herb steeped in cold water overnight. Bring to boil, strain, and add to sitz bath water.

COMBINATIONS: With Peppermint and Elder flower for fevers, colds, and flu, with Calendula and Plantain for wounds, with Raspberry leaf for menstrual problems, and with Hawthorn or Garlic for cardiovascular problems.

RESEARCH: Studies on patients with multiple sclerosis taking 250 mg. a day and 500 mg. a day Yarrow extract showed an increased time between relapses and decrease in severity of symptoms after 1 year, more pronounced with the higher dose. Showed effectiveness at protecting the stomach lining from acute and chronic ulcers.

CAUTION: Avoid using over a long period of time. Not advised during pregnancy.

YELLOW DOCK

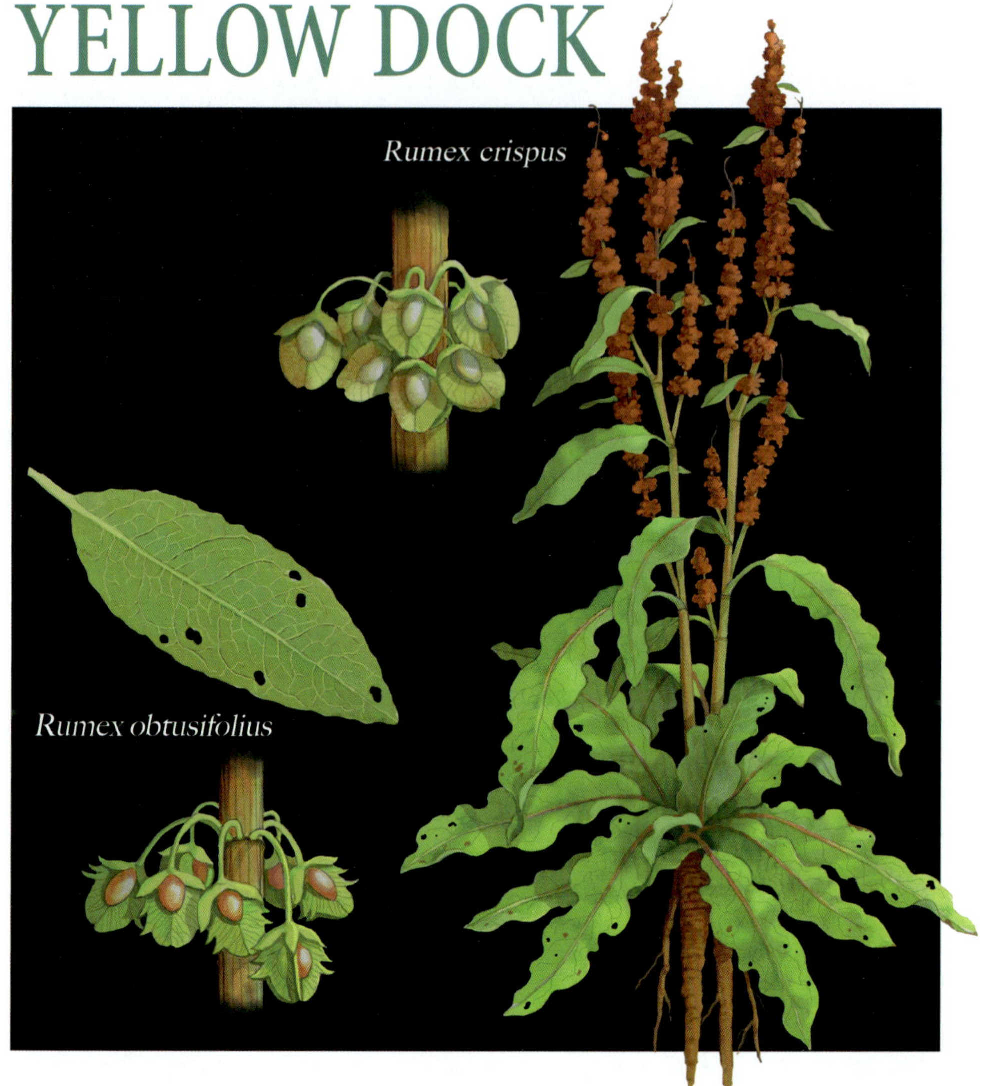

Rumex crispus
Rumex obtusifolius

FAMILY: Polygonaceae

OTHER NAMES: Curly Dock, Sour Dock, *Fr.* Oseille crépue, Patience crépue

PARTS USED: Primarily the root, but also stems, leaves, and seeds

CHARACTERISTICS: Bitter, cold, dry, sour

ACTIONS: Astringent, laxative, alterative, tonic, hepatic, cholagogue, anti-inflammatory, antimicrobial, diuretic

RANGE: Introduced across Canada except Nunavut, Saskatchewan

This common perennial weed is native to Europe and Africa but is now found throughout most of North America. As its names imply, it has broad, wavy, crinkled leaves, crisp around the edges, with a long taproot that's usually not forked, and yellow inside with thick rusty brown bark. Its close relative, *Rumex obtusifolius*, or Bitter Dock, has similar properties and is distinguished by its wider, flat leaves and tiny spikes on its seedpods. Both are tenacious weeds, often despised by gardeners, as each root must be dug out in its entirety since even the smallest piece left in the ground will produce another plant. The stem grows up to 90 cm. high, with green flower spikes branching off at intervals, producing an abundance of rust-coloured seed spikes in late summer and fall. The roots should be dug up in late summer or early fall; clean well and split lengthwise before drying.

MEDICINAL USES:

Liver sluggishness, constipation, skin irritations, anemia, throat and gum inflammation, eczema, arthritis

- This bitter digestive tonic contains tannins, acting specifically on the liver and gallbladder, promoting bile production, cleansing, assisting digestion of fats and proteins, and toning the digestive tract. This in turn improves conditions related to sluggish liver and build-up of waste, including skin problems, headaches, constipation, joint pain, and long-term chronic diseases of the intestinal tract. Liver congestion is often due to poor eating habits and alcohol consumption, so changes in diet are necessary for detoxification. A mild laxative, it contains anthraquinone glycosides, which stimulate peristalsis and increase mucous production in the colon, normalizing bowel movements and decreasing inflammation.
- Improves digestion, constipation, jaundice, hepatitis, and swollen lymph glands.
- Alterative and cleansing action when taken internally helps clear up skin problems like acne, boils, eczema, and psoriasis. Fresh leaves applied externally in a poultice are cooling and astringent, soothing heat from Stinging Nettle stings, burns, boils, bites, cuts, rheumatism, arthritis, and inflamed gums.
- Contains many nutrients, and is a good source of iron, but it also aids absorption when taken with iron supplements. Cleanses and nourishes the blood and is helpful in formulas as a remedy for anemia. Strengthens capillaries, helps hemorrhoids, varicose veins, internal bleeding.
- Decoction of the boiled stems or roots can be used in an ointment made with beeswax and olive oil to relieve itching, eczema, psoriasis, or other irritations. The decoction also works topically as an antiseptic and astringent to treat wounds, swellings, burns, hemorrhoids, and insect bites. Young shoots when rubbed on the skin will help soothe Stinging Nettle stings. The mashed root pulp is used as a poultice by Indigenous Peoples for swellings and sores.
- Young shoots are very nutritious and can be boiled and eaten. Good for rheumatism.
- Commonly used for inflammations of the nasal passages, throat, and gums as well as coughs and bronchitis.
- May decrease bone loss and increase mineralization in osteoporosis, although research is limited.

DECOCTION: 1 tsp. dried root in 1 cup water. Decoct 10–15 minutes, steep another 30 minutes. Take ½ cup 2–3 times a day.

SYRUP: For anemia or blood deficiency, add Stinging Nettles, Peony root, Red Clover, and molasses to decoction. Take 1 cup 3 times a day for no more than 3 months.

TINCTURE: Fresh 1:2, dried 1:5, in 50% alcohol. Take 1–3 ml. 3 times a day.

CAUTION: Should not be taken in combination with other diuretics, Lasix, or other drugs treating congestive heart failure or edema, as it can cause potassium depletion. Leaf contains oxalates and may cause digestive upset but cooking in water removes most oxalates. Avoid if pregnant or breastfeeding, if you have kidney stones or severe liver or kidney problems. Do not consume in large quantities or over a long period of time.

POISONOUS PLANTS

This section deals with those plants we must be extra careful to avoid, since it is very easy when wildcrafting to mistake one plant for another and sometimes this can have dire consequences. I focused on plants that are primarily toxic to handle, although many of them are also poisonous when ingested. Garden plants and the ones already mentioned have not been included.

Apiaceae family

Plants in this family are tricky to identify and include edible plants like Carrots, Parsnip, Parsley, Fennel, and Dill; however, there are many others that can be extremely toxic although they may closely resemble their edible relatives. Identification by the flowers, which are usually white and in clusters arranged in umbels or umbrella-like formations, is particularly confusing. These plants contain chemicals in the sap that cause phytophotosensitivity, or extreme sensitivity to sunlight if the skin comes in contact with them. A good rule is: if you're not 100% sure what it is, leave it alone!

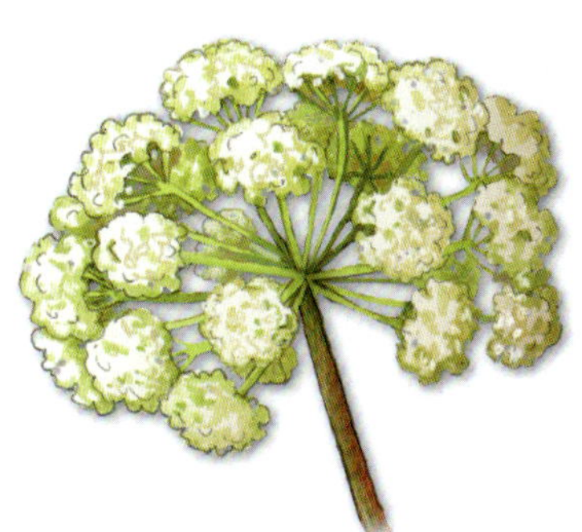

Treatment

If you accidentally touch any of these plants, immediately keep the skin away from sunlight and wash the area with cool running water. Avoid rubbing or using hot water as this will open the pores and allow the poison to go deeper. Do not touch other areas of the body, particularly the eyes. Use a mild soap to remove any remaining residue. If there is soreness, cover area with a cool, damp cloth. If there are open sores or blistering, apply an antibiotic cream and sterile bandage, changing at least twice a day. When a large area is affected, see a doctor.

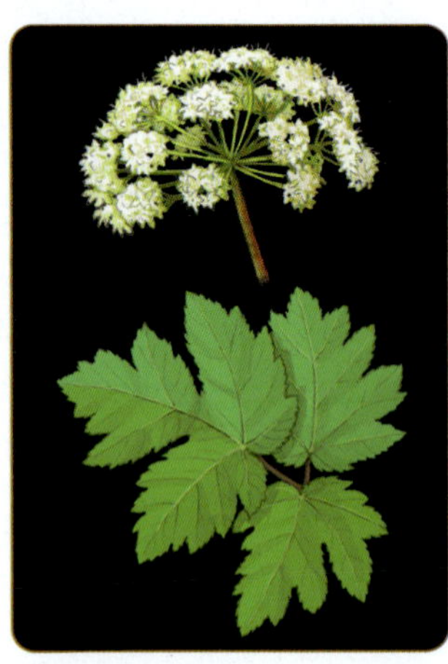

COW PARSNIP

Heracleum maximum (lanatum)

- Native from the Yukon to Newfoundland and Labrador
- Sap contains furanocoumarins, which will cause photo dermatitis; handle with gloves and use extreme caution when foraging or trimming. When exposed to sun, may cause rashes that could persist for months.
- Grows up to 3 metres tall. Flower umbels may be up to 20 cm. in diameter. Leaves are up to 60 cm. wide and hairy, and are divided into 3 deeply lobed leaflets. Lobes are more rounded than those of Giant Hogweed. Stem has some purple areas and deep ridges.
- Young leaves and flower pods may be eaten cooked, and seeds when dry and brown can be used as a spice. Plant is no longer toxic when dried or cooked. It is extremely important to properly identify before consuming, as it is similar to other poisonous plants.

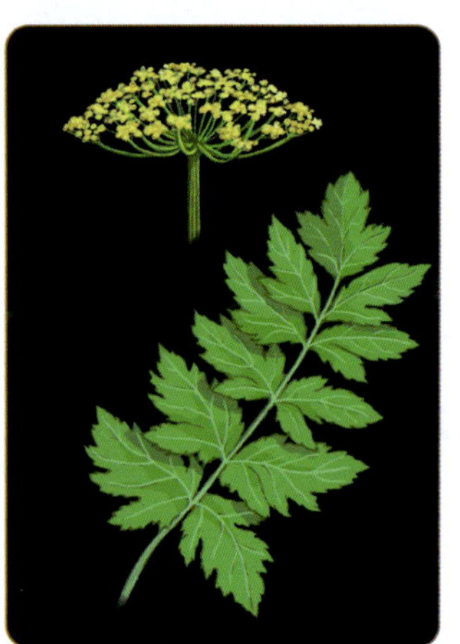

WILD PARSNIP

Pastinaca sativa

- Introduced in the Yukon to Newfoundland and Labrador, invasive
- Sap contains furanocoumarins, which will cause photo dermatitis. Handle only with gloves.
- In the first year it grows a rosette of basal leaves, the second year the tall flower stalk appears, and then the plant dies.
- Flowers grow in yellowish-green umbels. Grows up to 1.5 metres tall, its single smooth stem is deeply grooved with few hairs. Leaves are compound, its toothed leaflets arranged in pairs with a single leaf at the tip. Seeds are brown and flat.

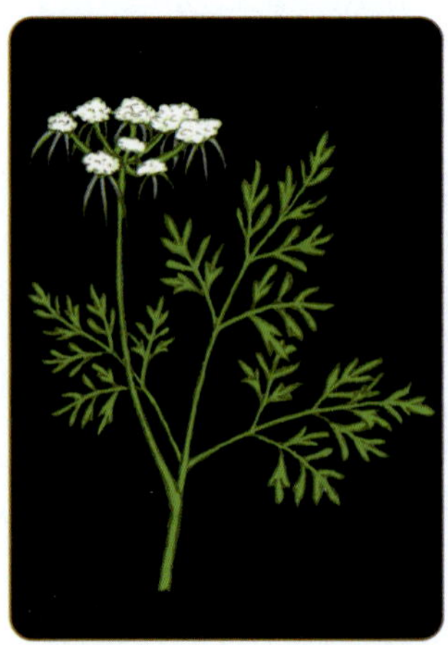

FOOL'S PARSLEY

Aethusa cynapium

- Introduced Ontario to Nova Scotia, annual or biennial.
- Hairless, smooth hollow, branched stem, up to 150 cm. in height.
- Leaves alternate, 2 or 3 times pinnate, triangular, similar to parsley but with a foul onion-like smell.
- Root shaped like a spindle, and tapered at each end.
- Flowers are white and appear in flat umbels; distinctive characteristic is 3 bracts or appendages hanging from each cluster.
- Dangerous if mistaken for parsley and ingested, for it contains poisonous alkaloids that cause burning in the digestive tract, vomiting, coldness, and even death.

GIANT HOGWEED

Heracleum mantegazzianum

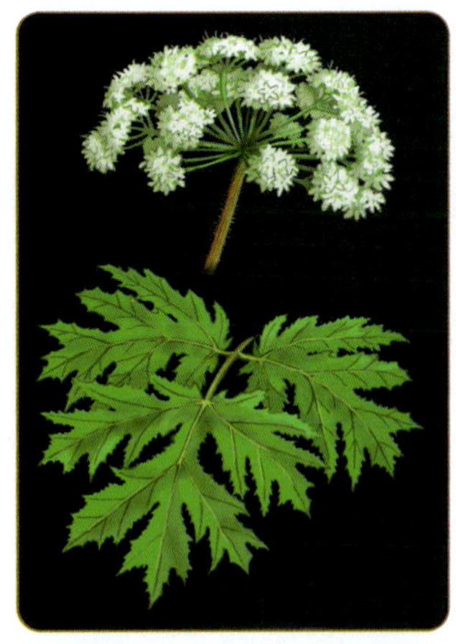

- Introduced, British Columbia, Ontario to Newfoundland and Labrador, invasive
- Sap contains furanocoumarins, which will cause severe photo dermatitis; avoid contact.
- Mature plant can reach 5 metres in height. Hollow stem is green with reddish-purple blotches or may be entirely purple, with a rough texture and stiff hairs. The compound leaves can be up to 1.5 metres long, are shiny and deeply divided into lobed leaflets with coarse, serrated edges. White umbels can be up to 60 cm. in diameter.

POISON HEMLOCK

Conium maculatum

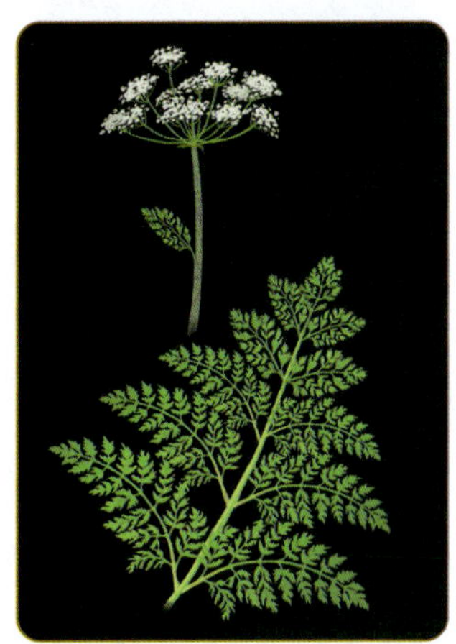

- Introduced, British Columbia to Saskatchewan, Ontario to Nova Scotia, invasive
- Biennial up to 3 metres tall in second year. Branching stem is hollow, red or purple spotted, smooth, and hairless. Leaves are compound with leaflets growing in pairs from opposite sides of leaf stalk, finely divided and feathery, much like Queen Anne's Lace or Parsley. They give off a strong musty odour when crushed. Flowers grow in rounded clusters 5–7.5 cm. in diameter.
- Contains the alkaloid *coniine*. All parts of the plant are poisonous and even remain toxic for up to three years after dying off. Eating the plant is the most dangerous, but the poisons can also effect the skin and respiratory system. Symptoms include dizziness, trembling, paralysis, and eventually death due to respiratory failure. Quick treatment can reverse the harm, but an immediate response is necessary.

WATER HEMLOCK

Cicuta maculata (Spotted), Cicuta douglasii (Western)

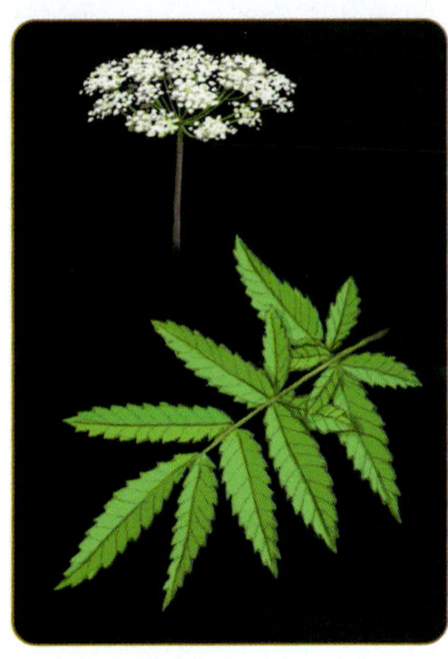

- *Cicuta maculata* is native across Canada except Newfoundland and Labrador. *Cicuta douglasii* is native to the Yukon, British Columbia, Alberta
- Contains cicutoxin, which is present in all parts of the plant. It is one of the deadliest plants in North America. A piece of the root the size of a walnut is enough to kill a cow.
- Perennial, grows up to 2 metres tall, typically in wetlands and along streams.
- Stem is smooth, mostly hairless and hollow, sometimes branching and usually with purple streaks or stripes. Leaves are two or three times pinnate with a single leaf at the top, have lance-shaped, sharply toothed leaflets with veins that terminate in notches, not at the tips. Flowers are white growing in compound umbels about 15 cm. across.

Other species to avoid

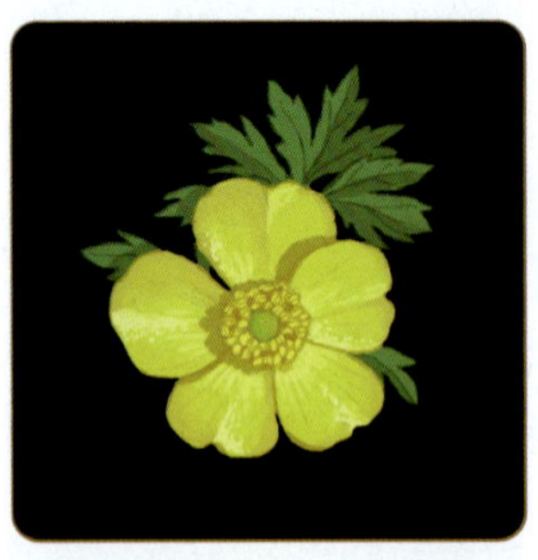

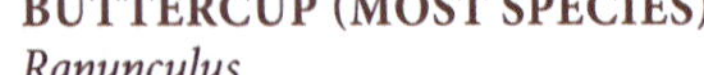

BUTTERCUP (MOST SPECIES)

Ranunculus

- Native across Canada
- Contains protoanemonin, an acrid, toxic oil that can cause itching and burning of the skin, irritate the eyes, and if chewed can create blisters in the mouth and on the face. If swallowed they can cause severe gastrointestinal irritation, spasms, and paralysis.
- Family consists of several hundred species, with varying levels of the toxic compound, including popular garden plants like *Clematis*, *Helleborus*, *Pulsatilla*, and *Anemone*. They have alternate, palmately veined leaves that may be entire, lobed, or finely divided. Flowers are usually yellow, but may be any colour, with 5 petals and can grow singly or in loose clusters.

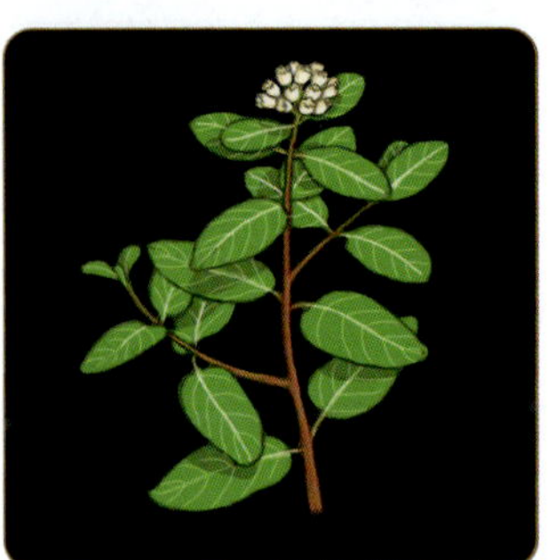

HEMP DOGBANE (INDIAN HEMP)

Apocynum cannabinum

- Native perennial, across Canadian provinces and Northwest Territories.
- Resembles Milkweed. Identify Hemp Dogbane by its red stem, often branched, and smaller cluster of whitish flowers, smaller narrower leaves, and narrow seedpod.
- Grows up to 1.8 metres tall; used by Indigenous peoples to make fibre for ropes and clothing.
- Leaves are elliptical, opposite, with light-green veins.
- Flowers are small, cylindrical, and greenish-white; milky white sap in stems and leaves.
- Contains cardiac glycosides and cymarin; consumption in humans and animals may cause rapid pulse, vomiting, blue mucous membranes, weakness, convulsions.
- Treatment suggestions in animals include emetics or activated charcoal. Humans who have been poisoned should seek immediate medical help.

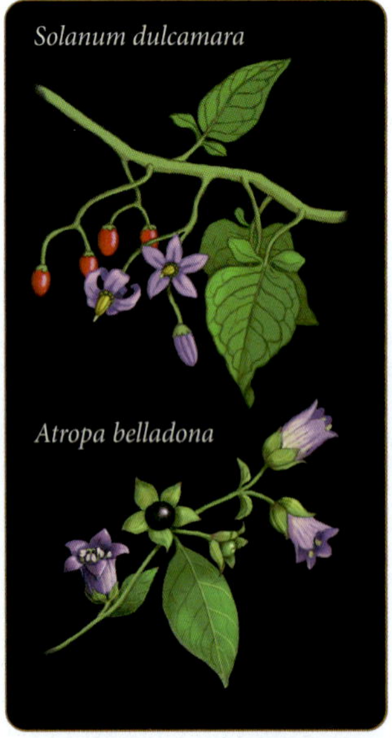

NIGHTSHADE

Solanum dulcamara (Bittersweet Nightshade)

Atropa belladonna (Deadly Nightshade)

- *Solanum dulcamara* was introduced in British Columbia, Saskatchewan, Ontario to Newfoundland and Labrador. *Atropa belladonna* was introduced in southern British Columbia (rare).
- *S. dulcamara* is a perennial vine or shrub with purple, star-shaped flowers and a prominent yellow centre growing in clusters along the vine. Berries are egg-shaped and green when unripe, changing to bright red as they ripen. Leaves are dark green, often with one or two lobes near the base, and emit an unpleasant smell

when crushed. The entire plant contains solanine, a toxin found in green potatoes and other nightshades, and dulcamarine, similar to the toxin found in Deadly Nightshade. Although not as toxic as Deadly Nightshade, the leaves, green berries, and even ripe berries can be poisonous if ingested.
- *A. belladonna* is a perennial that contains atropine, along with other toxic alkaloids, in all parts of the plant, particularly in the sweet, black berries, which can be confused with blueberries or black currants. Can cause increased heart rate, dilated pupils, hallucinations, vomiting, respiratory failure, and death. It grows as a shrub of up to 1.5 metres, with single, greenish-purple star-shaped bell flowers growing from the leaf axils. Leaves are dark green, alternate, smooth and oval. Contact a physician immediately if poisoning is suspected.

POISON OAK
POISON IVY
POISON SUMAC

Toxicodendron diversilobum (Western Poison Oak)
Toxicodendron radicans (Poison Ivy)
Toxicodendron vernix (Poison Sumac)

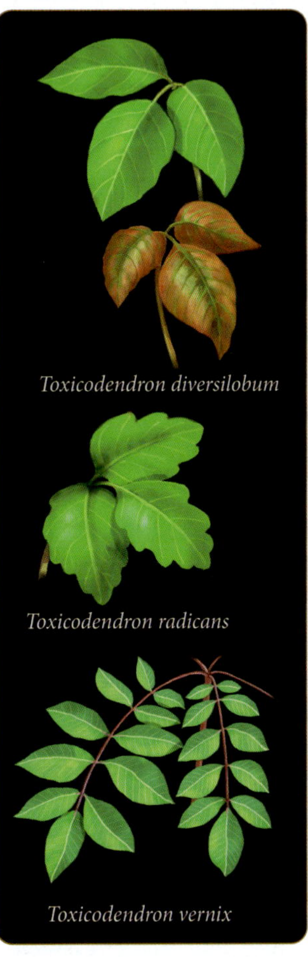

Toxicodendron diversilobum

Toxicodendron radicans

Toxicodendron vernix

- *Toxicodendron diversilobum* is native to British Columbia.
- *Toxicodendron radicans* is native from Yukon to the Maritimes, introduced to Newfoundland.
- *Toxicodendron vernix* is native to Ontario, Quebec and Nova Scotia.
- Poison Oak grows as a shrub, ground vine, or woody vine that wrap around trees for up to 30 metres; Poison Ivy grows only as a ground vine. Leaves vary in colour, from green with tinges of red in the spring to shiny green to red in the fall. Each leaf consists of three leaflets from 2.5 to 15 cm. long. Poison Oak leaves resemble Oak leaves with irregular, rounded lobes, whereas Poison Ivy has leaflets that may or may not be lobed and have pointed tips. Tiny flowers are greenish-white, growing in clusters on a stem, and the fruit are whitish glossy berries with ridges, that become dry with a papery shell when ripe.
- Poison Sumac is a woody shrub, growing in moist areas up to about 6 meters high, with reddish stems and opposite leaves that are smooth, not serrated like other Sumacs, and are more stout. The blooms are clusters of yellow-green flowers that hang down, unlike regular Sumacs, and turn to white or grey berries in the fall.
- They all contain the oil urushiol, which can be transferred to the skin from direct contact or contact with objects, clothing or other people or animals that have touched the plant. It can remain for long periods of time and can only be degraded by washing thoroughly with soap and water, however, it can even remain in the water or washing machine and be transferred to other clothing. Causes severe contact dermatitis, itching, swelling, and blisters. Inhalation of smoke from burning plants can cause respiratory tract inflammation that may require hospitalization.
- If you've been exposed, wash skin thoroughly with soap and water as soon as possible, trying not to spread the oil to other areas. Take an oral antihistamine to reduce itching, apply calamine lotion, or take oatmeal baths or compresses to soothe irritation. Avoid scratching or touching the area. Seek medical advice if large areas have been affected.

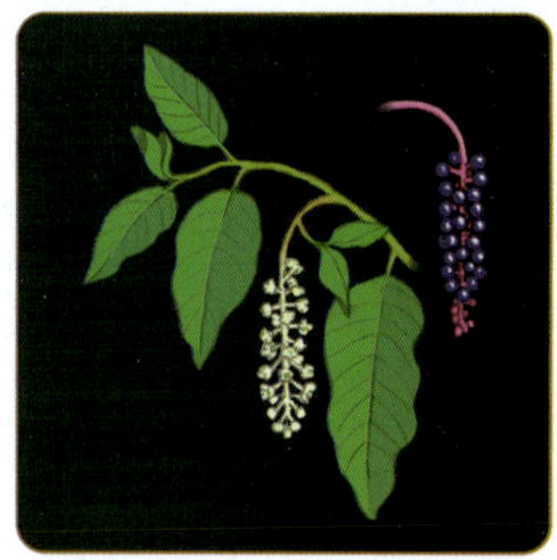

POKEWEED

Phytolacca Americana

- Native perennial, usually up to 2 metres high, and found only in New Brunswick and Quebec.
- Several stems growing out of a central taproot; stems are smooth, green to reddish, and the leaves are alternate with long petioles.
- Flowers grow in elongated racemes with bright-pink peduncles. The clusters of flowers are radially symmetric and white or greenish. Ripe berries are shiny dark purple.
- All parts are toxic to mammals, but not to birds. A violent emetic, Pokeweed causes cramps, bloody diarrhea, and/or paralysis of respiratory organs, depending on amount consumed. Plant juice may also be absorbed through the skin. If only ingested in a small amount, people or animals will recover in a day or two.

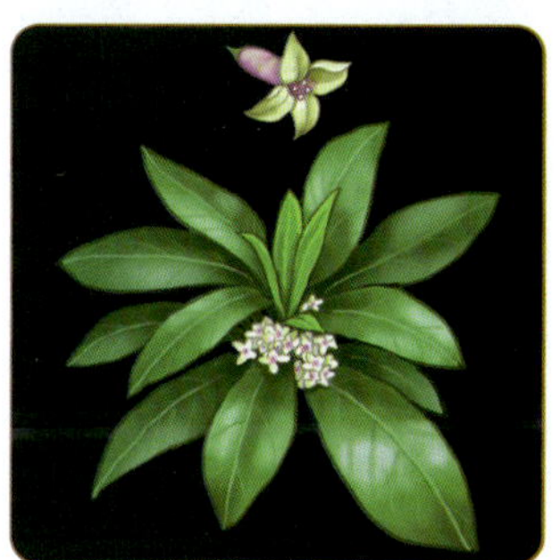

SPURGE-LAUREL

Daphne laureola

- Introduced in British Columbia; invasive
- Evergreen shrub that grows to a height of up to 1.3 metres. Dark green leaves are glossy, thick, oval shaped, and grow in a spiral pattern around the top of the stem. Twigs have a strong smell when cut. Small, fragrant flowers are light green with orange stamens and grow in clusters at the base of the leaves, followed by black berries in the early summer.
- Leaves, berries, and sap contain irritating toxins that cause severe skin irritation and blistering if touched, or burning of the mouth and lips and swelling of the tongue, difficulty swallowing, nausea, and diarrhea if berries are ingested. Flush with water if touched, and apply antihistamine cream to reduce irritation. Contact a physician immediately if ingested.

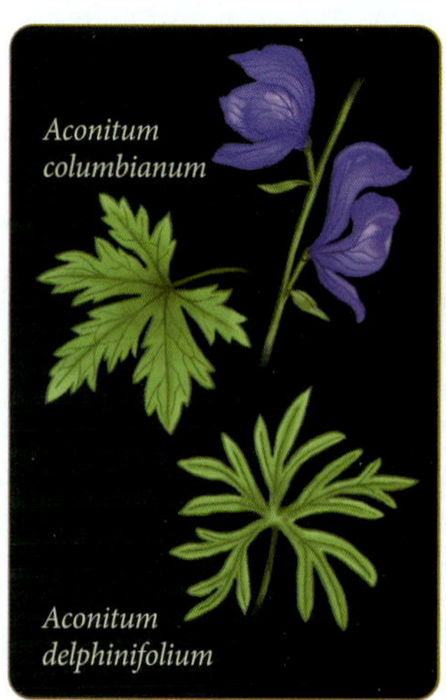

MONKSHOOD

Aconitum columbianum (Columbian Monkshood)

Aconitum delphinifolium (Mountain Monkshood)

- *Aconitum columbianum* is native to British Columbia. *Aconitum delphinifolium* is native to the Yukon, Northwest Territories, British Columbia, Alberta.
- Herbaceous perennial identified by the sepal or outer part of the flower that resembles a hood. They typically grow vertically on upright stems in racemes or groups and vary in colour from blue to white. Alternate leaves are usually 5-lobed and deeply cleft. Height of *A. columbianum* can be up to 2 metres tall, but *A. delphinifolium* is much smaller at 50 cm.
- All parts are poisonous, most severely from ingesting, but toxins can also be absorbed through the skin. Contains the alkaloid aconitine, which mainly affects the heart but can also cause nausea, chest pain, diarrhea, dizziness, shortness of breath. Seek medical help immediately.

GLOSSARY

Abortifacient A substance that brings on an abortion.

Adaptogen Herbs that work on the immune and neuro-endocrine systems, increasing the body's resistance and adaptability to stress while balancing the overall physiology without being toxic, even with long-term use. Tonic, antioxidant, and anti-inflammatory, not specific to any organ but helps regulate organ and system function in general and maintains homeostasis.

Adjuvant A substance that aids the action of a medicinal agent or medical treatment.

Alterative A medicine that favourably alters the course of an ailment, and gradually restores health.

Amenorrhea Absence of menstruation, usually due to either stress, weight gain or loss, excessive exercise, cysts or tumours, hormonal imbalance, pregnancy or lactation. May be erratic, occurring for short periods of time.

Analeptic An agent that has a restorative or stimulating effect, as on the central nervous system; may act as an anticonvulsant.

Analgesic An agent that relieves pain.

Anaphrodisiac An agent that reduces one's capacity for sexual arousal.

Anodyne An agent that relieves pain or promotes comfort, usually externally.

Anthelmintic A substance that kills and expels intestinal parasitic worms.

Anti-adipogenic A substance that inhibits fat cell formation.

Antibiotic An agent that inhibits the growth of or kills an organism, usually in reference to bacteria or microorganisms.

Antifungal An agent that kills or stops the growth of fungi or yeast that can cause infections in the body.

Anti-inflammatory An agent that reduces redness, heat, and swelling of inflamed tissues.

Antilithic A substance that dissolves or reduces the size of kidney stones.

Antioxidant An agent that helps protect the body from damage by free radicals, a major cause of disease and aging.

Antipruritic An agent that prevents or relieves itching.

Antipyretic An agent that prevents or reduces fever.

Antirheumatic A substance that is used in the treatment of arthritis.

Antiscorbutic A substance that prevents or cures scurvy.

Antitussive A substance that relieves coughs.

Aperient An agent that is mildly purgative or laxative.

Astringent Remedies that cause soft tissues to pucker or draw together, usually due to the presence of tannins. They are useful for reducing irritation and inflammation and create a barrier against infection in wounds and burns. They diminish secretions, check minor bleeding, and control diarrhea. Not recommended for long-term use.

Bitters Herbs having a bitter taste that stimulate digestive juices and bile production, and subsequently increase appetite. They may also stimulate peristalsis and help repair damage in the gastrointestinal wall.

Carminative Soothes the gut, easing pain, and causing release of stomach or intestinal gas. This action is due to the presence of volatile oils, which have anti-inflammatory, antispasmodic, and antimicrobial effects on the lining of the intestines.

Catarrh A condition where the mucous membranes of the nose and breathing passages are inflamed, often chronically.

Cathartic A purgative or laxative causing evacuation of the bowels.

Cholagogue An agent that increases the flow of bile from the gallbladder, which in turn facilitates fat digestion and works as a natural laxative. Should not be used with toxic liver disorders, acute viral hepatitis, painful gallstones, or other acute liver problems.

Cystitis A urinary tract infection characterized by inflammation in the bladder, most commonly in women.

Decoction A herbal preparation of roots or woody plant material boiled in water.

Demulcent Herbs that tend to become slimy in water and work to form a barrier on irritated tissues, soothing inflammation of the mucous membranes. They reduce irritation all through the digestive tract, easing muscle spasms and sensitivity to gastric acids, as well as easing coughs, sore throats, and pain in the bladder and urinary systems.

Depurative An agent that has a purifying effect.

Diaphoretic An agent that usually works by relaxing the sweat glands and inducing a greater outward flow of blood, thereby increasing the amount of perspiration. This rids the body of offensive materials and aids the immune and endocrine systems.

Diffusive Having the effect of spreading every way by flowing and improving circulation of fluids.

Diuretic Agents that help the body get rid of excess fluids by increasing urine flow, helping with a wide range of disorders where too much fluid accumulates in the tissues (edema).

Dropsy An old-fashioned term for edema or lymph congestion.

Dysmenorrhea Painful menstruation with cramping, due to a variety of underlying causes.

Edema A build-up of fluids in the tissues causing swelling.

Emetic An agent that induces vomiting.

Emmenagogue An agent that regulates and stimulates normal menstruation, as well as having a toning effect on the female reproductive system.

Emollient Having the ability to soften and moisturize the skin.

Expectorant An agent that facilitates the expulsion of phlegm from the respiratory tract by irritating and stimulating the bronchioles to liquefy and move thick sputum upwards so it can be cleared more easily by coughing, or by relaxing and loosening thinner mucous as in a dry cough.

Febrifuge An agent that relieves fever.

Galactagogue An agent that promotes the flow of milk.

Hemostatic An agent that controls or stops bleeding.

Hepatic Remedy that supports the liver by toning, strengthening and in some cases detoxifying and increasing the flow of bile, which in turn affects the entire digestive system.

Hyperglycemia When there are high levels of glucose or blood sugar in the blood due to too little insulin or inability to use insulin properly. Typical in people with diabetes.

Hypertensive An agent that causes a rise in blood pressure.

Hypnotic Herbs that promote sleep and have a relaxing effect on the nervous system.

Hypoglycemia When the level of glucose or blood sugar drops to levels that are unhealthy, most common in people with diabetes.

Hypotensive An agent that reduces elevated blood pressure.

Infusion A herbal preparation made by soaking it in hot or cold water to be drunk as a tea.

Leukorrhea Thick, white vaginal discharge.

Lymphatic System in the body that consists of a network of delicate tubes or vessels that drain fluid (lymph) that has seeped from the blood vessels into the tissues and returns it to the bloodstream through the lymph nodes. Includes the tonsils, spleen, and thymus. An important part of the immune system.

Mastitis Inflammation of the breast tissue due to infection, mainly affecting breastfeeding women, that results in pain, swelling, and redness, and sometimes fever and chills.

Menorrhagia Excessive menstrual bleeding, in younger women usually as a result of fibroids, tumours, polyps, endometriosis, or blood-clotting problems, in older women typically caused by erratic hormones due to perimenopause.

Mucilaginous Containing a gel-like, slimy substance called mucilage which can be helpful to soothe inflammation.

Nervine An agent that has a beneficial effect on the nervous system. Depending on the plant, this can work as a tonic, which repairs damage to the nervous system in cases of trauma or stress; as a relaxant, which eases anxiety and relaxes the peripheral nerves, muscles and organs of the body; or as a stimulant, which helps enhance vitality where the body is sluggish.

Neuroprotective An agent that protects nerve cells from damage or degeneration by pathogens in neurodegenerative diseases.

NSAIDS Non-steroidal anti-inflammatory drugs.

Pectoral Relating to the chest or thorax, between the neck and abdomen.

Peristalsis A series of wave-like involuntary contractions of the muscles that move food along the digestive tract.

Parturient A substance that aids in the birthing process.

Poultice A warm mass of plant material, or a cloth wrapped in plant material, that is applied to the skin to cause a medicinal action.

Purgative An agent that acts as a strong laxative, cleansing the bowel, often with cramping and pain.

Restorative An agent or medicine that is able to restore health, strength, and well-being.

Rubefacient Causes localized reddening of the skin.

Saponin A compound in some plants that has a foaming or soapy action when shaken with water.

Scrofula Swellings of the lymph glands in the neck, caused by tuberculosis.

Sialagogue An agent that promotes the production of saliva.

Styptic A substance that slows or stops bleeding by contracting the blood vessels; astringent.

Stomachic An agent that aids the stomach and digestion.

Sudorific An agent that causes sweating.

Tincture A herbal medicine prepared by soaking plant material in alcohol, cider vinegar, or glycerine over a period of time and then straining, in order to extract the medicinal compounds.

UTI Urinary tract infection.

Vermifuge An agent that rids the body of worms (anthelmintic).

Vulnerary A remedy that promotes healing of wounds.

Yin and Yang In Chinese philosophy these two forces are symbols of the balance existing in the universe, Yin being the feminine principle of darkness, receptivity, dampness, concealed, fluid, and lunar, whereas Yang is masculine, contracted, dry, overt, rigid, and solar. We all contain a mixture of these energies within us, often one is in excess and this throws our bodies out of balance.

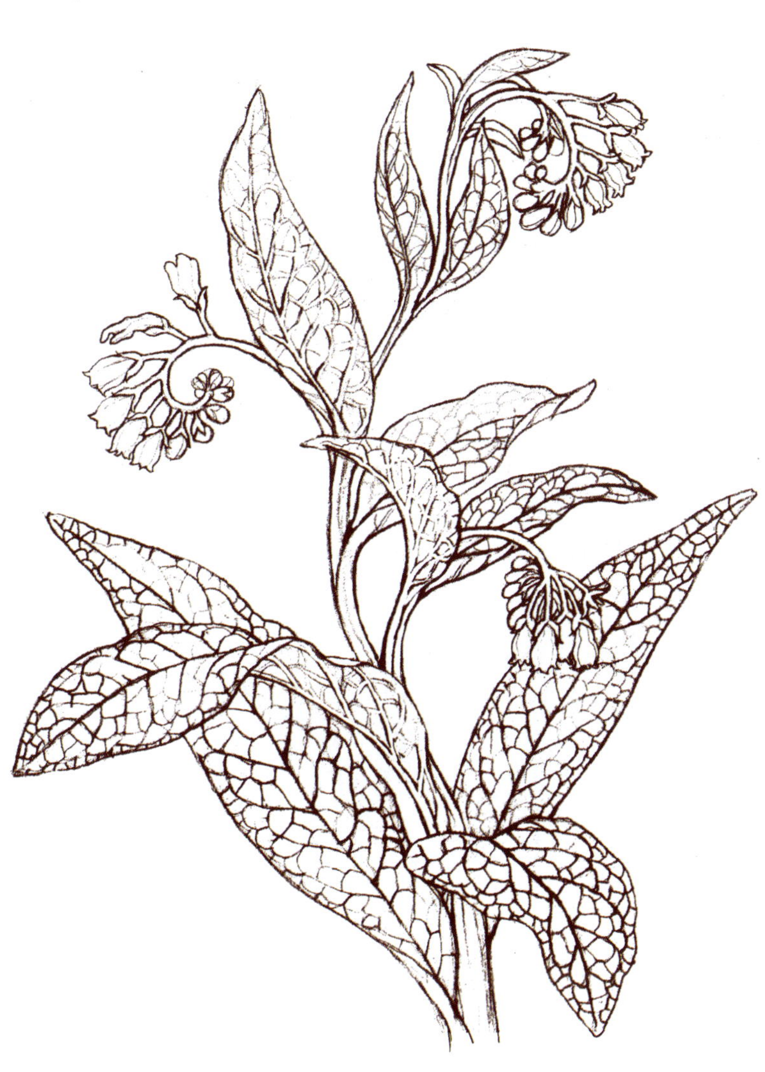

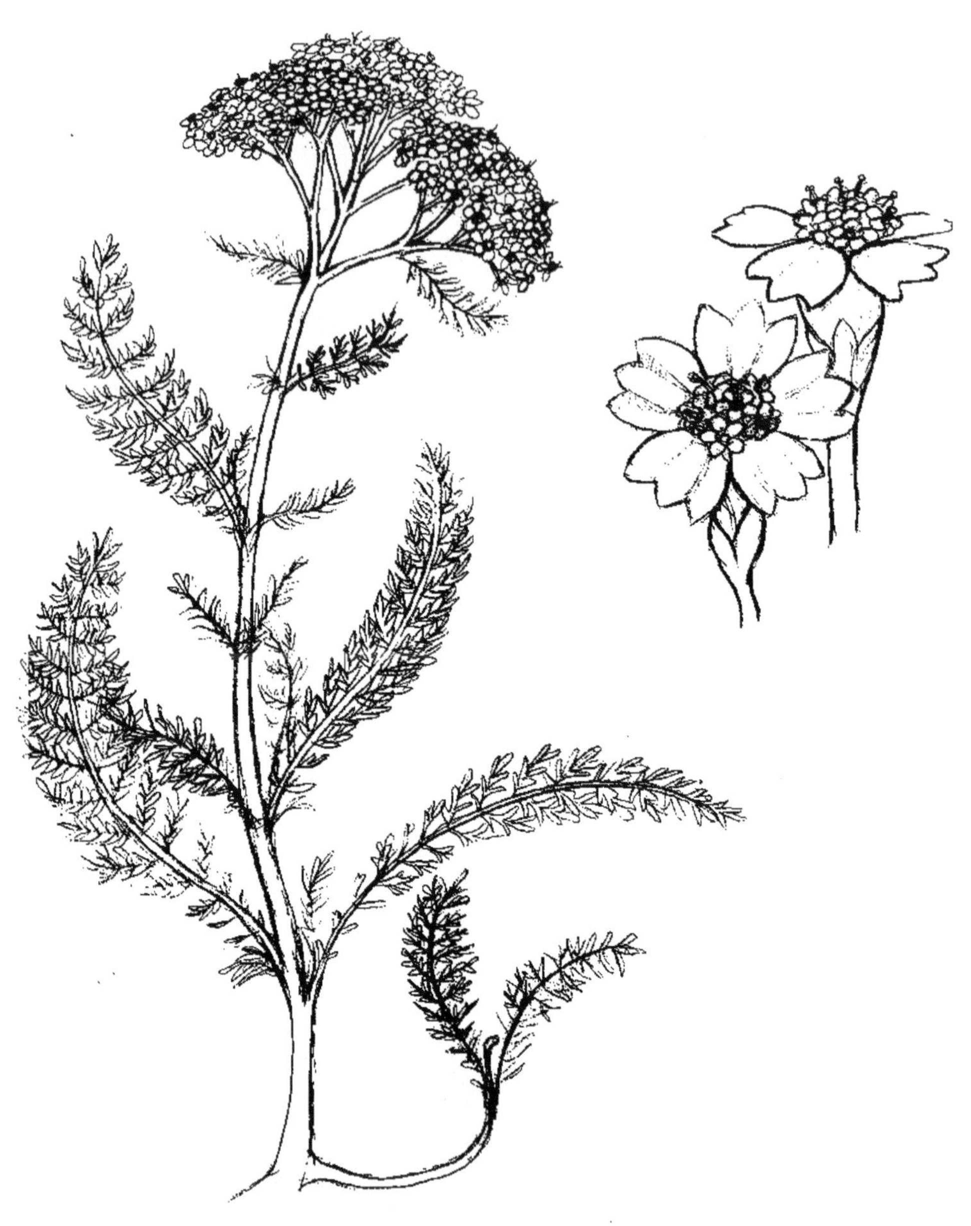

BIBLIOGRAPHY

Boxer, Arabella and Philippa Back. *The Herb Book*. London: Octopus Books Limited, 1981.

Buhner, Stephen Harrod. *Sacred Plant Medicine: The Wisdom in Native American Herbalism*. Rochester, Vermont: Bear & Company, 2006.

Bunney, Sarah. *The Illustrated Encyclopedia of Herbs, Their Medicinal and Culinary Uses*. London: Chancellor Press, 1992.

Burke, Nancy. *The Modern Herbal Primer, A Simple Guide to the Magic and Medicine of 100 Healing Herbs*. Alexandria, Virginia: Time-Life Books (Old Farmer's Almanac Home Library), 2000.

Castleman, Michael. *The Healing Herbs, The Ultimate Guide to the Curative Power of Nature's Medicines*. Emmaus, Pennsylvania: Rodale Press, 1991.

Clough, Katherine. *Wildflowers of Prince Edward Island*. Charlottetown, Prince Edward Island: Ragweed Press, 1995.

Duke, James A. *The Green Pharmacy*. Emmaus, Pennsylvania: Rodale Press, 1997.

Easley, Thomas and Steven Horne. *The Modern Herbal Dispensary, A Medicine-Making Guide*. Berkeley, California: North Atlantic Books, 2016.

Foster, Steven and James A. Duke. *Eastern/Central Medicinal Plants and Herbs of Eastern and Central North America*. New York: Houghton Mifflin Company (Peterson Field Guide Series), 2000.

Foster, Steven and Rebecca L. Johnson. *Desk Reference to Nature's Medicine*. Washington, DC: National Geographic Society, 2006.

Gray, Beverley. *The Boreal Herbal, Wild Food and Medicine of the North*. Whitehorse, the Yukon: Aroma Borealis Press, Co-published by Canadian Circumpolar Institute, 2011.

Grieve, Maud. *A Modern Herbal*. London: Tiger Books International, 1973 (Originally published in 1931).

Hoffmann, David. *The Complete Illustrated Holistic Herbal*. London: Element (An Imprint of Harper Collins), 2002.

Kloos, Scott. *Pacific Northwest Medicinal Plants*. Portland, Oregon: Timber Press, Inc., 2017.

Lacey, Laurie. *Mi'kmaq Medicines, Remedies and Recollections*. Halifax, Nova Scotia: Nimbus Publishing, 2012.

MacKinnon, Andrew A. *Edible & Medicinal Plants of Canada*. Edmonton, Alberta: Partners Publishing, and Lone Pine Media Productions (BC), 2014.

Pahlow, Mannfried. *Healing Plants*. Hauppauge, New York: Barron's Educational Series, Inc., 1993.

Reader's Digest. *Magic and Medicine of Plants.* Pleasantville, New York: Reader's Digest Association, Inc., 1989.

Redfield, Edmund. *Wildflowers of the Maritimes: A Guide to Identifying 150 of the Region's Wild Plants.* Halifax, Nova Scotia: Nimbus Publishing, 2016.

Scott, Peter J. *Edible Plants of Atlantic Canada.* Portugal Cove-St. Philip's, Newfoundland and Labrador: Boulder Publications, 2010.

Tierra, Michael. *The Way of Herbs.* New York: Pocket Books (Simon and Shuster), 1998.

Vermeulen, Nico. *The Complete Encyclopedia of Herbs.* Lisse, The Netherlands: Rebo Publishers, 1998.

Walker, Marilyn. *Wild Plants of Eastern Canada.* Halifax, Nova Scotia: Nimbus Publishing, 2008.

Wood, Matthew. *The Earthwise Herbal Repertory.* Berkeley, California: North Atlantic Books, 2016.